Biomechanical Modeling of the Cardiovascular System

IPEM–IOP Series in Physics and Engineering in Medicine and Biology

About the Series

Series in Physics and Engineering in Medicine and Biology will allow IPEM to enhance its mission to 'advance physics and engineering applied to medicine and biology for the public good.'

Focusing on key areas including, but not limited to:

- clinical engineering
- diagnostic radiology
- informatics and computing
- magnetic resonance imaging
- nuclear medicine
- physiological measurement
- radiation protection
- radiotherapy
- rehabilitation engineering
- ultrasound and non-ionising radiation.

A number of IPEM–IOP titles are published as part of the EUTEMPE Network Series for Medical Physics Experts.

Biomechanical Modeling of the Cardiovascular System

Ricardo L Armentano
Bioengineering R&D Group (GIBIO), Universidad Tecnológica Nacional,
Buenos Aires, Argentina
Department of Biological Engineering, Universidad de la República, Uruguay

Edmundo I Cabrera Fischer
Favaloro University, IMETTyB-CONICET, Argentina

Leandro J Cymberknop
Bioengineering R&D Group (GIBIO), Universidad Tecnológica Nacional,
Buenos Aires, Argentina

IOP Publishing, Bristol, UK

ISBN 978-0-7503-1281-3 (ebook)
ISBN 978-0-7503-1282-0 (print)
ISBN 978-0-7503-1283-7 (mobi)

DOI 10.1088/2053-2563/aafb0d

Version: 20190401

IOP Expanding Physics
ISSN 2053-2563 (online)
ISSN 2054-7315 (print)

British Library Cataloguing-in-Publication Data: A catalogue record for this book is available from the British Library.

Published by IOP Publishing, wholly owned by The Institute of Physics, London

IOP Publishing, Temple Circus, Temple Way, Bristol, BS1 6HG, UK

US Office: IOP Publishing, Inc., 190 North Independence Mall West, Suite 601, Philadelphia, PA 19106, USA

This book is dedicated to René Gerónimo Favaloro (July 12, 1923–July 29, 2000), the Argentine cardiovascular surgeon who revolutionized the field with his pioneering contributions, among which the most remarkable one is the standardization of the coronary artery bypass surgery, performed for the first time in the Cleveland Clinic 1967. He centered his attention on human resources, creating a team of young students, engineers, medical doctors, physicists, mathematicians and other specialists in order to disseminate his latest advances in medicine and engineering. This book is focused on the main findings emerged from that enormous and magnificent experience.

Contents

Preface

The systemic circulation plays a significant role, in which blood vessels (arteries) contribute in the regulation of the blood flow periodically imposed by cardiac ejection. The heart is usually considered the main element, the only one which has an actual relevance in the operation of the system, thus neglecting blood vessels, which are considered simple conduits that connect the cardiac pump with the organs. Such a basic approach underestimates the prominent role shown by blood vessels in general, and by arteries in particular (especially the aorta), in the regulation of the blood flow periodically imposed by cardiac ejection. The study of the arterial system is therefore very important, be it to understand its intrinsic operation or to evaluate the conditions for optimal coupling with the heart. The arterial hydraulic load exhibited by the circulation towards the left ventricle may be divided into three main components: systemic vascular resistance, arterial elasticity and the reflected wave present in the circulation since it is a distributed system. This conceptual framework of cardiovascular engineering, which integrates elements from biology, engineering, mathematics and physics to describe and understand the cardiovascular system has the main objective to develop, verify and validate a predictive and quantitative detailed comprehension of the cardiovascular system and to apply such concepts to the solution of various diseases. This discipline leads to the development of a higher level of specificity to address the study of the phenomena related to the arterial wall–blood interface, where the main causes of cardiometabolic diseases emerge. The purpose of this book is to address one of the many approaches for modeling the mechanical properties of the cardiovascular system to contribute to the evaluation and follow-up of factors involved in the physiopathology of cardiometabolic diseases and human aging.

The use of *in vivo* models remained a need in research concerning certain physiologic phenomena, especially those related to the pathophysiologic mechanisms of disease. Traditional small animal models (e.g., rats, mice, guinea pigs, hamsters, and rabbits) have provided the scientific community with access to physiological *in vivo* models to study mechanisms relating to human disease and basic biological processes. When considering appropriate animal models for research, the researcher and sponsoring institution should first assess their responsibilities with respect to existing regulations. All laboratories using animals must recognize and comply with current definitions of humane animal care and use. In this sense, the closer the *in vivo* assessment parallels a clinical situation, the more clinically applicable are the results of the assessment. Particularly, the sheep is often the superior model in cardiovascular research, as it is relatively easy to control many variables. A chronically instrumented animal is an animal which has undergone a surgical procedure, under strict asepsis standards, during which measurement instruments were implanted (pressure transducers, intravascular or intra-cardiac catheters, dimension sensors, devices for altering or interrupting blood flow through a certain vessel, etc) at a first stage, and which, after a postoperative recovery period, is studied using such instruments. Since instrumentation is performed in advance, the researcher has direct and immediate access to the variables to be studied without the need to anesthetize the animal, allowing the studies to be performed while the animal is conscious. A conscious animal is defined as an animal that completely maintains its relation with its environment, without any sedation and in a state of wakefulness, that is, whose central nervous system and autonomous nervous system are functioning normally during experimental sessions. This is very important when studying the cardiovascular system given the active participation of the nervous system in hemodynamic regulation. It is important to stress that this is an integrative physiology model, in which the physiological compensatory mechanisms are operating and intact. Although this impairs 'variable control', it facilitates the extrapolation of the results to the clinical situation.

The authors of this book have been doing research for the development of techniques to measure the arterial dynamic properties locally and accurately. The strength of this joint work is based on extensive experience in the fields of biomedical engineering, physiology, biomechanics, biomaterials, numerical methods and non-invasive measurement techniques. The multidisciplinary approach taken in this book makes it possible to complete virtually all the stages of a modern scientific research process— mathematical modeling, numerical simulation, 'customized' equipment, and technological innovation and physiopathology, leading to direct applications in the field of tissue engineering. The latter emerges as a futurist alternative starting to gain relevance, moving from the laboratory to the patient, creating the field of regenerative medicine. It can be defined as the application of principles and methods of engineering and the life sciences to the understanding of the structure–function relationships under normal or pathological conditions. This multidisciplinary technology is currently being used to develop biological substitutes to repair or regenerate functional tissues and organs.

The approach of this book was focused on the mechanics of the cardiovascular system, in the conceptual framework of the application of biomechanics to life sciences in a realistic environment, aimed at the domains of integrative physiology. This challenge comes to fill the gap in the specialized literature, which could be attributed to the fact that living organisms are highly complex dynamic systems (multi-feedback, non-linear) and with some hierarchical organization. These conditions, which refer to the study of the rheological properties of living things, pose a series of specific problems and often require an approach different from that used in the exact sciences. The relationships between measurable quantities and the parameters that describe the mechanical properties of the materials are extremely complex and consequently impose more or less complicated mathematical models, based on approximations that tend to be more realistic as the measurement techniques become more precise. For this reason, the theoretical approach articulated with the experimental approach must be considered as a whole—a single conceptual unit. In this idea, the great advantage is provided by *in vivo* studies derived from animal experimentation, since the latter constitutes the closest approximation to the human being in the testing of new drugs, the improvement of therapeutic approaches and non-orthodox diagnoses, avoiding subjecting the patient to risk procedures.

It is through extensive work in scientific experimentation and collaboration with international interdisciplinary groups that the authors discovered the immense wealth of this unconventional research. This book is intended to be positioned within a broader context, more fundamental than that of immediate application, given the formal nature of the chapters that comprise it. This quality makes it possible to contribute in answering this constantly renewed question about the particularities of the mechanisms of nature placed at the service of man, but which man has not yet put at his service.

Acknowledgments

The authors would like to thank Dr Jaime Levenson, Dr Alain Simon, Dr Ramiro Sánchez and all the colleagues from Favaloro University (Argentina), University of the Republic (Uruguay), Mar del Plata National University (Argentina), Polytechnic University of Madrid (Spain), Pierre and Marie Curie University (France), Paris Descartes University (France) and Georges-Pompidou European Hospital (Paris Descartes Faculty of Medicine, France).

Author biographies

Ricardo L Armentano

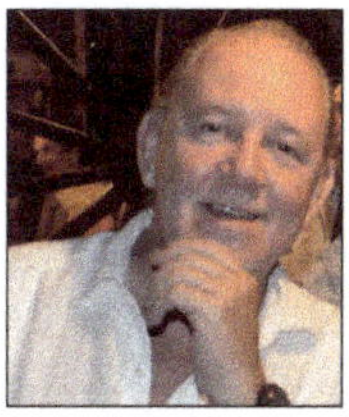

Ricardo L Armentano received his Engineering degree in 1984. He earned his degree as Doctor in Physiological Sciences from the University of Buenos Aires (1994) and in 1999 he obtained the PhD degree from Université de Paris VII Diderot, for the Doctorat de Biomecanique: Mecanique de Systèmes Biologiques. He is currently a Distinguished Professor of Biomedical Engineering Director of the Biological Engineering Department and Principal Investigator of UNPD/84/002 at Universidad de la República (Uruguay). He is also Director of the PhD program on signal processing and head of the Bioengineering R&D group (GIBIO) at Universidad Tecnológica Nacional, Buenos Aires (Argentina). He has acquired international recognition in the field of cardiovascular hemodynamics and arterial hypertension. He has taught in the fields of cardiovascular dynamics and in the broad area of engineering in medicine and biology and has extensive experience in PhD supervision and examination of local and international higher degree theses. He is on the editorial board of journals of cardiovascular research and is a reviewer for 25+ international scientific journals. He has 250+ publications, including a book, book chapters and peer-reviewed articles. Currently he is a member of EMBS IEEE Technical Committee on Cardiopulmonary Systems and EMBS Distinguished Lecturer.

Edmundo I Cabrera Fischer

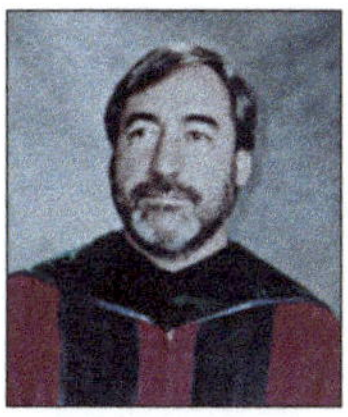

Dr Edmundo I Cabrera Fischer is a physician (La Plata University, 1972–1978), former cardiology chief resident (Team of Dr René G Favaloro, 1978–1981), cardiologist (El Salvador University, 1981–1983), PhD in Medicine (Buenos Aires University, 1985), PhD in Medical Humanities (Buenos Aires University, 2011), and professor (School of Medicine, Buenos Aires University, 1997–2003). Between 1980 and 1982 he was chief of the clinical area and staff of the Hemodynamic Equipment at the Favaloro Foundation. He completed internships in: Mount Sinaí Hospital (Florida, USA), Saint Joseph Hospital (Atlanta, USA) and Hospital Ramón y Cajal (Madrid, Spain). Since 1983, he has been a full-time researcher in 'Cardiovascular dynamics and circulatory assistance'. From 1986 to 2002 he worked in the Brussaiss Hospital of Paris(France) as part of a Franco–Argentine cooperation agreement (INSERM–CONICET). In this period, the results obtained in animal models were reported jointly with the research groups headed by Drs Michel Safar and Alain Carpentier. In 1994 he was admitted to the National Council of Scientific Research of Argentina (IMETTYB-CONICET-UF), where he remained until today. He has published around 150 papers, 22 book chapters, 117 abstracts in scientific meetings, 31 books—edited in Spanish, English, Portuguese and French. He has reviewed articles in several journals, notably the *Artificial Organs* journal (UK). He is an editor of the *High Blood Pressure and Cardiovascular Prevention* journal (Italy). He is a Fellow of the American College of Cardiology, Member of the European Society of Cardiology, Membre Société Française de Cardiologie and member of the International Society of the History of Medicine.

Leandro J Cymberknop

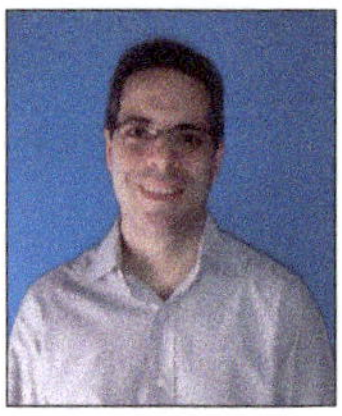

Dr Leandro J Cymberknop received his engineer's degree in electronics engineering and PhD in signal and image processing from Universidad Tecnológica Nacional, Buenos Aires, Argentina. He is currently developing his research activities as a researcher and assistant professor at the Bioengineering R&D Group (GIBIO) of the same institution, where he also serves as the coordinator. He is also a member of the PhD program committee and current chairman of the Argentine chapter of IEEE-EMBS. His research interests are focused on biomedical signal processing, modeling and simulation of systems mostly applied to the arterial biomechanics field.

Introduction

The purpose of this introduction is to comment on theoretical and practical topics concerned with cardiovascular modeling in human and animal research. Scientific research has developed different models that mimic those phenomena that require investigation concerning different fields of life sciences and technological developments in many sectors.

Modeling of the cardiovascular function is a great chapter of scientific research and constitutes a useful tool to confirm scientific hypotheses in the field of biological discoveries and the development of new technologies. In an attempt to reduce the number of deaths worldwide, medical research has developed physical and mathematical models in order to mimic the global and partial function of cardiac and vascular structures.

Animal models were used for physiological research in ancient Greece and afterwards by Arab and European physicians (Ericsson *et al* 2013). The fact that humans share biological characteristics with different animal species is the basis for the use of models to study normal and modified physiology. On the other hand, mathematical models can mimic any aspect of the world surrounding the researcher. Numerical modeling can represent many things, such as a volcanic eruption, or the function of a human organ. Simulation of the circulatory function has replaced a good number of physical models and at present mathematical models, *in vitro* setups and *in vivo* animal experimentation are complementary methods utilized in almost all biomedical laboratories.

Models of cardiovascular function have different purposes and can be hydraulic, mechanical, electrical or numerical, all of them being useful tools incorporated not only in scientific research but also in teaching and the testing of prototypes emerging from technological research. Moreover, modeling cardiovascular function facilitates interdisciplinary research and links physicians, biomedical engineers and mathematicians, among others.

At present, there are cardiovascular system models ensuring the simulation of any constitutive circulatory element. However, it is difficult to obtain results with mathematical accuracy due to the geometrical complexities of the heart and vessels and the nonlinear behavior of the measured variables that characterize cardiovascular function. This is one of many explanations regarding the origin of mechanical and mathematical model complexity, which in all cases tries to reflect a real condition characterized by interaction between systems and subsystems. Moreover, local and external regulations that ensure the adaptation of cardiovascular function to the human environment take into account a multiplicity of factors interacting with each other and provide data of isolated variables, as in associations chosen by the researcher that use a specific modeling approach. On the other hand, the complexity of cardiovascular modeling compels the validation of any model using real data obtained from *in vitro* and *in vivo* experimental research and clinical practice through invasive and non-invasive measurements.

Modeling has provided not only answers to questions related to normal or pathological function but can also predict multiple adaptations of the total and individual dynamic structures that are included in cardiovascular research.

Physical modeling

In vitro *experimentation*

In humans, blood circulates in a closed-loop system assuming that the intraluminal fluid is incompressible. Therefore, hydromechanical models using closed-loop hydraulic structures enable a complete analysis of functional parameters including large changes that are not possible in *in vivo* experimentation. This not a new modality; hydraulic simulation has been used to study cardiovascular function since the nineteenth century (Zimmer 2002).

Many setups using hydraulic parameters have been developed since the earlier studies of fluid dynamics reported by Hagen (1839) and Poiseuille (1840), as widely mentioned in different scenarios (Nichols and O'Rourke 1998). Moreover, signal recording was developed for the first time in the Karl Ludwig Institute in Germany in 1847 (Zimmer 1999). This type of experimentation is frequently performed in parallel with numerical simulation. Both are complementary resources to investigate similar biological functions.

A mechanical model of the heart and blood vessels should incorporate basic components such as a pump, pipes, valves and a control system that enables adjustments of cardiovascular parameters in order to imitate both normal and pathological states. All variables included in a research that uses a circulating loop should be in consonance with the clinical variables used in medical practice.

Hydraulic models and electrical analogies sometimes are very easy to understand, as in the case of the Windkessel system that can be easily visualized looking at an air chamber positioned in a circulating loop. On the other hand, electrical simulation allows one to replicate hemodynamic parameters corresponding to cardiac chambers and vascular structures. Observational studies promoted the search of electrical analog elements (voltage, current, diode, resistor, inductor and capacitor) in order to complete an ***electrical circuit simulating*** blood circulation.

In vivo *experimentation*

An *animal* model destined to mimic a specific human disease should consider the range of variation of measured variables used in medical practice or biology. These models can be acute or chronic, depending on the research chosen. Both modalities involve activities protected by legal and ethical regulations concerning the physical environment and training of the qualified personnel of the institution in which the investigation is performed. A careful selection of the animal species, transportation, housing, pain control, anesthesia and euthanasia should be also taken into account.

The dynamics of cardiovascular structures involves concepts of blood pressure, volume, pulse wave velocity, flow and a high number of indicators and indexes that should be included in the records obtained in the experimental animal.

To understand the complexity of cardiovascular modeling development, it is important to consider that circulatory dynamics has a high number of variables controlled by nerves and hormones. Both neural and humoral control systems determine changes in any cardiovascular parameter, which is barely isolated. In fact, circulatory variables are continuously interacting and influenced by each other.

The complexity of the cardiovascular system forces one to take into account not only changes in diameters and thickness of hollow structures that characterize the itinerary of the human blood pathway, but also the different components of the intraluminal constituents, as for instance, blood viscosity, a variable capable of changing arterial wall elasticity.

Hemodynamic variables have well known values that characterize healthy and pathological states within ranges that identify populations, including humans and animals. Moreover, the mentioned states are continuously changing in order to adapt cardiovascular function to daily activities. Cardiovascular modeling should take into account all these parameters in order to obtain faithful data originating in animal and *in vitro* simulation.

At present, animal experimentation is also performed to test cardiovascular prostheses (including synthetic vessels and heart valves) and assist devices (such as axial and pneumatic pumps) before utilization in humans. In this case, animal research would be placed between *in vitro* experimentation in a first step using a prototype and the clinical utilization of new devices applied to save a human life.

Animal models have advantages and disadvantages with respect to *in vitro* experimentation, in terms of ethical limitations and care destined to ensure handling within legal and ethical regulations, which are included in manuals such as the 'Guide for the Care and Use of Laboratory Animals' (NRC 2011).

Mathematical modeling

Isaac Newton is considered to be a pioneer in the utilization of mathematical models to analyze nature according to the concepts included in his *Philosophiæ Naturalis Principia Mathematica*[1] (1687). Models developed by this pioneer contributed to the understanding of planetary motion and initiated a long pathway that benefited the comprehension of biological systems.

On the other hand, Poiseuille was a medical doctor in the first half of the nineteenth century who is identified as the creator of cardiovascular modeling (Ethier and Simmons 2007). Afterwards, in 1899, Otto Frank developed the concept of Windkessel models to mimic the elastic characteristics of the arterial wall (Frank 1899).

At present, mathematical models not only allow the analysis of cardiovascular anatomy, but also the adaptive variability in normal and pathological states. Nonetheless, mathematical models face a system with a high degree of complexity and variability. Consequently, many future endeavors are needed to accomplish results in this interesting field of knowledge and technological development.

[1] *Mathematical Principles of Natural Philosophy*.

The word 'experiment' has been defined as the action that produces changes in a variable that takes part in a research, in which a hypothesis is to be verified. Cardiovascular experimentation has been performed since the nineteenth century, usually using *in vitro* specimens and *in vivo* animals. *In vivo* and *in vitro* experimentation remains the mainstay for investigating normal and abnormal human physiology, developing a great number of therapies that contribute to improving survival and quality of life. On the other hand, since 1970, development of informatics has allowed the execution of numerical experiments, expanding the field of cardiovascular research from clinical practice to molecular levels.

Hydraulic modeling, mathematical models and numerical simulation of normal and abnormal cardiovascular states provide quantitative data, establishing bonds among different circulatory variables in conditions that are impossible to obtain in clinical practice and in *in vivo* experimental animals. For instance, the use of mathematical models applied to the cardiovascular system provides a detailed analysis of the pressure–volume–flow relationship and precise answers about diseases and a way to decrease morbidity and mortality. Moreover, cardiovascular simulation is a very important tool that aims to help in the comprehension of circulatory dynamics and contributes to the evaluation of technological advances such as left ventricular assist devices.

Linked to the development of cardiovascular models, it is necessary to validate any simulation in the field of mechanical or mathematical simulation. At present, the methods of computational mechanics offer precise answers in prognosis and therapeutic decisions allowing the prevention and treatment of cardiovascular diseases. Validation of any model should be performed against animal physiological and clinical data. Special attention should be paid to the analysis of nonlinear systems used in the field of event prediction.

Validation of mathematical models also involves the use of statistics in order to confirm findings that could be obtained in nature, in experimental setups or observation of natural processes, and in the field of pathologies affecting large populations, such as atherosclerosis and systemic arterial hypertension. Once a mathematical model is validated, the combination of computer modeling and adequate signal processing techniques allow, for instance, understanding of the correspondence between cardiovascular function and indices developed to be used in clinical practice.

Final comments

In vivo experimentation is a useful tool largely and widely used in biology and medicine; however, the paradigms in the use of animals to model human systems are changing. More than fifty years ago, Russell and Burch published '*The Principles of Humane Experimental Technique*' (Balls 2010), in which a radical change was proposed in the use of animals for research purposes. In essence, the principles state that animal experimentation should consider three 'Rs': refinement, reduction and replacement.

Refinement: aims to provide human care by specialized personnel decreasing damage due to procedures applied to laboratory animals.

Reduction: tends to decrease the number of animals destined to experimental series for basic and applied research.

Replacement: is directed to avoid the use of animals and encourage their replacement with inanimate systems, mathematical modeling being a proposed option.

The concept of the three 'Rs' is included in the Guide for the Care and Use of Laboratory Animals' (NRC 2011).

Finally, according to the above description, mathematical models are destined to replace earlier or later experimentation, reducing the gap between the *in vitro* laboratory and clinical practice. Although mathematical models do not exactly coincide with nature, they can answer many questions and verify scientific hypotheses.

References

Balls M 2010 The principles of humane experimental technique: timeless insights and unheeded warnings *ALTEX* **27** 19–23

Ericsson A C, Crim M J and Franklin C L 2013 A brief history of animal modeling *Mo Med.* **110** 201–5

Ross Ethier C and Simmons C A 2007 *Introductory Biomechanics: From Cells to Organisms* (Cambridge: Cambridge University Press) ch 3, pp 119–61

Frank O 1899 Die Grundform des arteriellen Pulses. Erste Abhandlung: Mathematische Analyse *Z. Biol.* **37** 485–526

Hagen G 1839 On the flow of water in narrow cylindrical tubes *Ann. Phys. Chem.* **46** 423–42

NRC: National Research Council (US) 2011 Committee for the update of the guide for the care and use of laboratory animals *Guide for the Care and Use of Laboratory Animals* 8th edn (Washington (DC): National Academies Press)

Nichols W W and O'Rourke M F 1998 McDonald's blood flow in arteries *Theoretical, Experimental and Clinical Principles* (London: Arnold) ch 2 pp 11–53

Poiseuille J L M 1993 Recherches experimentales sur Ie mouvement des liquides dans les tubes de tres petits diametres; 1. *Annu. Rev. Fluid Mech.* 1–20; downloaded from Influence de la pression sur la quantite de Iiquide qui traverse les tubes de très petits diametres *C. R. Acad. Sci.* **1** 961–67

Zimmer H G 1999 The contribution of Carl Ludwig to cardiology *Can. J. Cardiol.* **15** 323–9

Zimmer H G 2002 Who discovered the Frank–Starling mechanism? *News Physiol. Sci.* **17** 181–4

IOP Publishing

Ricardo L Armentano, Edmundo I Cabrera Fischer and Leandro J Cymberknop

Chapter 1

Structural basis of the circulatory system

Edmundo I Cabrera Fischer

1.1 Introduction

Blood circulation is possible by means of a central pump—the heart and a conduit system—arteries and veins. This circulation system ensures human body cell survival by carrying all the necessary nutrients and removing the waste products of tissue metabolism. The study of blood and the cardiovascular structure is called *hemodynamics*, and can be analyzed from a biophysical point of view. Similarly, cardiac and vessel structures can be studied from a mechanical point of view (Feher 2012, Fung 2004, Peterson and Bronzino 2008, Ross Ethier and Simmons 2011).

In this chapter, the heart and blood vessels will be described anatomically, with emphasis on the mechanical role of each one.

1.2 Cardiac structure

The constituents of cardiac structures and blood vessels are mostly muscle cells and extracellular elements, such as collagen and elastin. Smooth muscle cells can be found in the vessel wall, and myocardial cells in the atrial and ventricular chambers of the heart.

Knowledge of cardiac structures provides the essential basis for an understanding of circulatory dynamics. Figure 1.1 shows large vessels towards the top and the right, and ventricular structures towards the bottom and the left (Netter 1997).

The diagram of the frontal view of a normal heart shows the superior vein cava and the aortic and pulmonary arteries at the top, while the inferior vein cava and the right and left ventricles appear at the bottom (Iaizzo 2005). The right margin of the cardiac silhouette is formed by superior and inferior vein cavae, which are joined to the right atrium (see figure 1.1). On the contralateral side, the left atrium and left ventricle complete the cardiac silhouette. It is important to remember that the cardiac apex belongs to the left ventricle and the left anterior descending artery runs approximately between the left and right ventricles. The left atrium is an *a posterior* structure that only appears as a small appendage in a frontal view, whereas the right

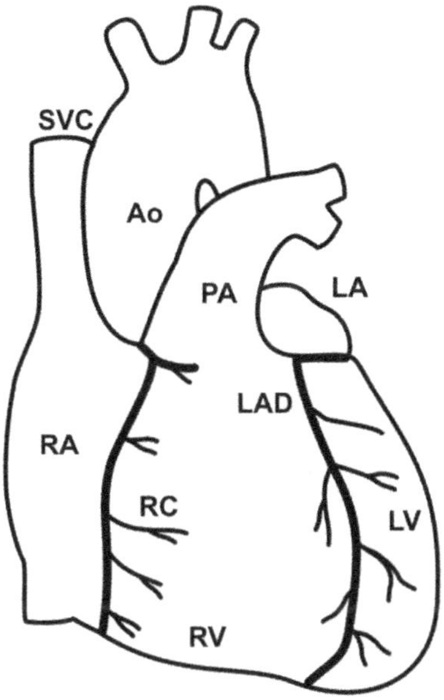

Figure 1.1. Structure of the heart and its main vessels. SVC: superior vein cava, Ao: aorta, PA: pulmonary artery, RA: right atrium, LA: left atrium, RV: right ventricle, LV: left ventricle, RC: right coronary artery and LAD: left anterior descending artery.

ventricle appears in an anterior position. The cardiac apex lies, approximately, in the intersection of the left midclavicular line and the fifth intercostal space (Iaizzo 2005).

The heart is located above the diaphragm, between the right and left lungs, and behind the sternum and costal cartilages. A pericardial sac surrounds it. The esophagus and the descending aorta are found behind the pericardium. The pericardium has two serous layers: *visceral* and *parietal*, separated by a lubricating fluid that facilitates the movement of the heart during its contraction and relaxation. The inferior parietal pericardium is fused to the diaphragm (Netter 1997).

The heart is a double pump that receives blood from vessels and circulates it to the left and right atria; blood volume is periodically passed through valves to the corresponding ventricles (see figures 1.1 and 1.2). Blood received by the right ventricle is pumped towards the lungs, and the blood collected by the left ventricle is ejected towards the aorta.

The cardiac structure can be represented as two separate atria followed by two separate ventricles. The heart can be considered as a pair of pumps, a right one and a left one, each of them with one atrium and one ventricle. Deoxygenated blood reaches the right atrium from the cava and coronary veins. This blood is delivered to the right ventricle through the tricuspid valve and arrives at the pulmonary artery after a right ventricular contraction that produces a pressure that allows the opening of the pulmonary valve. Oxygenated blood from the lung vessels is received through the left atrium and reaches the left ventricle through the mitral valve. Once a left ventricular contraction has occurred, oxygenated blood is pumped to the aortic artery through the aortic valve (Burton 1965).

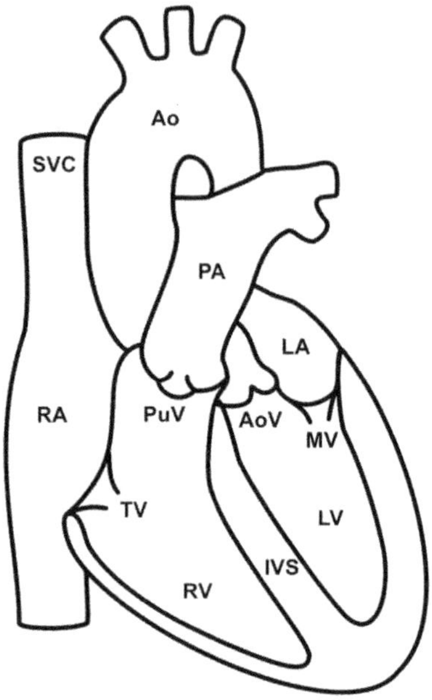

Figure 1.2. A frontal view of the heart, its valves and main vessels. SVC: superior vein cava, Ao: aorta, PA: pulmonary artery, RA: right atrium, LA: left atrium, RV: right ventricle, LV: left ventricle, TV and MV: tricuspid and mitral valves, PuV and AoV: pulmonary and aortic valves, IVS: interventricular septum.

The heart has a fibrous structure with four annuli for the mitral, tricuspid, pulmonary and aortic valves, i.e. each valve is inserted into a fibrous ring that serves as an anchorage mechanism. Furthermore, the upper interventricular septum has a short membranous extension that acts as anchorage for the tissues of the atrial and ventricular chambers.

Summarizing, the heart is a muscular structure that consists of two atrial chambers connected to two ventricles. The arteries are communicated to the ventricles through valves. There are no valves between the right and left atria and the entering veins. All heart valves are unidirectional and prevent blood flow from the arteries into the ventricles (aortic and pulmonary valves) and from the ventricles into the atria (tricuspid and mitral valves) (Kroemer *et al* 2010).

1.2.1 Heart valves

The mitral valve (figures 1.2 and 1.3) has a complex and dynamic anatomical structure and it is important to consider all its constituents. The mitral annulus acts as anchorage for the antero-septal and posterior leaflets. Each mitral leaflet is connected to both papillary muscles through the chordae tendineae (Burton 1965, Netter 1997).

Similarly, the right atrium is connected to the right ventricle through the tricuspid valve, which has three leaflets, one more than the mitral valve.

The aortic valve is positioned between the left ventricle and the aorta in order to prevent blood reflux during diastolic muscular relaxation. On the contralateral side,

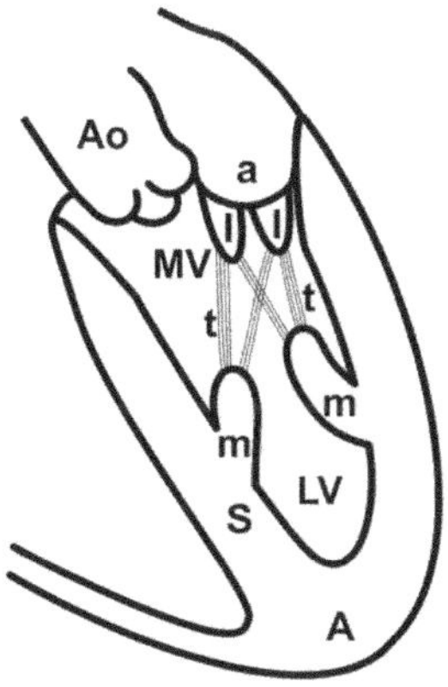

Figure 1.3. Cross-section of the left ventricle. The mitral valve (MV) includes an annulus (a), two leaflets (l) attached to papillary muscles (m) through chordae tendineae (t). A is the apex of the left ventricle, S is the interventricular septum, and Ao is the aorta.

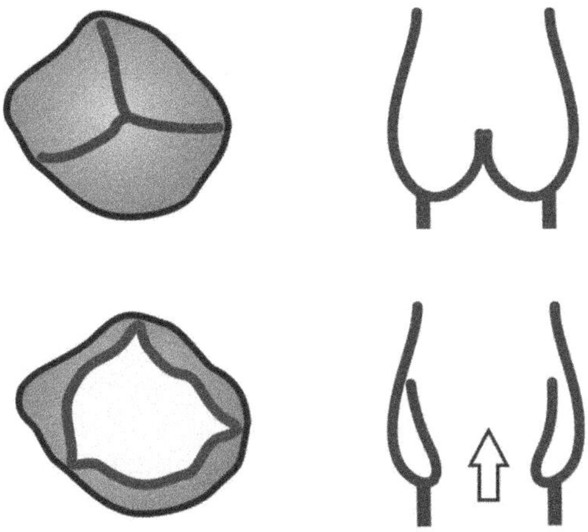

Figure 1.4. Cross-sectional (left panel) and lateral (right panel) views of the ventriculo-arterial valves. Three leaflets can be observed, in the closed position (upper panel) and in the open position (lower panel) during ventricular ejection.

the pulmonary valve has a similar role between the pulmonary artery and the right ventricle (Iaizzo 2005).

Both the aortic and the pulmonary valves have three leaflets or cusps that remain closed during the diastolic period, and open towards to the arterial wall during systole (see figure 1.4).

Describing the heart valves before the cardiac chambers seems inconsistent. However, considering the cardiac structure includes annulus for the valves, the pedagogic strategy is clearer. Thus, the atrial and ventricular structures are described as follows.

1.2.2 Cardiac chambers

The left atrium receives blood from four pulmonary veins that arrive from the left and right lungs. There are two right and two left pulmonary veins. The left atrium has an *a posterior* position and is separated from the right atrium by the interatrial septum. The thickness of the left atrium wall is approximately 3 mm.

The right atrium lies between the superior and inferior cava veins. Its wall thickness is slightly smaller than the left atrium (Lunkenheimer *et al* 1985).

The ventricular structures are made of striated muscular cells, similar to skeletal muscle cells, except control of the former is involuntary.

The ventricles have an inflow and an outflow tract. The input and output valves are placed laterally to each other, which means that the ventricular contraction must start distally to the output valve.

The left ventricle muscular walls are about 10 mm thick, and its geometry is generally described as hemi-ellipsoidal. The left ventricular lumen is not at all smooth: a great number of trabeculae are observed.

The right ventricle is in the cardiac midline, and has an anterior (ventral) position. It has thinner walls (3–4 mm) than the left ventricle because of the lower pressures involved. The right ventricle has a complex shape, which could be described as a crescent moon in cross-section. As in the left ventricle, a great number of trabeculae can be observed in the inner surface of the right ventricle (Lunkenheimer *et al* 1985).

1.2.3 Microscopic structures

The heart has a fibrous skeleton in which the mitral and tricuspid annuli are lodged. The muscular cells of both the auricular and ventricular chambers are attached to this collagenous structure. Even though the heart walls contain elastin and collagen fibers, it is considered a muscular structure from a quantitative point of view. The cardiac architecture includes pacemaker cells and non-pacemaker cells.

Muscular cells, *miocytes*, are the most important constituents of ventricles. They are combined with elastic and collagen fibers that contribute to a complex architecture, together with fibroblasts, endothelium and pacemaker cells. Myocytes have nuclei in a central position, contractile fibers and a large number of mitochondria surrounded by a membrane called sarcolemma. The contractile apparatus is formed by filaments of actin and myosin. These protein molecules are responsible for the muscular contraction that occurs by a sliding mechanism in which actin and myosin filaments take part (Iaizzo 2005, Feher 2012). The ends of the thin actin filaments are attached to structures called Z lines. The sarcomere is the segment of myofibrils between Z lines, and is recognized as the contractile structural and functional unit of muscular cells. The length of a sarcomere changes according to the degree of muscle contraction and relaxation (Fung 2004). The degree of overlap of actin and myosin fibers determines the distance between the Z lines, which ranges between 2.2 (during contraction) and 3.3 microns (during relaxation); see figures 1.5 and 1.6.

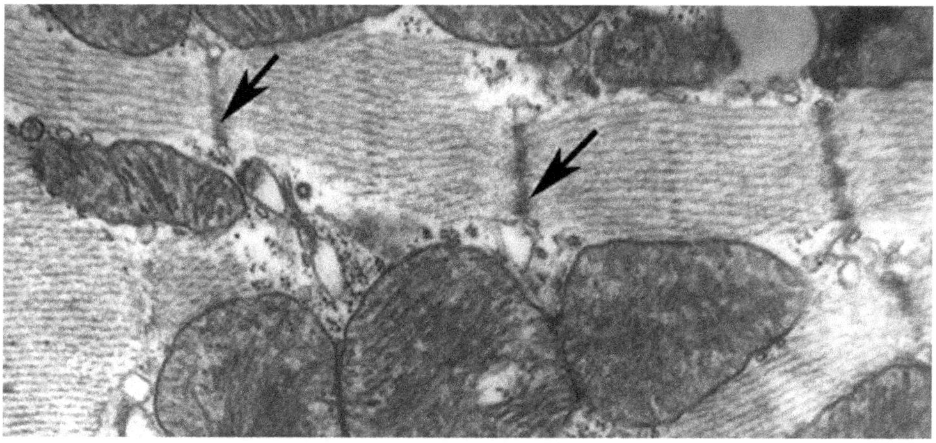

Figure 1.5. Mitochondrial and sarcolemmal structures viewed through electron microscopy. The arrows indicate the dark lines Z of the sarcomere (the contractile units of heart muscle). Between them, actin and myosin fibers that determine the distance between the Z lines range between 2.2 and 3.3 microns.

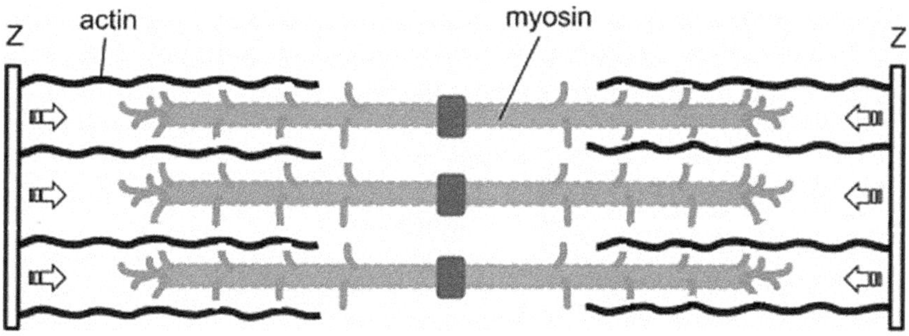

Figure 1.6. Diagram showing vertical Z lines that limit the sarcomere. The sliding of actin and myosin filaments determines a shortening of the distance between Z lines (arrows) during muscular contraction.

1.2.4 Electrical system

The dynamic function of the heart begins with a biologically generated electrical signal that contracts the atria first, and then the ventricle. The stimuli that determine cardiac muscle contraction are synchronized by an automatic system that produces and conducts electrical signals. This is the cardionector system, made up of specialized cells that generate electrical activity in pacemaker cells. The electrical impulse is generated by an action potential, and is rapidly transmitted through a specific conduction system, towards the myocardial muscle mass to cause rhythmic contraction. It is true electrical wiring (Iaizzo 2005).

Anatomically, the nerve fibers of the heart begin in the right atrium and end in the ventricles. The impulse originates in the junction between the superior vein cava and the right atrium, where a cellular node of pacemaker cells is found (also called Keith and Flack node). From this sinoatrial node, in physiological conditions, rhythmic

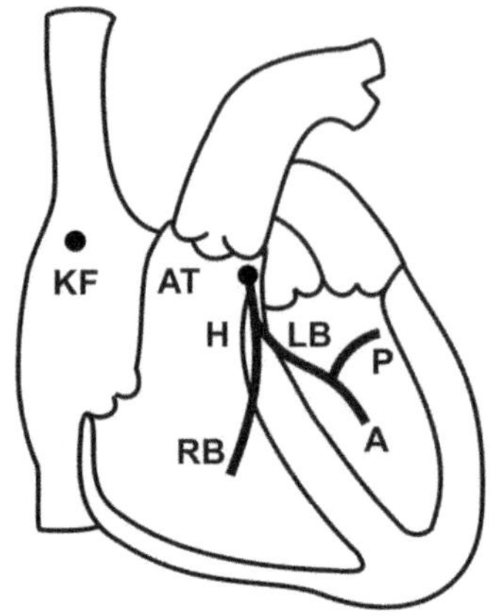

Figure 1.7. Electrical impulses begin in the Keith and Flack node (KF), then spread towards the right and left atria. Then, the impulse arrives at the Aschoff–Tawara node (AT), also called the atrioventricular node. Next, the impulse passes to the bundle of His (H), which diverges into a right branch (RB) and a left branch (LB). The latter has two divisions: posterior (P) and anterior (A) branches.

pulses are generated, which travel to the left atrium and connect to the atrioventricular node (see figure 1.7). The impulse is delayed before going towards the ventricles. This delay determines that the atria contract before their respective ventricles, achieving optimal ventricular filling (Feher 2012).

The atrioventricular node (also called the Aschoff–Tawara node) in the cardionector system is followed by the His bundle. It is a one-centimeter long collection of cardiac cells that is divided into a right and a left branch. The latter is divided into two branches: anterior and posterior.

The terminal branches of the above-described divisions are called Purkinje fibers. It is the peripheral specialized conduction system that provides the stimulation for the cardiac muscle cells to contract. The Purkinje fibers are in direct contact with the myocardial contractile cells (Iaizzo 2005).

1.3 Vessel structure

It is important to consider that a ventricle acts as a pump in a truly hydraulic sense. This is particularly relevant when the left ventricular–aortic coupling is analyzed. Both the aortic and pulmonary arteries periodically receive blood from the left and right ventricles, respectively, determining a dynamic vascular adaptation that can be explained by a biophysical analysis (Li 2000). This function depends on the viscoelastic properties of the smooth muscle cells, elastin and collagen of the ***arterial*** wall.

A cross-section view of the aorta and pulmonary arteries shows an arrangement of three concentric zones, called tunicae: intima, media and adventitia. The thickness of these layers changes as the arterial diameter decreases (Clark and Glagov 1979, Ross 1992).

The inner layer has cellular and extracellular constituents between the endothelial cells (which are in contact with blood) and the internal elastic lamina (a tubular elastic structure). This innermost layer is called ***tunica intima*** and contains collagen, laminin and fibronectin. The tunica intima is thinner than the media layer. The endothelial cells are arranged as a single monolayer and they have no structural role whatsoever. On the other hand, these cells are capable of modifying the entire arterial wall dynamics, as will be explained in the next chapter (Rhodin 1980).

Between the tunica intima and the adventitia layer, is the ***tunica media***, a complex structure linked to the mechanical properties of the arterial wall. The most important constituent of the aortic wall is elastin, followed by collagen fibers. Smooth muscle cells are approximately 15% of the dry weight of the aortic wall. The amount of collagen, elastin and smooth muscle varies along the arterial tree, with a significant increase of smooth muscle cells distally to the heart (Clark and Glagov 1979); see figure 1.8.

Arteries have the ability to retain their tubular shape, even when they are empty; the opposite happens to veins, which collapse. However, in humans the physiological diameter is given by the relationship between intraluminal pressure and smooth muscle tone.

In elastic arteries (i.e. the aorta and the brachiocephalic trunk), most of the elastin is arranged in the walls of these structures in the form of tubes of different diameters, as shown in figure 1.9. These tubular structures are called lamellar units and are fenestrated. The number of elastic lamellae is in the range of 50–80 in the aorta but only 2 in the muscular arteries (figure 1.10). In the latter, only the internal and the external elastic lamellar unit limit the tunica media (Bia *et al* 2014, Zócalo *et al* 2013).

The space between the elastic lamina is occupied by smooth muscle cells and collagenous fibrils. Vascular smooth muscle cells have two important physiological roles: (a) to determine the arterial diameter and (b) to produce elastin and collagen. Smooth muscle cells are oriented longitudinally, circumferentially and obliquely, which impact on the mechanical role of the vessel (Wolinsky and Glagov 1969, Fischer *et al* 2009).

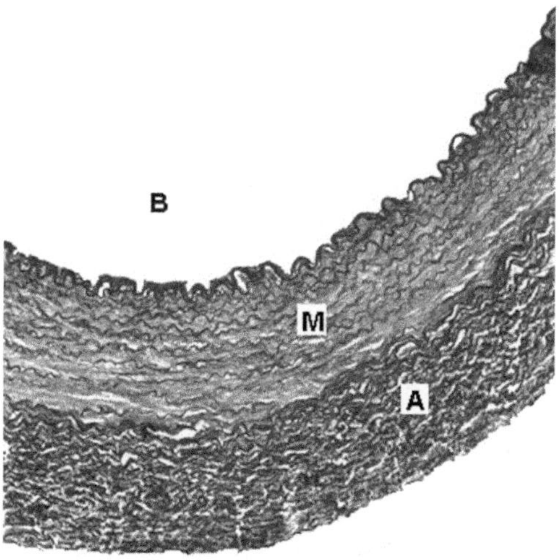

Figure 1.8. The arterial lumen is shown at the top (B), the inner layer is the intima, followed by the media (M) and adventitia (A). Several elastic lamellae are shown in the media. The stained artery is taken from a laboratory animal.

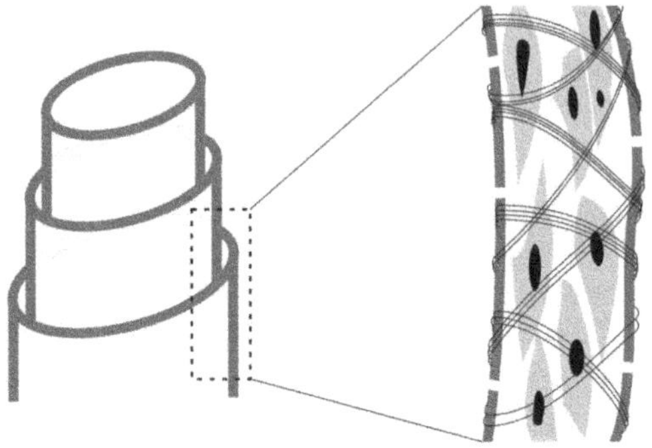

Figure 1.9. Left panel: schematic model of the structural constituents of the arterial wall, showing elastic lamellae. Right panel: smooth muscle cells are positioned between the tubular elastic structures. The right panel illustrates the structure of smooth muscle cells placed between two elastic fenestrated lamellae and collagen fibers (thin black lines).

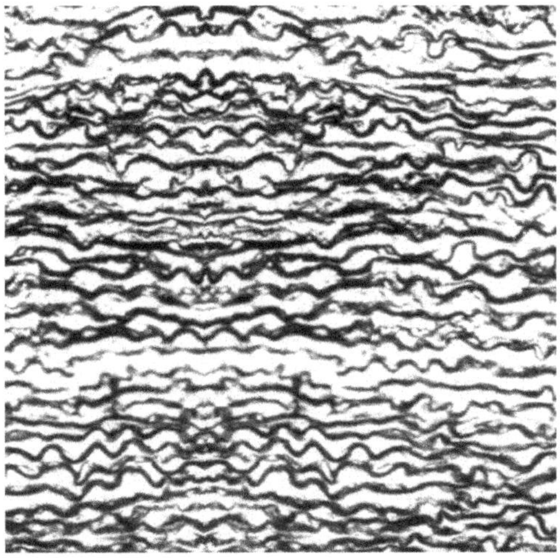

Figure 1.10. Image of a stained artery from a laboratory animal, showing the elastic lamellae in the tunica intima. The lack of distending intraluminal pressure explains the winding shape of the elastic units shown in figure 1.9.

Collagen fibers are made of the most abundant protein in the human body: collagen. There are several types of collagen, and in arteries it is, quantitatively, the most important constituent of the abdominal aorta (Fischer and Llaurado 1966, Fischer *et al* 1991).

The outermost tunica is the tunica adventitia, for which the thickness changes in the different arterial territories. This outermost tunica has a fibroelastic matrix and adipocytes. It also contains vasa vasorum and nerves that ensure vessel wall blood perfusion and innervation, respectively. Interestingly, the word 'adventitia' derives from *adventicius,* which means '*coming from abroad, foreign*' in Latin (Wolinsky and Glagov 1967, Fischer 2006).

Veins and arteries have similar constituents: elastin, collagen and smooth muscle cells. Nonetheless, there are quantitative differences and some anatomical details to take into account. Veins have thinner walls and a larger diameter than arteries. However, three layers can be differentiated in the walls of the veins (Zócalo *et al* 2013).

Since an important function of veins is the storage of large amounts of blood, the volume contained in the veins is close to 65% of the total content of the circulatory system. The venous wall is thinner than the arterial wall, and accordingly, venous pressure is lower than arterial pressure.

The most important difference between arteries and veins is possibly the existence of valves in the latter. Also, veins on the upper limbs are thinner than the lower limbs. Furthermore, veins have more connective tissue than arteries.

Blood supply in the vein wall is ensured by the vasa vasorum that can be found in the adventitia and media layers of medium-sized veins.

1.4 The circulatory system

The circulatory system can be considered as a single closed circuit whose beginning and ending is arbitrary, for example: starting in the left atrium, blood passes to the left ventricle and through the aortic valve to the aorta, the elastic arteries, the capillaries, the veins, towards the right atrium and ventricle, then to the pulmonary arteries, the capillaries and the pulmonary veins, to start over the same cycle. Evidently, any other point can be chosen as a starting point. Furthermore, two different subcircuits can be identified within the circulatory system: the pulmonary and the systemic systems (Li 2000); see figure 1.11.

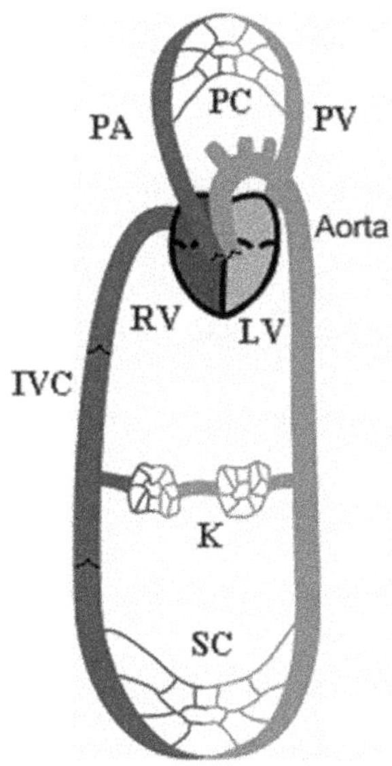

Figure 1.11. Schematic representation of the human blood circulatory system. IVC: inferior vena cava, RV: right ventricle, PA: pulmonary artery, PC: pulmonary capillaries, PV: pulmonary vein, LV: left ventricle, K: kidney showing artero-arterial portal system and SC: systemic capillaries.

The pulmonary circuit goes from the right ventricle to the left atrium, passing through the right pulmonary artery, capillaries and pulmonary veins. On the other hand, the systemic circulation goes from the left ventricle to the right atrium through arteries, capillaries and veins.

The above-described cardiovascular arrangement enables the maintenance of blood flow that ensures an adequate perfusion of all of the tissues of the human body. As shown in figure 1.11, pulmonary blood circulation is connected in series with systemic circulation.

The circulatory system determines the path used by the blood, but tissue fluid reabsorption is completed by the ***lymphatic vessels*** that carry the lymph to the veins. Lymphatic vessels have unidirectional valves. The lymph has a liquid nature and has no red blood cells. The lymphatic wall structure is similar to that of the capillary wall. This system carries the large molecules of the interstitial space including large proteins and lipids. The lymphatic fluid eventually drains into the venous system. The most important lymphatic vessel is the thoracic duct that is situated between the aorta and the esophagus, ending in the left confluence of the subclavian and jugular veins.

1.5 Human blood

Human blood has cells and plasma that can be separated using a simple technique that consists of centrifuging a sample obtained from a peripheral vein. Centrifugation allows one to separate the solid (cellular) from the liquid phase (plasma). The *Hematocrit* is the volume of erythrocytes expressed as a percentage of the total centrifuged blood volume. It is valuable data that helps one to diagnose blood diseases such as anemia. In humans, the normal value of the hematocrit ranges from 40% to 45%, and is higher in males than in females (Fung 2004).

1.5.1 Blood plasma

Plasma is a straw-colored fluid, with water being its most important constituent. As blood is considered a tissue, plasma would be a part of the interstitial space. The solutes present in plasma are: proteins (albumin, fibrinogen, globulin among others), ions (Na^+, Ca^{++}, Cl^-, K^+), metabolites, hormones, platelets, nutrients and waste products of cellular metabolism. Platelets are little pieces of bone marrow cells called megakaryocytes, which have a very important role in blood clotting formation. Platelets are formed elements of human blood whose concentration is in the range of $1.8–4.0 \times 10^5$ mm^3 of blood (Feher 2012).

1.5.2 Blood cells

There are two types of circulating cells in the blood: red (erythrocytes) and white (leukocytes) cells. In humans, blood cells originate in the bone marrow.

In a static condition, red cells are symmetrically disc-shaped. The most important intracellular constituent of an erythrocyte is hemoglobin, and it has no nucleus. Erythrocytes in humans range from 5 to 6×10^6 cells per mm^3 of blood (Fung 2004); see figure 1.12.

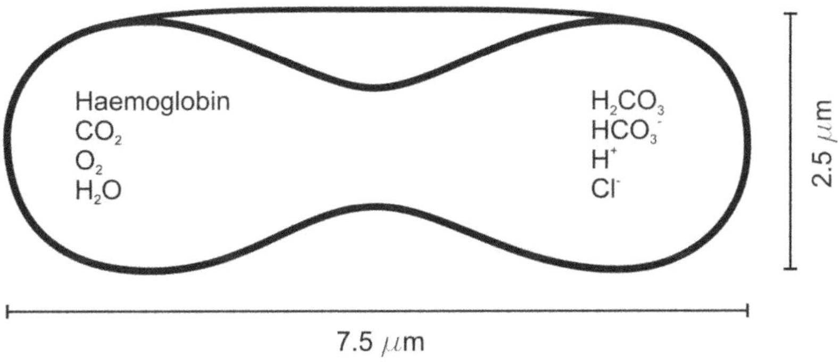

Figure 1.12. Diagram of a red blood cell; a biconcave shape can be observed. Erythrocytes have no nucleus and the mean diameter changes according to the vascular bed where the erythrocyte is traveling.

The different types of leukocytes account for only 1% of the cellular constituents of human blood; they have morphological and functional differences among them. Different leukocytes include neutrophils, basophils, eosinophils, lymphocytes and monocytes. Leukocytes in humans range from 5000 to 11 000 cells per mm^3 of blood.

In humans, blood distribution in the circulatory system is not uniform. Blood cells and plasma total a volume of approximately 5.5 l in a healthy adult human. This volume is distributed as follows: 64% is in the venous system, 15% in the systemic arteries, 9% in the lungs, 7% in the cardiac chambers and 5% in microcirculation. As can be seen, the larger volumes of blood are contained in the low pressure reservoirs (i.e. the venous system).

1.6 Microcirculation

The above-described cardiovascular structures are distributed in every human body territory in order to irrigate the perivascular parenchyma, i.e. the tissue that surrounds vessels. The general operating scheme is that of an artery entering an organ and then dividing itself into smaller arteries, arterioles and capillaries, followed by small venules and veins. The latter ensure that blood returns to the cardiac structures.

There are certain territories in which microcirculation shows particular characteristics. For example, lung capillaries are very close to the alveolus, which contain a modified atmospheric air (e.g. different pressure and relative humidity conditions); in kidneys, the arterial portal systems ensure tissue irrigation and urine formation; in the skin, vessels participate in body temperature regulation; in the digestive system a vein portal system enables the carrying of nutrients from the intestines to the liver lobules.

1.6.1 Capillaries

Capillaries are vessels that have two important characteristics: (a) they are the smallest vessels, with a 7–10 μm diameter, and (b) they provide the largest vessel wall area to communicate the circulatory system with the surrounding interstitial space of the different tissues of the human body. The capillary wall consists of endothelial cells surrounded by a tubular structure with no smooth muscle cells. The diameter values of capillaries differ from one tissue to another, and so do some other morphological characteristics. Three types of capillaries are described below (Tedgui 1994).

Continuous capillary: the wall of these capillaries is constituted of endothelial cells joined to each other with no fenestrations or gaps between them. Endothelial cells are arranged on a basement membrane. This is the most common type of capillary.

Fenestrated capillary: the capillary has certain small areas in which the wall has fenestrated endothelial cells. Fenestrae are pores of which the diameter is approximately 100 nm.

Discontinuous capillary: these capillaries have the largest diameter of all capillaries (from 30 to 70 μm). Endothelial cells have gaps that allow free communication between the intravascular space and the surrounding tissues.

1.6.2 Alveolar capillary barrier

Systemic circulation was adequately described for the first time by William Harvey, and pulmonary circulation was discovered and characterized by Ibn al-Nafis (1213–88), an Arab physician. The pulmonary circuit has several features regarding other organs of the human body. In fact, lungs are organs that receive the greatest amount of blood, since the right ventricle pumps the same volume as the left ventricle (Feher 2012, Despopoulos and Silbemagl 2003).

Lung parenchyma is perfused by oxygenated blood provided by the bronchial arteries, and blood that is involved in gas exchange is pumped by the right ventricle through the pulmonary artery. Oxygen contained in the lung alveoli is carried by red blood cells, while carbon dioxide is transported by plasma and erythrocytes. Carbon dioxide is a well-known product of the Krebs cycle that easily diffuses through the soft tissues of the human body.

Gas exchange takes place at the lungs alveoli, which are surrounded by pulmonary capillaries. The oxygen contained in an alveolus passes through several barriers in order to oxygenate the hemoglobin contained in the red blood cells (figure 1.13). The first barrier is the aqueous lining containing surfactant in the alveolus, the second is the pneumocyte type one cell, the third is the interstitial space, the fourth is the endothelial cell that is part of the capillary vessel, the fifth is the blood plasma and last, the erythrocyte membrane (see figure 1.13).

1.6.3 Portal venous system

There is a portal system between the intestines and the hepatic structures. The portal vein originates from anastomosis of the splenic vein and the superior and inferior mesenteric veins. In this way, the blood goes from the spleen and intestine to the liver. Other veins are also anastomosed to this system: the right and left gastric, gastro-epiploic, cystic and pancreatic-duodenal veins.

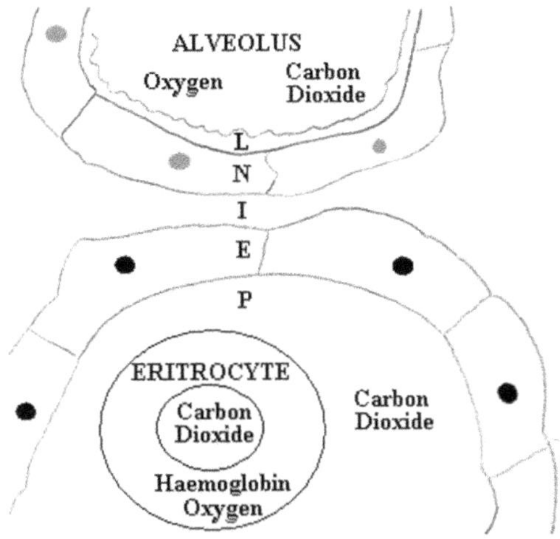

Figure 1.13. Barriers that the oxygen passes through from the alveolus to red blood cells (erythrocytes) to combine with hemoglobin molecules. L: aqueous lining containing surfactant, N: neumocyte Type 2 cell, I: interstitial space, E: Endothelial cell and P: blood plasma. Oxygen transport is linked to hemoglobin while carbon dioxide is transported by plasma and erythrocytes.

This venous portal system receives blood from the esophagus, the stomach, the spleen, the pancreas, the gall-bladder and the intestinal tract. The portal vein is a thick trunk divided into two branches that enters the liver and originates from the veins of the liver lobule. The blood supply to the liver lobule contains nutrients that are obtained from intestinal absorption and splenic activity. The latter is very important in the iron recycling process carried out by the splenic macrophages out of old erythrocytes. The portal vein blood received by the hepatic lobule goes to the central vein and finally joins the inferior vein cava. Summarizing, the blood that perfuses the digestive tract is the same as that which arrives at the liver, that is to say, there is a capillary barrier in the intestines and another one in the hepatic lobule (Feher 2012, Despopoulos and Silbemagl 2003).

The physiological role of this portal system is to provide a direct pathway for nutrients that are metabolized in the hepatic parenchyma. The relevance of this portal system is to avoid a large amount of blood from entering directly into the inferior vein cava bypassing the hepatic stage. In this case, blood supplied to the hepatic tissue has a very different function to that provided by systemic arteries to body tissues.

Another venous portal system is involved in the secretion of the hypothalamic-pituitary hormone. There are hormones secreted in the hypothalamus that regulate the anterior pituitary gland function after traveling through a portal venous system. The superior hypophyseal artery perfuses the median eminence and this blood enters the capillaries, which after merging into each other form a venous network that carries releasing hormones. These portal veins split into capillaries that perfuse the anterior pituitary gland, stimulating or inhibiting the production of several hormones. Later, these hormones are released into the systemic circulation and travel to specific organs in order control physiological functions.

1.6.4 Arterial portal system

The basic function of kidneys is to produce urine. This complex liquid is produced in the *nephron,* which is the basic structural and functional *unit* of the *kidney*. A nephron has basically two components: tubular and vascular structures. Histologically, the nephron begins in the glomerulus that is a tuft of capillaries that originate from afferent arterioles. These capillaries drain blood onto the efferent arteriole; see figure 1.14.

Each glomerulus is embraced by a Bowman's capsule, which is followed by the proximal convoluted tubule. The Bowman's capsule receives a filtrated modified plasma from the glomerulus. The proximal convoluted tubule is continued by the loop of Henle. The loop of Henle is followed by the distal convoluted tubule, which ends in the collecting duct. At the end of the collecting duct, the fluid contained in the tubular lumen is urine.

With respect to blood vessels, the glomerulus receives blood from the afferent arteries and the constitutive capillaries; in other capillary beds they are followed by a venule, but in this case they are continued by the afferent arteriole. Efferent arterioles perfuse the renal parenchyma including the tubules and loop of Henle through the vasa recta. Blood contained in the capillaries that constitute the peritubular network is drained by venules (Schrier 2008).

The arterial portal system described above has a set of capillaries (glomerulus) that filtrates plasma into the Bowman's capsule. This capillary network is continued by the efferent artery that originates from the peritubular capillaries. As can be seen, there are two capillary networks before the drainage of venules.

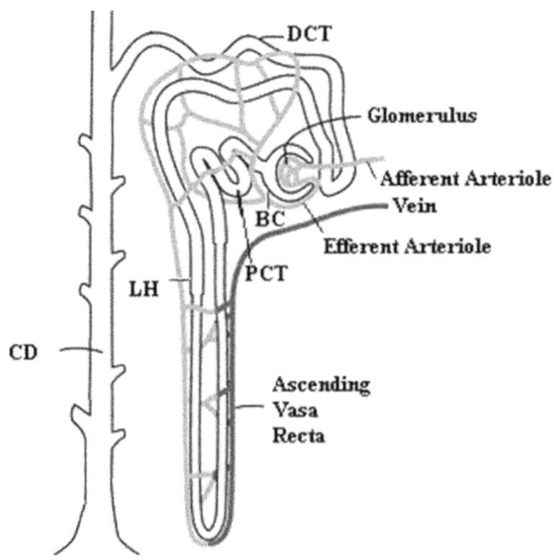

Figure 1.14. BC: Bowman's capsule, PCT: proximal convoluted tubule, LH: loop of Henle, DCT: distal convoluted tubule, CD: collecting duct. Note that the peritubular capillaries originate from the efferent arterioles that drain in a vein.

1.6.5 Arteriovenous anastomoses

The capillary network starts in the arterioles, which drain their contained blood into the venules. However, there are certain territories in which arteriovenous shunts avoid the capillary network. These anatomical findings have physiological connotations and are usually linked to adaptive mechanisms. An example of a shunt is the skin, in which arterioles are anastomosed to venules, particularly in fingers. In this case, this dynamic shunt participates in the control of body temperature (Despopoulos and Silbemagl 2003).

According to several authors, another example of arteriovenous fistula is uteroplacental circulation.

In the lungs, there is a functional shunt in which blood provided by bronchial arteries to pulmonary parenchyma are drained in the pulmonary veins.

1.6.6 Splenic circulation

Capillaries that allow blood cells to go through the vessel wall are only found in splenic circulation and in bone marrow. As red blood cells are formed in the latter, they need a direct path to enter intraluminal space. Downstream, the old red cells are trapped by splenic structures.

After an approximate period of 120 days, the old erythrocyte is destroyed in the spleen. As an adult human being has a blood volume of 5 l and each mm^3 contains 5 000 000 erythrocytes, the production and elimination of blood red cells is a very dynamic process. This involves the erythrocytes passing through capillaries to enter the splenic tissue, where iron is recycled (Despopoulos and Silbemagl 2003).

An interesting physiologic phenomenon occurs during active physical exercise; hematocrit increases due to a splenic contraction that releases red blood cells into the circulatory system.

1.6.7 Myocardial circulation

As previously described, coronary arteries perfuse the myocardium and heart structures. This is the nearest and shortest circuit of the human circulatory anatomy; consequently, it is the blood of the human body recirculating (Despopoulos and Silbemagl 2003).

Usually, an artery is a vessel that enters an organ and branches into smaller vessels. This is impossible to attain in the myocardium of the left ventricle since it reaches 120 mmHg during the systolic period and the muscular contraction occludes the arterial lumen. Indeed, the coronary intraluminal pressure can never be higher than the ventricular pressure. Consequently, the large coronary vessels should be surrounding the left ventricular wall rather than being inserted in the muscle.

Intramuscular coronary arteries are a pathologic entity that sometimes determine ischemic episodes or myocardial infarction. There are cases in which coronary arteries have muscular 'bridges' and are partially intramuscular arteries. In this case, muscular contraction produces dynamic coronary stenosis that disappears during diastole.

In a normal heart, some intramuscular small arteries are called 'perforators'. This is the case of septal branches of the left anterior descending artery. The coronary flow is strongly influenced by anatomical factors due to left ventricular mechanical dynamics. This is not the case of the atria and the right ventricle, in which intramural pressures are lower than the coronary arterial pressure.

During myocardial contraction, the external compression of small coronary branches is maximal in endocardium, and decreases towards the epicardium. Since large coronary arteries are not surrounded by myocardial tissue, no lumen decreases are observed on them during heart contraction.

References

Bia D, Zócalo Y, Cabrera-Fischer E I, Wray S and Armentano R L 2014 Quantitative analysis of the relationship between blood vessel wall constituents and viscoelastic properties: dynamic biomechanical and structural *in vitro* studies in aorta and carotid arteries *Physiol. J.* 2014 Article ID 142421

Burton A C 1965 *Physiology and Biophysics of the Circulation* (Chicago, IL: Year Book Medical Publishers)

Clark J M and Glagov S 1979 Structural integration of the arterial wall. I. Relationships and attachments of medial smooth muscle cells in normally distended and hyperdistended aortas *Lab. Invest.* **40** 587–602

Despopoulos A and Silbemagl S 2003 *Color Atlas of Physiology* 5th edn (New York: Thieme)

Feher J 2012 *Quantitative Human Physiology: An Introduction Academic Press Series in Biomedical Engineering* (New York: Elservier)

Fischer G M and Llaurado J G 1966 Collagen and elastin content in canine arteries selected from functionally different vascular beds *Circ. Res.* **XIX** 394–9

Fischer E I C, Armentano R L, Levenson J, Barra J G, Morales M C, Breitbart G J, Pichel R H and Simon A C 1991 Paradoxically decreased aortic wall stiffness in response to vitamin D_3-induced calcinosis: a biphasic analysis of segmental elastic properties in conscious dogs *Circ. Res.* **68** 1549–59

Fischer E I C, Bia D, Zócalo Y and Armentano R L 2009 Smooth muscle-dependent changes in aortic wall dynamics during intra-aortic counterpulsation in an animal model of acute heart failure *Int. J. Artif. Organs* **32** 354–61

Fischer E I C 2006 Adventitia-dependent mechanical properties of brachiocephalic ovine arteries in *in vivo* and *in vitro* studies *Acta Physiol.* **188** 103–11

Fung Y C 2004 *Biomechanics. Mechanical Properties of Living Tissues* 2nd edn (New York: Springer)

Iaizzo P A 2005 *Handbook of Cardiac Anatomy, Physiology, and Devices* (New York: Humana Press)

Kroemer K H E, Kroemer H J and Kroemer-Elbert K E 2010 *Engineering Physiology. Bases of Human Factors Engineering/Ergonomics* (Berlin: Springer)

Li J 2000 *The Arterial Circulation: Physical Principles and Clinical Applications* (New York: Humana Press)

Lunkenheimer P P, Lunkenheimer A and Torrent-Guasp F 1985 *Kardiodynamik: wege zur strukturgerechten. Analyse der Myokardfunktion* (Erlangen, Germany: Perimed Fachbuch-Verlagsgesellschaft)

Netter F H 1997 *The Ciba Collection Of Medical Illustrations. Heart* vol 5 (New York: Elsevier)

Peterson D and Bronzino J 2008 *Biomechanics: Principles and Applications* (New York: CRC Press)

Rhodin J A G 1980 *Handbook of Physiology, The Cardiovascular System* Section 2 ed D Bohr, A Somlyo and H J Sparks (Bethesda, MD: American Physiological Society) ch 1

Ross Ethier C and Simmons C A 2011 *Introductory Biomechanics: From Cells to Organisms Cambridge texts in Biomedical Engineering* (New York: Cambridge University Press)

Ross R 1992 The vessel wall *The Heart and Cardiovascular System* 2nd edn ed H A Fozzard *et al* (New York: Raven Press Ltd)

Schrier R W 2008 *Diseases of the Kidney and Urinary Tract* 8th edn (Philadelphia: Lippincott Williams and Wilkins)

Tedgui L B 1994 Biologie de la paroi artérielle *Aspects normaux et pathologiques* (Paris, France: Masson)

Wolinsky H and Glagov S 1967 Nature of species differences in the medial distribution of aortic vasa vasorum in mammals *Circ. Res.* **20** 409–21

Wolinsky H and Glagov S 1969 Comparison of abdominal and thoracic aortic medial structure in mammals *Circ. Res.* **25** 667–86

Zócalo Y, Bia D, Cabrera-Fischer E I, Wray S, Galli C N and Armentano R L 2013 Structural and functional properties of venous wall: relationship between elastin, collagen, and smooth muscle components and viscoelastic properties *ISRN Physiol.* Article ID 906031

Chapter 2

Human circulatory function

Edmundo I Cabrera Fischer

In this chapter, the basic principles of blood circulation, the function of the left ventricle and vessel mechanics will be described.

2.1 Hemodynamics

The circulatory system ensures the transport of all the necessary elements for cell survival and the removal of waste products. A central pump (the heart) and a conduction system (the vessels) are continuously conveying all elements needed for life using blood as the vehicle. Blood, in physiological conditions, is a tissue that lacks a definite shape. Since blood is needed to connect each cell with all other systems of the human body, a dynamic component should be considered in the study of this tissue. In fact, blood is a type of connective tissue that should be analyzed considering it as a fluid. Consequently, the principles and laws of hydrodynamics are used to explain the dynamic behavior of human blood, and its study is called hemodynamics, which describes blood circulation and adaptive mechanisms (Feher 2012).

The cardiovascular function is mainly mechanical, and the best way to understand the heart and vessel dynamics is by performing a biophysical analysis. Throughout this chapter it will become evident that the cardiac chambers, vessels and blood are in constant movement during the entire existence of a living human. Curiously, the word ‘heart’ is etymologically related to the dynamic characteristic of this organ. In Sanskrit, *hrid* or *krid* means ‘jumping’, from which the words ‘heart’, ‘Herz’ (German) and ‘kardia’ (Greek) derive. On the other hand, the word ‘artery’ implies a terrible mistake, since it derives from the Greek words *aer* (‘air’) and *terein* (‘to contain’), implying that an artery contains air, according to the etymology of this old word (Fischer and Barmak 2005).

The heart begins its mechanical function with a biologically generated electrical signal that causes the atria to contract in the first place, followed by the ventricles. Blood is conveyed through a circuit that starts at the left ventricle, and ends at the

doi:10.1088/2053-2563/aafb0dch2

right atrium passing through all of the *systemic circulation*, and then through another circuit from the right ventricle to the left atrium through the *pulmonary circulation*. An *artery* is any vessel carrying blood away from the heart and a *vein* is any vessel that conveys blood towards the heart (McCulloch 2008).

Blood is responsible for cellular survival, since it carries all of the substances needed to maintain vital functions. This is why blood as a liquid-state tissue has a great number of static and dynamic characteristics. Blood is considered to be a non-Newtonian fluid, and therefore understanding its dynamic behavior requires further knowledge. This is particularly useful when *in vitro* studies are carried out using hydraulic loops that mimic the human cardiovascular system (Ross Ethier and Simmons 2011).

Blood circulation has multiple purposes that are analyzed depending on their characteristics. Some of the body functions are: temperature control, hormone transport, PH regulation, waste excretion, cellular respiration, immunologic response to foreign organisms, and others involved in the maintenance of the integrity of the circulatory system, such as blood clotting. Since the scope of this book is focused on mechanical analysis, some of the previously mentioned body functions, when necessary, will be superficially commented on in the following sections.

2.2 The left ventricular function

To understand cardiovascular dynamics, a thorough understanding of basic sciences, which describe the principles and laws of bodies under motion, is needed. A basic physiology background and minimal handling of the instruments required to measure biological signals are also needed.

Left ventricular performance depends on intrinsic and extrinsic variables, which should be identified to understand the normal and abnormal functions of this muscular chamber. This has physiological and medical connotations linked to technologies developed for diagnostic or therapeutic purposes (Loushin and Iaizzo 2005).

In a cardiac cycle, the filling period is followed by the cardiac contraction. During the filling of the ventricular chamber, the volume rises from 50–79 ml (end systolic volume) to 120–140 ml (end diastolic volume). The Frank–Starling law states that the more the ventricular chamber is filled, the more blood will be ejected, which is concomitant with the fact that the energy of contraction is a function of the length of the muscle fiber. The physiological meaning of the Frank–Starling law is that increases of diastolic left ventricular volume and pressure just before contraction will determine an augmentation of the length of the myocardial fibers, which will accordingly increase the stroke volume and systolic pressure developed during the ventricular contraction (Valentinuzzi 2001, Lunkenheimer *et al* 1985). After the filling stage, i.e. the *end of* systole, the mitral valve closes and the contraction of the heart muscle determines an increase in the pressure, from 0 mmHg to 120–140 mmHg. ***Preload*** is defined as the left ventricular pressure at the end of the filling period.

Aortic blood pressure is a determinant factor in left ventricular function. Indeed, the aortic valve opens when the left ventricular pressure is higher than the aortic pressure. This is called ***afterload***, and it means that increases of arterial pressure will determine decreases in the systolic left ventricular volume ejected during the systolic period (Loushin and Iaizzo 2005). The increase in afterload directly changes the end systolic left ventricular volume (i.e. the volume at the beginning of the diastole) and indirectly changes the end diastolic volume and pressure of the next beat. These increased diastolic volumes induce an increase of contractility, producing higher systolic left ventricular pressures. These changes in left ventricular contraction have been described as a 'homeometric autoregulation' (Folkow and Neil 1971).

The left ventricular function can be studied using pressure–volume diagrams, which have been used since the nineteenth century. In 1824 a text was published, called 'Réflexions sur la puissance motrice du feu et sur les machines propres a développer cette puissance' ('Reflections on the Motive Power of Fire') by Sadi Carnot. In this text, the power of steam machines with respect to changes in volume was analyzed (Carnot 1824). Later, Otto Frank obtained left ventricular pressure–volume loops during *in vitro* studies, describing the ventricular mechanical behavior (Crottogini *et al* 1987).

The dynamic concepts thus described help to explain left ventricular function using a model of the cardiac cycle of four phases, as follows.

2.2.1 Filling phase

Each ventricular contraction is preceded by a filling period in which the blood contained in the atria goes through an auriculo-ventricular valve called the *mitral valve*. A left atrial contraction determined by electric stimulus produced in the Keith and Flack node forces a mitral blood flow towards the ventricle. This phase begins when the mitral valve opens and lasts until before the left ventricular myocardial contraction begins, which closes the mitral valve (Burton 1965).

2.2.2 Isovolumic contraction

Myocardial contraction is triggered by the electrical signals that come from the pacemakers of the sinus node, which travel towards the auriculo-ventricular pacemaker node and then to the bundle of His and Purkinje tissue. The aortic valve is closed at this stage, and a sudden increase of intraluminal pressure ensures the closing of the mitral valve (Burton 1965).

2.2.3 Ejection period

The ejection period begins when intraluminal left ventricular pressure is higher than the aortic pressure and ends at the beginning of diastole, when the aortic valve is closed due to the impossibility of the myocardium to maintain the pressure gradient blood flow (Burton 1965).

2.2.4 Isovolumic relaxation

When the aortic valve closes, the myocardium of the left ventricle relaxes. This *isovolumic* relaxation phase is maintained during the time it takes the left ventricular pressure to fall below the left atrial pressure. At this stage, the mitral valve opens (Burton 1965).

2.2.5 Myocardial contractility

The left ventricle myocardial contraction can develop intraluminal pressures that could eventually be raised due to increases in the volume of the ventricular filling (Frank–Starling law). Myocardial contractility is the force developed by the left ventricular wall independently of the myocardial fiber length, i.e. independently of the end diastolic left ventricular volume; see figure 2.1.

Left ventricular contractility can be quantified using several indices such as the first derivative of the intraventricular pressure with respect to time, *dp/dt*. The most reliable index that allows one to obtain accurate measurements of left ventricular myocardial contractility are the values of the slopes of the straight lines that connect the end systolic pressure–volume points (Fischer and Barmak 2005).

It is noteworthy that the slope of the end systolic instantaneous pressure–volume relationship is not modified by changes of preload or of afterload. Furthermore, during physiological and pathological states it is a straight line with a slope that represents the maximum elastance. Increases in left ventricular contractility tend to increase the slope of the end systolic pressure–volume relationship (figure 2.2). On

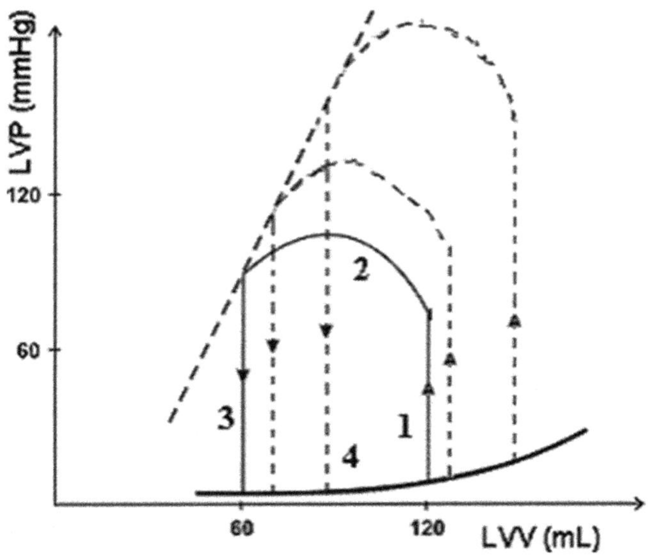

Figure 2.1. Left ventricular phases of the cardiac cycle. 1: isovolumic contraction and 2: ejection during systole, 3: isovolumic relaxation and 4: filling period during diastole. LVP: left ventricular pressure. LVV: left ventricular volume.

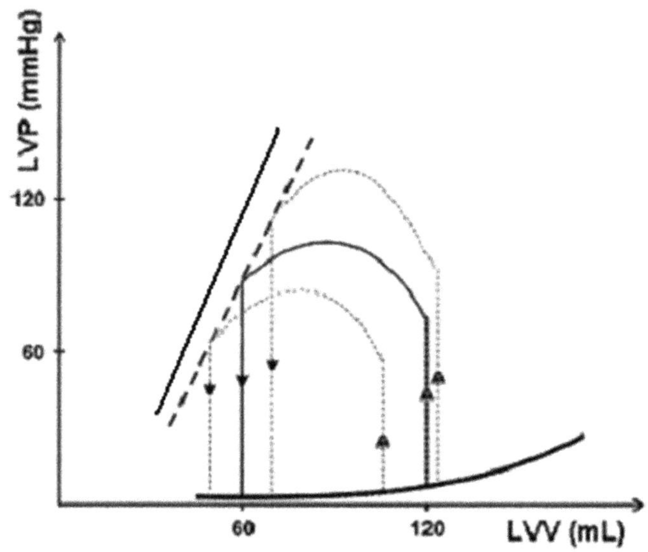

Figure 2.2. Three pressure–volume loops. The dotted lines connect the end systolic pressure–volume relationship in control state. The bold line shows a similar line obtained after a pharmacologically induced increase of myocardial contractility. The left ventricular pressure–volume relationship loop has a counter-clockwise sense of rotation.

the other hand, a decrease in left ventricular contractility determines a decrease in the value of this maximum elastance, indicating a lower inotropic state (Fischer *et al* 1988, Fischer and Barmak 2005).

2.2.6 Diastolic function

The measurement of left ventricular diastolic pressure usually shows positive values during the isometric relaxation period, during the time that the mitral valve is open and until the end of the diastole. However, the left ventricular structure is able to develop low pressure values ranging from 6 to −7 mmHg. These near-vacuum pressure values have been observed during left ventricular relaxation at the beginning of the filling phase. This 'suction effect' is explained by the sudden decreases of the left ventricular volume at the end of the systolic period, and it is simultaneous with a quick aspiration of blood from the left atrium. Thus, this physiological condition may be produced by elastic forces that promote a quick dilatation of the left ventricle when the end systolic volume has been suddenly decreased. In other words, when the muscle fibers of the left ventricular myocardium are shorter during systole, the potential energy stored at the end of the systolic period is then released at the beginning of the diastole, determining this 'sucking effect' due to the rapid ventricular expansion (Fischer *et al* 1991a, Fischer and Barmak 2005).

2.3 Vessel function

2.3.1 Arteries

The ventricular–aortic interaction is a fundamental aspect of the systemic blood circuit; its quantitative evaluation is vital. As left ventricular function is assessed using the pressure–volume relationship, the study of arterial wall function in this book will include a similar pressure–diameter relationship analysis.

Intraluminal blood pressure in arteries can be measured instantaneously using two well-known instruments: (a) solid state catheter, and (b) fluid-filled catheters. The physical basis of these widely used techniques are explained later in this chapter. These ***pressure*** measurement techniques are often complementary. Aortic pressure can be measured, for example, using a pressure microtransducer (1200 Hz frequency response). This catheter is calibrated using a fluid-filled polyvinyl chloride catheter inserted in the same artery. Both pressure sensors are implanted in the arterial lumen through a collateral branch. The fluid-filled catheter should be previously calibrated *in vitro* in saline solution at 37 °C against a pressure digital caliper (Xcaliber, Viggo-Spectramed, Oxnard, CA). The traditional technique to calibrate pressure sensors was to use a mercury manometer and both mentioned techniques use mmHg as units (Fischer *et al* 2002).

External instantaneous arterial diameter can be accurately measured using a pair of ultrasonic piezoelectric crystals (5 MHz, 4 mm diameter) sutured to the adventitia of an artery. This is a simple technique of minimal dissection; two external sensors are implanted: one for the emission and the other for the reception of an ultrasonic signal. The velocity of the ultrasonic signal traveling through tissues is considered to be $1580\,\mathrm{m\,s^{-1}}$. The distance between crystals, i.e. the arterial external diameter, is calculated by the sonomicrometer, measuring the time the signal takes to travel between the emisor crystals and the receptor (Fischer *et al* 2002).

After arterial pressure and diameter analogical signals are obtained, both of these periodic waves can be digitized to allow an online visualization. Pressure and diameter signals change when measured in different arterial territories. There is a pressure gradient between the aortic root and capillaries that ensures blood flow in tissues. The external diameters of the aorta and large arteries vary within the cardiac cycle between 7% and 10%. On the other hand, it is important to remember that arteries are subjected to longitudinal changes during the cardiac cycle, which sometimes are greater than 20% in larger vessels (Nichols and O'Rourke 1998, Feher 2012).

As seen in figure 2.3, a complete cardiac cycle can be represented in a graph with the diameter and pressure in the axes and a clockwise loop constructed. As arteries are modeled as viscoelastic solids, three moduli are used to describe the stress–strain or pressure–diameter relationships: elastic, viscous and inertial moduli. As would be the case of elastic pure material in ideal conditions, the pure-elastic behavior of arteries is nonlinear. Additionally, the viscous and inertial phenomena determine a hysteresis loop, a typical expression of viscoelastic materials. While elastin fibers have an elastic behavior, the smooth muscle and collagen that make up the arterial wall have a viscoelastic behavior. Acute changes in viscous phenomena are mainly related to the smooth muscle dynamics (Fischer *et al* 2006).

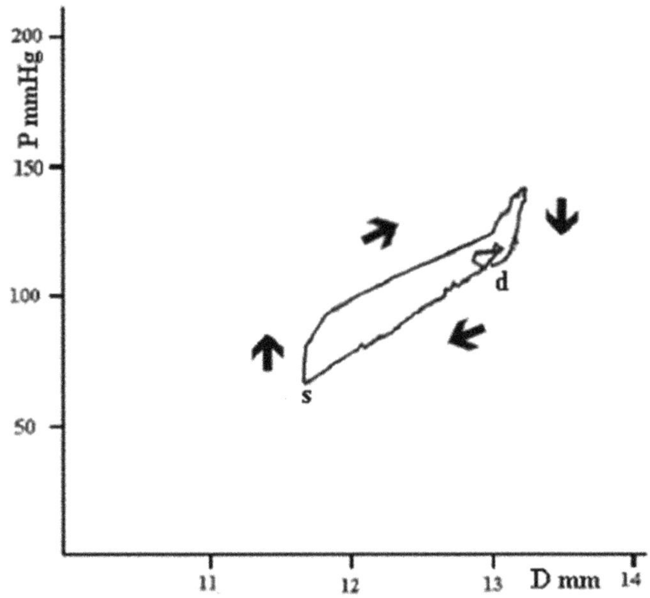

Figure 2.3. Arterial pressure (P) and diameter (D) loop. A clockwise rotation during one cardiac cycle is observed, opposite to the ventricular cycle. The diastolic period begins in 'd' and ends in 's'.

Under very stable conditions (i.e. without respiratory movements), the constitution of the above-described pressure–diameter loop should be overlapped cycle after cycle, but this regularity is hardly ever observed. Normally, the aortic pressure–diameter loop is constantly shifting, due to breathing movements, changing body positions, during walking tests and many other physiological situations (Von Frey 1911).

The arterial wall should be modeled as a viscoelastic material under physiological (i.e. cyclical) conditions, since this model explains the time-dependant properties of these types of materials. On the other hand, quasi-static (i.e. slow enough to ignore time-dependent effects) *in vitro* testing is used to model the pure-elastic behavior of arteries. As arteries are made up of components of different mechanical properties, the stress–strain relationship will not be linear. Collagen fibers have a Young's modulus of 1×10^{10} dynes cm^{-2}. This is higher than that found in bones in which the Young's modulus is 1×10^{11} dynes cm^{-2}. On the other hand, elastin has a lower Young's modulus: 6×10^{6} dynes cm^{-2}. Smooth muscle is a contractile tissue, and therefore has two different Young's moduli, one when contracted (2.5×10^{6} dynes cm^{-2}) and another one when relaxed (0.1×10^{6} dynes cm^{-2}). At low pressures, collagen fibers are coiled. As pressure rises, they merely uncoil and therefore have little to no mechanical response to stress; instead, elastin fibers take the load and deform accordingly. At higher pressures, collagen fibers uncoil and become completely recruited. Since they are more rigid than elastin fibers, they bear the entire load. This explains the nonlinear elastic behavior of arteries in quasi-static conditions and the break-point of two different slopes (i.e. Young's moduli) in figure 2.4 (Fung 2004).

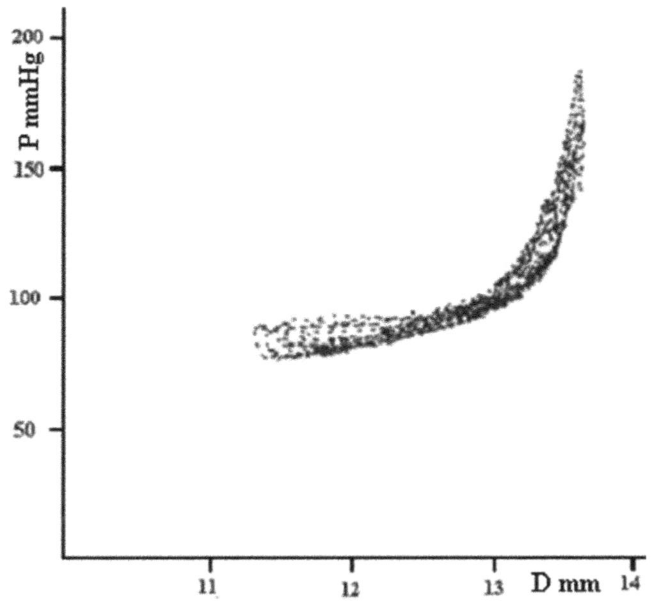

Figure 2.4. Loops obtained using blood pressure (P) and aortic diameter (D) signals during several beats and increases of left ventricular afterload. A displacement towards higher pressures exists when the diameter increases. There is a maximum reachable diameter, when all of the collagen fibers are recruited and stretched.

As described in chapter 1, arteries have different proportions of elastin, collagen and smooth muscle cells in each territory of the human body. These changes are the determinants of viscoelastic differences among vessels (Fischer *et al* 1991b, Fischer *et al* 2010).

While elastin and collagen determine the passive viscoelastic behavior of the vessel wall, the smooth muscle tissue is the only active component that can quickly react to electrical stimuli and/or chemical stimuli. In basal conditions, there is a state of semi contraction or semi relaxation called 'smooth muscle tone'. This vascular tone is an important determinant of vascular geometry, including diameter values (Barra *et al* 1993).

The elasticity of the arterial wall can be modified by three main factors: (a) changes in blood pressure, (b) heart rate and/or (c) smooth muscle tone. Smooth muscle tone depends on the stimuli originated in the intima layer (endothelial cells) or in the adventitia (Bia *et al* 2011, Fischer *et al* 2013). As can be seen, the changes in the biomechanics of the arterial wall are determined not only by pressure-dependent (i.e. passive) mechanisms but also by vascular smooth muscle-dependent (i.e. active) mechanisms.

The endothelial cells, situated in the intima layer, actively regulate the arterial diameter through changes of smooth muscle tone. Our group demonstrated that endothelial cells are able to detect changes in blood composition and modulate accordingly the smooth muscle tone, achieving a physiological diameter adaptation (Fischer *et al* 2002).

Considering the active role of smooth muscle vascular tissue, stimulation of the arteries during experimental surgeries determines changes in the pressure–diameter loop, similar to those observed in figure 2.4 but shifted to higher levels of pressure, as seen in figure 2.5. These smooth muscle changes are observed after the infusion of phenylephrine (Barra *et al* 1993).

2.3.2 Veins

Human blood is contained mainly in the veins (64%), which act as capacitance vessels. As explained in chapter 1, there are no valves between the cava and pulmonary veins and the right and left atria, respectively. Thus, approximately the same amount of blood arrives at each atrium in one cardiac cycle. This is called *venous return* and is dependent of pressure gradients that are not uniform. The left atrial pressure signal profile is determined by the amount of blood that comes from the lungs (wave v) and by the contraction of the atrium during systole (wave a). Mean right atrial pressure is a hemodynamic parameter largely measured in order to assess the clinical status of a patient during and after surgery (Feher 2012).

Blood pressure and flow in veins are not homogeneous, and they change depending on the vascular territory and vessel caliber. These parameters are determined by biochemical and neurologic stimuli triggered by tissue requirements. The relatively low pressure values in veins with respect to systemic arteries are the source of important changes during physiological variations during human daily

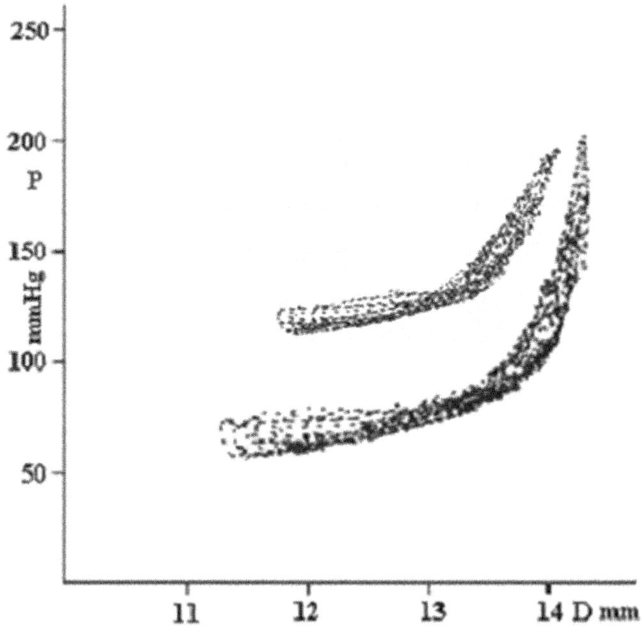

Figure 2.5. Loops of blood pressure (P) and artery diameter (D) with displacement to the right and above, experimentally obtained by increasing left ventricular afterload. At the bottom of the preparation are the basal conditions and higher results were obtained after stimulation of arterial smooth muscle with a vasoconstrictor.

activity. For example, the transition between supine and standing positions shifts the blood from the vena cava territory towards the veins of the lower limbs. Because of this blood displacement, central vein pressure decreases, while it increases in the lower limbs.

The viscoelastic properties of the vein wall allow rapid adaptations, protecting the vessel by attenuating the effects of blood pressure waves during walking and active exercise. The veins in the lower-limb territory have internal valves that prevent backflow, helping the blood to return to the heart more easily. This system is particularly efficient when the individual is in a standing position, and the contractions of skeletal muscles compress the veins, driving the blood upwards, and enabling venous return. This is the reason why this system is thought of as a *skeletal muscle pump*.

2.4 Blood rheology

The circulatory system has basic functions such as (a) transport of nutrients, gases and final products of the Krebs cycle, (b) organ function regulation through hormone supply and PH control, (c) temperature regulation, and (d) immune response.

Nutrients needed to fulfill aerobic cellular metabolism are transported from the intestine and the liver towards all cells. On the other hand, blood flow in the tissues has a scavenger function, removing urea, uric acid, carbon dioxide and other final products of cellular metabolism. The transport in this case goes from the tissue towards the lungs and kidneys, where they are excreted. Moreover, liver blood perfusion allows several metabolic transformations of waist elements, contributing to clean human plasma.

Gas transport is an important task for cell respiration, ensuring a quick renewal of oxygen and carbon dioxide. The oxygen is carried from the lungs to the tissue by the hemoglobin contained in the erythrocytes, and carbon dioxide is transported from the tissues to the lungs, both, in plasma and in red blood cells.

Vitamins, hormones and chemical function mediators are also transported by blood flow from the cells in which they are synthesized to the targeted tissues, in which they participate in the general control of corporal functions.

Body temperature depends on cellular metabolism, which is under neuro-hormonal control. Moreover, some fine adjustments are made through vasodilatation and vasoconstriction of vessels located under the skin, which determines changes in blood flow. This produces an increase and decrease of heat loss.

The protection of the human body against external agents is provided by white blood cells. There are two main mechanisms: cellular (phagocytes) and humoral response (antibodies). Monocytes, lymphocytes and neutrophils fight against external microorganisms that invade human tissues through phagocytosis (and other mechanisms), while basophils are responsible for the release of factors mediating the inflammatory response (bradykinin, heparin, histamine, serotonin among others). The lysis of products derived from the antigen–antibody reaction is carried out by eosinophils.

Blood function includes cellular and chemical factors that are required by tissues according to specific roles determined by the nature of the human body. One of them is oxygen supply, which must be provided continuously, while others, such as the growth hormone (somatotrophin) acts in much larger scales of time and should be provided following an age-dependent plan. Moreover, some chemical mediators maintain specific concentrations of certain substances in the blood, which may include daily variations.

2.4.1 Blood pressure

As mentioned previously, intraventricular blood pressure and volume allow one to characterize the left ventricular function. In the case of intraluminal pressure, there are several available methods that allow an accurate measurement of this variable in any territory of the circulation system. Arterial pressure is a well-known parameter that was measured for the first time by Reverend Stephen Hales in a mare in 1733. Reverend Hales was also a physicist.

A pressure is defined as the force per unit area exerted on a perpendicular surface, $P = F/A$, where P is pressure, F is force and A is surface area. As force has units of mass (M) times length (L) over time squared (T^2), and the unit of surface is length squared (L^2), pressure has units of ($M\ L^{-1}\ T^{-2}$). In medicine and experimental biology the use of millimeters of mercury (mmHg) as units for pressure is extended, although sometimes, in veins and the right atrium, pressures are reported in centimeters of water.

Pressures in the circulatory system are measured invasively using two different techniques: using a fluid-filled catheter or a solid state catheter (figure 2.6). The main limitation of the first method is its ability to respond to quick changes. Thus, it is important to avoid connectors between the catheter and the transducer and regular flushing is recommended whenever bubbles appear. It is possible to avoid the aggregation of fibrin and platelets inside the catheter, which would otherwise reduce the internal diameter and hinder the frequency response. Heparin has been widely used to avoid clot formation. The diameter and length of the catheter influence the measured values, therefore large-caliber catheters, >6 F, are recommended (1 F = 0.33 mm).

This methodology allows one to obtain accurate measurements of blood pressure and it is easily calibrated.

Solid state catheters have a piezoelectric sensor on their tip, which is placed in the area of interest. Its main advantage over fluid-filled catheters is that it has no viscous inertial effects. The intrinsic high frequency determines the low damping property, which reduces the delay of the pressure recording. This method does not need a fluid column but it is not easy to calibrate. The main advantage of the tip catheter is its high capacity to assess changes in the phasic pressure waveform. Furthermore, this method does not require flushing. The surgical procedure for the implantation of a tip catheter is similar to that used for a fluid-filled catheter.

Once the signals are acquired and recorded, the analysis of the pressure waveform can be completed by digitizing the analogic signal, but there are some important characteristics that should be taken into account in both experimental research and

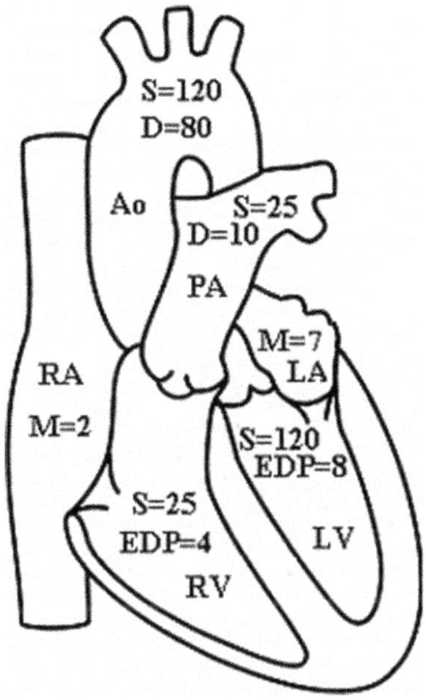

Figure 2.6. Cardiac and large-vessel pressure values in mmHg. *S*, D and M are the systolic, diastolic and mean values. EDP: end diastolic pressure, measured in the ventricle. RA: right atrium, LA: left atrium, Ao: aorta, PA: pulmonary artery, RV: right ventricle, LV: left ventricle.

hemodynamic evaluations. To evaluate the left ventricular function it is important to measure the systolic, diastolic and end diastolic pressures. The reason is that these values are important to characterize physiological and pathological conditions. The aortic pressure values to be obtained are the systolic, diastolic, mean and pulse pressures. The pulse pressure is the difference between the systolic and diastolic values. The mean pressure is calculated by integrating the instantaneous pressure throughout a whole cardiac cycle, but in clinical practice it is useful to use a simple calculation, by adding 1/3 of the difference between the systolic and diastolic pressures to the diastolic pressure. Some variables are indicators of normality or malfunction of the circulatory system (Lieber 2008).

The devices destined to measure intraluminal pressures in the circulatory system should accomplish certain requirements to operate efficiently: *stability*, *sensitivity*, *linearity* and adequate *frequency response*. Stability is the ability to maintain a steady or uniform output when the input is another steady value. Sensitivity is the ability to detect small changes in the input. Linearity is the measurement of the linear relationship between the input and output values. The frequency response is the ability to detect quick changes in the input.

Intraluminal blood pressure determines a parietal stress that depends on wall thickness and the internal diameter of the cardiovascular structures. The explanation of ***Laplace's law*** is the best way to understand the real effects of the intraluminal pressure on the surrounding structures, i.e. the wall of the ventricles, auricles and vessels. The blood contained inside the structures tends to push the wall outwards (figure 2.7), exerting a pressure on the walls. This pressure is equilibrated by a parietal stress inside the walls.

If wall thickness and internal diameter are constant all along the walls, the wall thickness is small and the ventricle is still, the stress is uniform across the wall. According to Laplace's law:

$$p^*\pi^*Ri^2 = \sigma^*(\pi^*(Ri + Th)^2 - \pi^*Ri^2),$$

where p is the internal pressure, Ri is the internal radius, Th is the wall thickness and σ is the stress. Then,

$$p^*Ri = \sigma^*th^*\left(2 + \frac{Th}{Ri}\right).$$

If wall thickness is much smaller that the internal radius, wall stress σ is equal to:

$$\sigma = \frac{p^*Ri}{2^*Th}.$$

This formula could be used to model the circumferential stresses in the left ventricle. But Laplace's law could also be applied to a tubular structure, such as an artery. In this case the derivation of the formula has little changes, as we will see in the following:

$$p^*2^*\pi^*Ri^*l = \sigma^*(2^*\pi^*(Ri + Th) - 2^*\pi^*Ri)^*l,$$

where p is the intraluminal pressure, Ri is the internal radius, l is a specific longitude of the vessel and Th is the wall thickness.

In arteries, blood exerts a pressure onto the wall and there must be an opposing stress in order to equilibrate the position of the vessel. This is the arterial wall stress. Thus, if the area of a cylindrical structure is $2^*\pi^*Ri^*l$, the arterial circumferential stress can be calculated as:

$$\sigma = \frac{p^*Ri}{Th}.$$

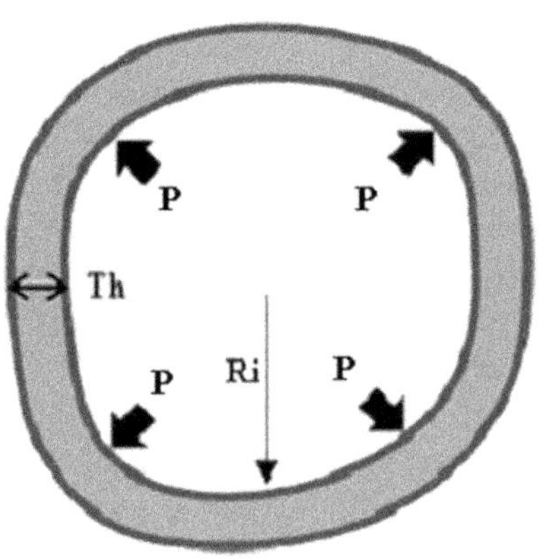

Figure 2.7. Intraluminal pressures (p) act on the chamber wall and the stress will depend on internal radius (Ri) and wall thickness (Th).

This formula contributes to understanding the physiological consequences of blood pressure periodic changes during the cardiac cycle. Furthermore, the pathological consequences are very important and involve therapeutical maneuvers in order to restore the lost function.

2.4.2 Blood volume

Blood volume in some structures of the cardiovascular system is not as easy to measure as it appears. In vessels, the intraluminal diameter and length can be easily measured and the cylindrical geometry allows the use of a simple formula: $\pi \times r^2 \times L$, where r is the internal radius and L is the length. On the other hand, calculating the ventricular or atrial volumes has several problems: in ventricles, the limit between the blood chamber and the myocardial wall is not uniform; moreover, the ventricular geometry does not help one to find a formula to be used. Furthermore, the systolic and diastolic cyclic periods determine constant changes that require one to consider the precise time in which intraventricular volume is calculated.

The use of the ultrasonic microcrystal technique allows one to accurately measure the diameter and length of cardiac and vascular structures. In vessels, this technique is used by suturing two crystals on diametrically opposite sides, thus measuring the external diameter. One of these ultrasonic crystals emits a signal after being excited with high voltage pulses. The ultrasonic signal has a velocity of 1540 m s^{-1} across the tissues and arrives at the opposite crystal (i.e. the receiver) sending a signal to the sonomicrometer. As instantaneous ultrasonic velocity is considered to remain constant, changes in the transit time to reach the receiver microcrystal can only be attributed to diameter variation (Fischer and Barmak 2005).

Left ventricular volume can be calculated using ultrasonic crystal techniques in experimental animals (Fischer *et al* 1988). This ellipsoidal structure can be modeled by measuring the longitudinal axis and two diameters using three pairs of ultrasonic crystals. Two microcrystals are positioned on the left ventricle measuring apex–base length. Another pair is placed measuring the distance between the interventricular septum and the lateral wall of the ventricle, and the third pair measuring the antero-posterior diameter. Once the ultrasonic signals are calibrated and data is acquired, the left ventricular volume can be calculated using the following formula:

$$LVV = \pi/6 \cdot ABL \cdot SLWD \cdot APD$$

Where LVV is the ventricular volume, ABL is the apex–base length, $SLWD$ is the interventricular septum-lateral wall diameter value and APD is the antero-posterior diameter.

As ultrasonic signals are obtained instantaneously, left ventricular volume changes can be measured at any stage of the cardiac cycle, enabling the detection of physiological and pathological modifications.

In humans, several versions of ultrasonic techniques such as two-dimensional and three-dimensional echocardiography are used; moreover, the use of impedancimetric and invasive techniques enables the estimation of left intraventricular volume (Fischer *et al* 1988).

The use of non-invasive techniques, such as radionuclides and cardiac resonance imaging allow one to obtain left ventricular volume and other deriving left ventricular function indexes.

The above-mentioned impendancimetric technique could be applied using conductance catheters. This technique uses the electrical conductance of blood to evaluate left ventricular volume. Changes in left ventricular volume are accompanied by variations in blood conductance: this is the biophysical base of the conductance catheter that can be used both in humans and in experimental animals, allowing one to quantify left ventricular volume and changes along the cardiac cycle (Fischer *et al* 1988).

The placement of the catheter into the left ventricular chamber is extremely invasive, if the measurement of volume is the sole purpose of the intervention. That is the case of the left ventriculography procedure and the insertion of conductance catheters.

2.4.3 Blood flow

Blood is ejected from the left ventricle during the systolic phase until the diastolic phase begins, but tissues require a continuous flow.

Blood flow is the volume of fluid that passes through a given section of the circulatory system during a certain amount of time, usually measured in liters per minute.

Blood flow in the cardiovascular system can be estimated using Poiseuille's law that has been developed in tubular structures and to be applied under certain physical requirements. At present, blood flow (Q) can be calculated using the Hagen–Poiseuille equation:

$$Q = \frac{\Delta P \cdot \pi \cdot r^4}{8 \cdot L \cdot \mu}$$

where ΔP is the difference in pressure that promotes the flow, r and L are the radius and the length of the tube, respectively, and μ is the viscosity of the fluid.

This model, which is applied to hydraulic circuits, assumes rigid tubes, uniform diameter, laminar flow with constant velocity, and constant viscosity. As all models simplify reality, they represent it to a certain extent; the above-mentioned conditions are not possible in human vessels, and therefore the results derived from the Hagen–Poiseuille equation are an approximation to the real value when applied to the circulatory system (Nichols and O'Rourke 1998).

The Hagen–Poiseuille equation shows the higher the pressure difference between any two points or the bigger the internal radius, the higher the flow. Conversely, the higher the fluid viscosity the lesser the flow (Nichols and O'Rourke 1998).

In a **laminar flow,** the velocity in the center of the tube is the highest, and it decreases towards the periphery. This behavior can be explained if flow is thought of as a series of concentric flow laminae. The force per unit area necessary to put in motion the fluid layer is the **shear stress,** and the velocity gradient between layers is the **shear rate** (see figure 2.8).

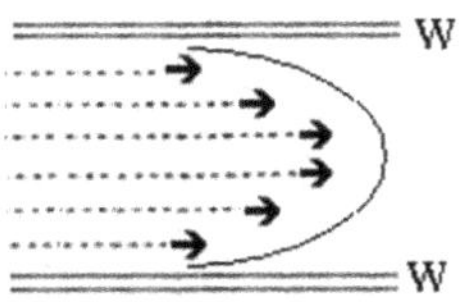

Figure 2.8. Laminar blood flow in a tubular structure. Note the arrows indicate velocity that is maximal in laminae at the centerline. W: arterial wall.

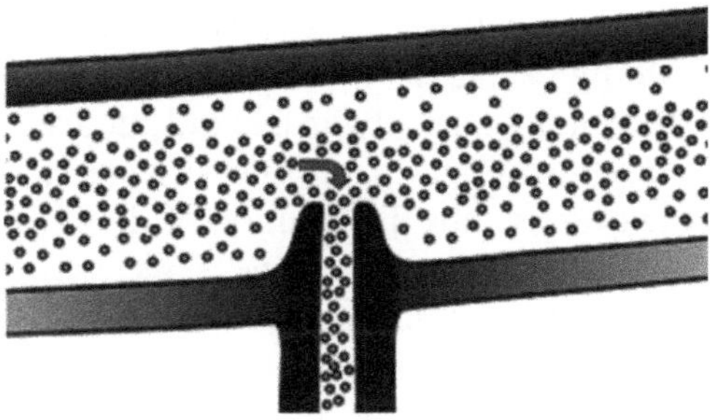

Figure 2.9. Axial accumulation of erythrocytes and the origin of a uterine rat artery near the axis of the aorta.

Fluid viscosity is defined as the friction between adjacent concentric lamellae, and can be expressed as: viscosity = (shear stress/shear rate). The apparent blood viscosity at 37° is 4.0 centipoise. Blood viscosity increases when a higher hematocrit is induced (Fischer *et al* 2002) and decreases as the vessel diameter decreases. However, in arteries of diameters smaller than 0.4iμm, blood viscosity increases. This phenomenon is called the **Fahraeus–Lindqvist** effect.

Blood viscosity is also associated with flow: increases in the former determine decreases in the latter. The explanation of this phenomenon is the **axial accumulation** of blood red cells (figure 2.9). In other words, hematocrit in the center of the artery will be higher than the hematocrit near the vascular wall. This biophysical phenomenon has anatomical connotations, as pointed out by Burton when describing the uterine artery from a rat's aorta (Burton 1965).

The opposite of a laminar flow is turbulent flow. An example of this is flow hitting an obstacle and a vortex appearing. Several factors are involved in the generation of a turbulent flow. These variables are summarized in the **Reynolds number** (Re), a dimensionless number whose value describes the nature of the flow (i.e. if it is laminar or turbulent). When the Reynolds Number is approximately 2000 (dimensionless) laminar flow turns on in turbulent.

The Reynolds number can be calculated as:

$$\mathrm{Re} = \frac{v^*\rho^*r}{\eta}.$$

In which, v is the average fluid velocity, ρ is the fluid density, r is the radius, and η is the viscosity of the fluid. The Reynolds number for blood in an artery is around 1540 for a mean flow, which means that for higher values a turbulent blood flow occurs.

2.4.4 Cardiac output

Cardiac output is defined as the amount of blood ejected by the left ventricle in a minute, and it is most commonly expressed in liters per minute. The left ventricle has a volume of 120–140 cm^3, and in basal state it ejects 70–80 cm^3 per beat. Thus, considering a heart rate of 70–75 beats/min, the normal volume per unit of time (i.e. the cardiac output) is 4.9–6.0 l min^{-1}.

The basal value of cardiac output increases four times during active exercise and is mainly due to heart rate increases. However, increases in heart rate determine decreases in the cardiac cycle duration and as this shortening reduces the diastolic time the left ventricular filling decreases.

As mentioned before, normal values of cardiac output are around 5–6 l min^{-1} in healthy adults. The distribution differs from one vascular territory to another, as seen in figure 2.10. During exercise, the distribution of the cardiac output changes in absolute and relative values, e.g. at rest, kidneys receive around 1–1.20 l min^{-1} (20%), while during active exercise is 0.22–0.64 l min^{-1} (2%–4%).

Cardiac output measurements are currently used as indicators of heart function, and are quantified using both invasive and non-invasive techniques. The ventriculography allows one to obtain cardiac output values using the concepts described above. In intensive care units and experimental research, cardiac output can be measured with a Swan–Ganz catheter positioned in the pulmonary trunk. This technique is minimally invasive. The operator injects a bolus of cold saline solution (i.e. the indicator) in the right atrium. Changes in blood temperature of the bolus are measured downstream with a thermistor in the tip of the catheter. As the cardiac output value is inversely related to the area under the temperature dilution curve, a reliable value could be obtained using specific software (Drobinski and Eugene 1982).

Other methods used to measure cardiac output include the use of radionuclides, ultrasonic techniques, the indicator dilution method and the Fick method.

Cardiac output is a widely used indicator of heart function in men, women and children. To be able to compare cardiac output values among subjects of different age, race and size, a normalization of values is usually adopted. The cardiac index is calculated by dividing the cardiac output by the body surface [l min^{-1} m^{-2}]. In experimental *in vivo* animals cardiac output is usually normalized by using body weight [l min^{-1} kg^{-1}].

2.4.5 Resistance and impedance

A conduit that contains a certain flowing liquid at any pressure opposes that flow. In blood vessels, this is called *vascular resistance*, a variable used to characterize the opposition to steady or constant flow. In the human circulatory system, the highest resistance to blood flow is found in the arterioles. There is more than one way to quantify arterial blood resistance and the simplest one is by dividing the gradient of pressure by flow (Nichols and O'Rourke 1998, Despopoulos and Silbernagl 2003).

From the Hagen–Poiseuille equation, resistance can be calculated as:

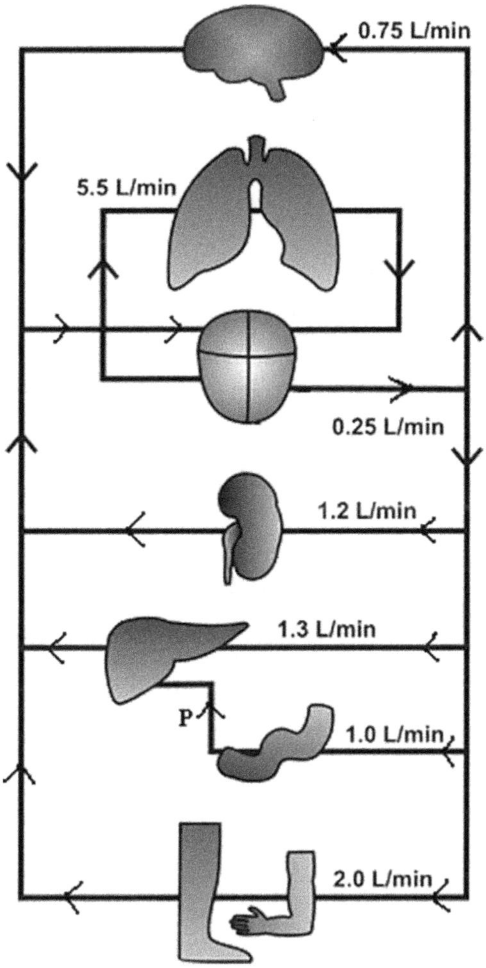

Figure 2.10. Distribution of cardiac output of a healthy adult at rest. Top to bottom: brain, lungs, heart, kidney, liver, intenstines, limbs. P is the hepatic portal system.

$$R = \frac{8\mu L}{\pi r^4},$$

where R is the resistance, μ is the viscosity of the fluid, L is the length of the tube and r is the internal radius. The most commonly used units are [dyn s cm^{-5}].

In the arterial tree the conduits are in series, and the total resistance is calculated as the sum of the resistance of each vascular territory. The resistance formula derived from the Hagen–Poiseuille equation, makes it is easy to understand that small increases in internal radius determine high decreases in resistance. This is the case for arterioles, which are responsible for more than 40% of the total peripheral resistance and are capable of changing the cross-sectional area through parietal smooth muscle tone variations. Capillaries are another source of resistance (27% of the total peripheral resistance), but the lack of smooth muscle cells in the vessel wall precludes any possibility to produce section changes. However, blood flow can be adjusted by a precapillary sphincter that allows changes in microcirculation in order to accomplish tissue requirements.

The above-described resistance to flow equation derived from Poiseuille's law has been developed for a steady flow, which is not exactly the case in the human arterial tree. However, the existence of a mean flow allows one to use the formula for vascular resistance to characterize blood flow in systemic and pulmonary arteries.

The concept of arterial impedance was developed to quantify the resistance to flow in pulsatile vessels.

When blood flow has a pulsatile behavior, its frequency determines changes in the conduit function. *Vascular impedance* is the resistance to pulsatile blood flow. Its units are the same as for resistance (e.g. dyn s cm^{-5}). There are four types of arterial impedance, but in this chapter only the characteristic impedance will be described.

Characteristic impedance is the resistance to pulsatile flow calculated without taking into account wave reflection. Assuming a cylindrical geometry for the arteries, the characteristic impedance (Z_c) can be estimated using the Water–Hammer equation:

$$Z_c = \frac{\rho \cdot \text{PWV}}{\text{arterial diastolic cross-sectional area}},$$

where ρ is the blood density (assumed as $1.055\ \text{g ml}^{-1}$) and PWV is the pulse wave velocity.

In the arterial tree, increases in Z lead to an augmented resistance to pulsatile blood flow, resulting in a decreased capacity to conduct blood. Therefore, by inverse reasoning, the conduit function can be defined as the inverse of the characteristic impedance = $1/Z_c$.

2.4.6 Bernoulli principle

Left ventricular ejection involves an important loss of energy, which is transferred into the circulatory system, mainly in the form of blood pressure and flow that is received by systemic vessels and distributed towards all body tissues. In other words, during left ventricular contraction there is potential energy that transforms into kinetic energy (Downey 2003).

Potential energy is calculated as: $\rho \cdot g \cdot h$, where ρ is the fluid density, g is the gravitational force and h is the height of the liquid column. During diastole, the left ventricle receives blood through the mitral valve, reaching the end diastolic point just before myocardial contraction. This event can be detected in the pressure–volume diagram towards the end of the diastolic filling and the beginning of the isometric systolic phase. A few milliseconds later, the myocardial contraction determines an increase in intraluminal pressure, i.e. the development of potential energy, which is transformed into kinetic energy once the aortic valve opens and blood begins to flow into the aorta. This kinetic energy per unit of blood volume in motion is equal to: $(\rho \cdot v)^2/2$, where ρ is the fluid density $[M\,L^{-3}]$ and v is the velocity of the fluid $[L\,T^{-1}]$.

The displacement of blood ejected in each left ventricular systole determines changes in aortic flow, heat loss and pressure.

Bernoulli's principle is a means to visualize energy changes in terms of blood pressure and flow changes. This principle states that the higher the velocity of a fluid moving along a conduit, the lower the pressure (von Frey 1911).

Bernoulli's principle can be explained considering that the total energy, which remains constant, is the sum of potential and kinetic energy. This can be written as:

$$\rho \cdot g \cdot h_1 + \frac{1}{2} \cdot \rho \cdot v_1^2 = \rho \cdot g \cdot h_2 + \frac{1}{2} \cdot \rho \cdot v_2^2.$$

The first terms in the left-hand and right-hand side correspond to the gravitational potential energy, and the second term on both sides corresponds to the kinetic energy. Increases in velocity occur simultaneously with decreases in pressure, to maintain a state of dynamic equilibrium.

In the human circulatory system, small arteries and arterioles are considered to be the major contributors to increases in peripheral vascular resistance. At this point it is important to take into account that the relationship between a pressure difference and a flow reflects the vascular resistance. Hence, an increment of caliber or the opening of new vascular channels (i.e. the augmentation of cross-sectional vascular area), results in a decrease of vascular resistance and an increase of blood flow. In figure 2.11, decreases in diameter (e.g. arterioles) are represented in R, where an increase in resistance to flow is expected. On the other hand, increases of diameter are shown between R and Po. An analogy in the arterial system is the increase in the cross-sectional area in the capillaries. Increases in flow at smaller diameters are synchronic with lower than expected pressures (dotted line). The lowest pressure observed at the right hand side of the schema figure mimics the right atrium, where venous blood return starts off the pulmonary circuit (Downey 2003).

2.4.7 Capillary function

Capillaries are responsible for mass transfer between arterial blood and the fluids surrounding cells in the near vascular territory. This function enables the delivery of elements (nutrients and oxygen) and the absorption of others (carbon dioxide and urea). The latter function is also carried out by venules and lymphatic vessels (Li 2000).

As there are three types of capillary vessels, the filtration function has different characteristics, depending on the vascularized territory. For example, capillaries in the skin participate in body heat control, capillaries in the bone marrow are involved in hematopoiesis, liver capillaries exhibit a bidirectional macromolecular exchange and capillaries of the small intestine absorb amino acids, glucose, water and minerals, among other elements (Despopoulos and Silbernagl 2003).

2.4.8 Skin blood circulation

Tissues are perfused by small vessels, arterioles, venules and capillaries. Fluid and oxygen flow across the endothelial cells of capillaries. The capillary network starts in

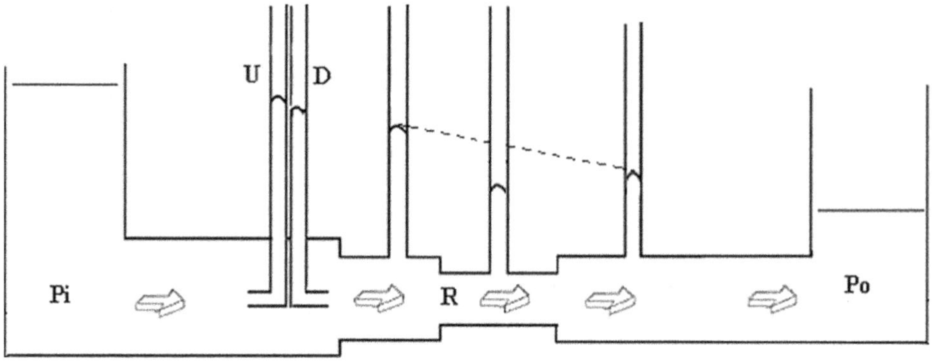

Figure 2.11. Pi: is the potential energy that changes transforms into kinetic energy determining a constant flow towards Po, in which the pressure drop is maximal. R is resistance, U is the dynamic pressure measured with a pitot tube, and D is the pressure measured downstream. The dotted line shows static pressures. Increases in flow velocity are concomitant with decreases in pressure. Hydrostatic pressure is measured by any lateral column, while the pitot tube measures both the hydrostatic and the kinematic pressures.

the arterioles, which eventually drain their contained blood into the venules. However, there are certain territories in which arteriovenous shunts bypass the capillary network.

The human circulatory system transports heat in order to maintain body temperature. Cutaneous vessels partake in the temperature control of human beings through increases in cutaneous blood flow in response to a rise in temperature. On the other hand, decreases in cutaneous blood flow limit heat loss (Feher 2012).

Temperature control through cutaneous vessels is dynamic and depends on the relaxation or constriction of the smooth muscle of vessels. Arteriolar blood flow to the skin is neutrally controlled, and is responsible for increases and decreases of perfusion in cutaneous capillaries and venous network. Furthermore, smooth muscle relaxations open the arteriovenous shunts, contributing to cutaneous heat loss.

2.4.9 Coronary circulation

As mentioned above, coronary arteries perfuse the myocardium and the heart structures. This is the consequence of a pressure gradient between the aortic root and the small arteries that nurture the myocardium. However, the irrigation of the parenchyma of the heart is not uniform (Despopoulos and Silbernagl 2003, Feher 2012).

Since the left ventricle generates 120 mmHg during the systolic period, the small arteries that travel through the ventricular parenchyma become collapsed and occluded, thus the left ventricular myocardium is perfused during the diastolic period (see figure 2.11).

The small coronary branches of the right coronary territory are not compressed during systole since the intraventricular pressures of the right heart are normally less than 25 mmHg. Consequently, the right ventricular wall is perfused in both the systolic and diastolic periods (see figure 2.12).

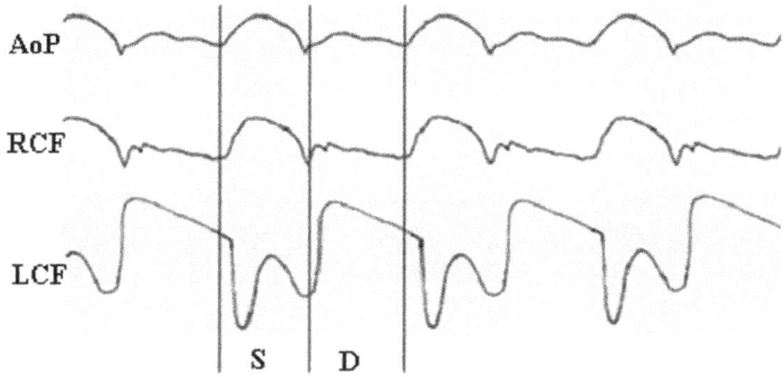

Figure 2.12. Upper panel: aortic pressure signal (AoP). This pressure determines a systolic (S) and a diastolic (D) right coronary flow (RCF) and a left coronary flow (LCF). Note that diastolic blood flow prevails in the latter.

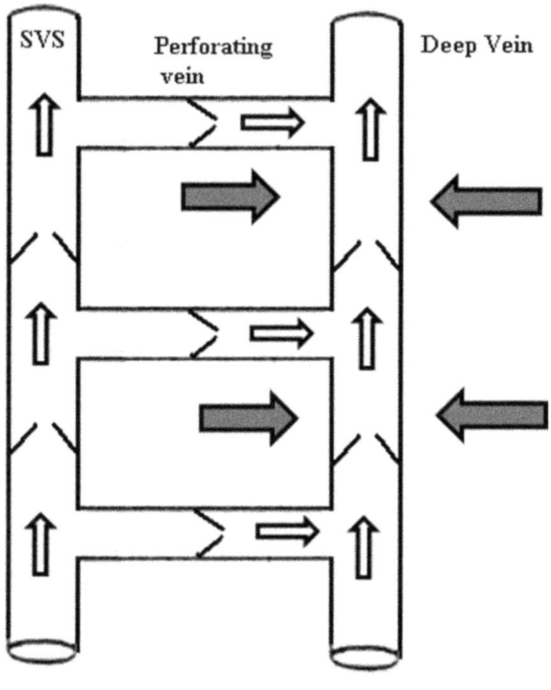

Figure 2.13. Vein blood flow in the superficial system (SVS), in the perforating vessels and in deep veins. The dark arrows indicate skeletal muscle compression. White arrows show blood flow direction. Note that valves in the perforating system ensure a blood flow towards the deep veins and prevent a reverse blood flow.

2.5 Venous return to right atrium

A large amount of blood flowing through the capillaries returns to the right atrium. In peripheral veins, such as legs and arms, there are valves that ensure one-way blood flow towards the heart during skeletal muscle compression. Moreover, the venous system is aided by a 'respiratory pump': when breathing, pressure differences are created and blood is drawn towards the right atrium by compression of the veins (Shoukas and Rothe 2008).

A standing subject tends to have a reverse blood flow towards the lower limbs. Large veins have one-way valves placed each 2–4 cm that prevent backflow and assist blood flow towards the right atrium. The absence of vein valves would determine venous pressures of approximately 90 mmHg in the lower limbs in a standing position, but in healthy adults this pressure is around 20 mmHg.

Veins in the lower limbs are distributed in a deep venous system (i.e. beneath the skeletal muscles), and a superficial system (i.e. subcutaneal veins). Both systems are connected by perforating veins that ensure blood flow from the superficial system to intramuscular veins, through one-way valves (see figure 2.13).

During skeletal muscle contraction, the deep venous system is alternatively compressed and decompressed. This compression opens the proximal valves while distal valves remain closed. Valves of the perforating veins prevent blood flow towards the superficial venous system during skeletal muscle contraction (Downey 2003, Feher 2012).

References

Barra J, Armentano R L, Levenson J, Fischer E I C, Pichel R and Simon A 1993 Assessment of smooth muscle contribution to descending thoracic aortic elastic mechanics in conscious dogs *Circ. Res.* **73** 1040–50

Bia D, Fischer E I C, Zócalo Y and Armentano R L 2011 The endothelium modulates the arterial wall mechanical response to intra-aortic balloon counterpulsation: *in vivo* studies *Artif. Organs* **35** 883–92

Burton A C 1965 *Physiology and Biophysics of the Circulation* (Chicago, IL: Year Book Medical Publishers) pp 129–40

Carnot S 1824 *Réflexion sur la puissance motrice du feu et sur les machines propres a développer cette puissance* (Paris, France: Bachelier) pp 1–38

Crottogini A J, Willshaw P, Barra J G, Armentano R, Cabrera Fischer E I and Pichel R H 1987 Inconsistency of the slope and the volume intercept of the end-systolic pressure-volume relationship as individual indexes of inotropic state in conscious dogs: presentation of an index combining both variables *Circulation* **76** 1115–26

Despopoulos A and Silbernagl S 2003 Cardiovascular system *Color Atlas Physiology* (New York: Thieme) ch 8, pp 186–221

Downey J M 2003 Hemodynamics *Essential Medical Physiology* 3rd edn ed L R Johnson (London: Elsevier Academic) ch 10, pp 157–74

Drobinski G and Eugene M 1982 *Exploration hémodynamique cardiovasculaire* (Paris: Masson)

Feher J 2012 The cardiovascular system *Quantitative Human Physiology: An Introduction* (New York: Elsevier) Unit 5, pp 417–550

Fischer E I C, Spinelli J C, Willshaw P, Crottogini A J, De Forteza E, Clavin O, Valentinuzzi M E and Pichel R H 1988 Detection of left ventricular regional myocardial ischaemia in dogs by intraventricular conductance catheter *Cardiovasc. Res.* **22** 185–92

Fischer E I C, Armentano R L, Pessana F M, Graf S, Romero L, Christen A I, Simon A and Levenson J 2002 Endothelium-dependent arterial wall tone elasticity modulated by blood viscosity *Am. J. Physiol. Heart. Circ. Physiol.* **282** H389–94

Fischer E I C, Bia D, Camus J M, Zocalo Y, de Forteza E and Armentano R L 2006 Adventitia-dependent mechanical properties of brachiocephalic ovine arteries in *in vivo* and *in vitro* studies *Acta Physiol.* **188** 103–11

Fischer E I C and Barmak W 2005 Left ventricular dysfunction *Cardiovascular Failure: Pathophysiological Bases and Management* 4th edn ed E I C Fischer, A Juffé Stein and J M Balaguer (Buenos Aires: FURGF) pp 13–33

Fischer E I, Bia D, Zócalo Y, Camus J M, de Forteza E and Armentano R 2010 Effects of removing the adventitia on the mechanical properties of ovine femoral arteries *in vivo* and *in vitro Circ. J.* **74** 1014–22

Fischer E I C, Chachques J C, Garcia A, de Fortezza E, Haab F, Cron C and Carpentier A 1991a Effect of cardiomyoplasty on left ventricular diastolic function *BAM* **1** 253–8

Fischer E I C, Armentano R L, Levenson J, Barra J, Morales M C, Breitbart G, Pichel R and Simon A 1991b Paradoxically decreased aortic wall stiffness in response to Vitamin D3-induced calcinosis. A biphasic analysis of segmental elastic properties in conscious dogs *Circ. Res.* **68** 1549–59

Fischer E I C, Bia D, Zócalo Y, Wray S and Armentano R 2013 The adventitia layer modulates the arterial wall elastic response to intra-aortic counterpulsation: *in vivo* studies *Artif. Organs* **37** 1041–8

Folkow B and Neil E 1971 The heart as a pump; myocardial metabolism *Circulation* (New York: Oxford University Press) pp 170–98

Fung Y C 2004 Bioviscoelastic solids *Biomechanics: Mechanical Properties of Living Tissues* (New York: Springer) pp 242–320

Li J K 2000 Physiology and rheology of arteries *The Arterial Circulation: Physical Principles and Clinical Applications* (Totowa, NJ: Humana Press) ch 2, pp 13–32

Lieber B B 2008 Arterial macrocirculatory hemodynamics *The Biomedical Engineering Handbook* ed D R Peterson and J D Bronzino (Boca Raton, FL: CRC Press) ch 10, pp 10.1–10

Loushin M K and Iaizzo P A 2005 Mechanical aspects of cardiac performance *Handbook of Cardiac Anatomy, Physiology, and Devices* (Totowa, NJ: Humana Press) pp 203–22

Lunkenheimer P P, Lunkenheimer A and Torrent Guasp F 1985 *Kardiodynamik: Wege zur strukturgerechten Analyse der Myokardfunktion. Beiträge zur Kardiologie* Band 33 ed K A Zölch (Heppenheim, Erlangen, Germany)

McCulloch A D 2008 Cardiac biomechanics *Biomechanics: Principles and Applications* ed D R Peterson and J D Bronzino (Boca Raton, FL: CRC Press) pp 8.1–26

Nichols W W and O'Rourke M F 1998 Properties of the arterial wall: practice *McDonald's Blood Flow in Arteries: Theoretical, Experimental and Clinical Principles* ed W W Nichols and M F O'Rourke (London: Arnold Publishers) pp 73–113

Ross Ethier C and Simmons C A 2011 Hemodynamics *Introductory Biomechanics: From cells to organisms* (Cambridge texts in Biomedical Engineering) (New York: Cambridge University Press) pp 119–61

Shoukas A A and Rothe C F 2008 The venous system *Biomechanics: Principles and Applications* ed D R Peterson and J D Bronzino (Boca Raton, FL: CRC Press) ch 12, pp 12.1–6

Valentinuzzi M E 2001 Left ventricular function cardiovascular failure *Pathophysiological Bases and Management* ed E I C Fischer, A I Christen and J C Trainini (Buenos Aires: FURGF) pp 21–46

Von Frey M 1911 Die Arbeit des Herzens *Vorlesungen über Physiologie* ed M von Frey (Berlin: Springer)

IOP Publishing

Biomechanical Modeling of the Cardiovascular System

Ricardo L Armentano, Edmundo I Cabrera Fischer and Leandro J Cymberknop

Chapter 3

Mathematical background for mechanical vessel analysis

Ricardo L Armentano and Leandro J Cymberknop

The circulatory system is the result of the evolution of the species in response to the more intricate specialization and organization of tissues. In unicellular or primitive pluricellular organisms, the fluid distribution needed to exchange O_2, CO_2 and nutrients from the intracellular space towards the environment and vice versa was possible due to their small size. In these organisms, the transport of gases or small molecules is possible through diffusion or other direct mechanisms that involve transport proteins in the cellular membrane, since each cell is in direct contact, or almost direct contact, with the external environment (Scher 1974). Natural selection has given reproductive advantages to those organisms that better adapted to their environment to profit from the available resources. Occasionally, the alteration in copies of the genome (i.e. mutations) were not always a drawback, but a way of expressing new features that enabled certain advantages in the exploitation of the environment, that were then transmitted to the next generation. In this manner, evolution was possible (Dawkins 1985). The evolutionary process promoted the increase in size of individuals, since this represented a reproductive advantage over other subjects of the same species. Simultaneously, the fact that most cells in a multicellular organism lost contact with the external environment, from where they used to obtain nutrients, resulted in the evolution of a contained medium that flows within the organism in a network of vessels that facilitate the transport of substances towards the inner cells. This is how the circulatory system was developed (Martin and Johansen 1965, Scher 1974, Dawkins 1985, Faury 2001).

The circulatory system has had an entity since the evolution of annelids, arthropods and mollusks, which have a fluid distribution system with vessels that flow into a coelomic compartment, or celom, with a contractile heart (in some species, more than one), and since the fluid is only partially confined in the vascular chamber, it is considered an open circulation. The celom progressively evolved in arthropods and mollusks by narrowing and by exhibiting an internal coating of

doi:10.1088/2053-2563/aafb0dch3

differentiated epithelium, which is major progress from a circulatory point of view with respect to annelids, in which the celom only became larger. Resistance to flow is low in open circulation, since the vascular network opens into a large chamber. These characteristics make for a slow flow and a low system pressure, both of which satisfy the needs of the organism (Martin and Johansen 1965). On the other hand, in more evolved species, the increase in size and in the specialization of the functions of the organs called for the need of a more efficient vascular system. In order to supply to a larger number of cells, vessels branched and capillary networks were developed; this resulted in an excessive increase of vascular resistance which led to a closed circulatory system. The evolution from an open to a closed circulatory system was simultaneous with changes in the efficiency of the heart, and fundamentally with the development of a high-pressure regime, to make flow possible faced with a higher resistance (Johansen and Martin 1965). The circulatory system can be represented simply as a pump (the heart) and a set of conduits (vessels) where a certain fluid flows (blood). The heart contracts cyclically and, therefore, the developed pressure produces a flow of a pulsatile nature. On the other end of the system are the cells, which are the final targets of blood supply, and require a continuous flow to nurture them and collect their metabolic waste.

Stephen Hales (1677–1761) was the first to measure arterial pressure in a horse, and the one to deduce the damping function of arteries, when observing the pulsatile nature of arteries versus the constant flow in veins. In his book *Haemostaticks*, published in 1733, he suggested that artery distensibility allows for an 'elastic reservoir' to be created during the ventricular systole, damping the systolic discharge. In the first translation of his work to German, the term 'elastic reservoir' was translated as *Windkessel*, or *wind chamber* by analogy with the air chamber used in old fire engines. This term was widespread by Otto Frank *et al.* Hales also introduced the concept of peripheral resistance, inferring that greater resistance is found in arterioles (McDonald 1974). The resistance imposed by arteries and their ramifications progressively decrease blood pressure along the system. Both the design and the structure define the mechanical properties of the vascular walls, such as the elastic, viscous and inertial characteristics. Elasticity is the major contributor towards the conservation of the amount of work needed to pump the blood across the entire body, also reducing the pulsatile nature of the cardiac cycle towards the periphery. Large arteries act as reservoirs that distend during systole and narrow during diastole. Even though the vascular wall has a mass and is viscous, the elasticity of the wall and the aortic valve make flow through capillaries possible, even after cardiac ejection (Bergel 1961b, Patel *et al* 1961, Peterson *et al* 1960, Alexander 1983). However, flow distribution is not only a result of parietal elasticity, viscosity or inertia, but of a more complex phenomenon: flow in arteries is also affected by reflection phenomena. Cardiac ejection produces a pressure wave that generates the flow (incident wave). These incident waves do not travel with ease: they collide against the arterial bifurcations, the narrowings and the arterioles, and these collisions cause reflected waves that travel back towards the heart (reflected waves) and interfere with the primary wave (Milnor 1982).

The heart releases kinetic and potential energy into the arterial system in each beat. Kinetic energy is expressed as blood flow and its acceleration, and potential energy as wall distensibility, i.e. the radial expansion of the aorta during the ventricular systole. In each systolic cycle almost 50% of the ejected volume by the heart remains transiently stored in the aorta, the pulmonary artery and other large arteries (Dobrin 1978). However, a share of the energy delivered by the heart is dissipated as heat, due to the viscous characteristics of the vascular wall. This lost energy is 15%–20% of the input energy. This means that most, but not all the energy delivered by the heart is elastically recovered each time vessels are distended (Shadwick 1999). Large arteries also transmit pressure waves and are a major site of vascular impedance, i.e. the dynamic resistance to the oscillatory components of blood flow (Dobrin 1978). During the diastolic period, the elastic energy stored in the vascular wall is released and blood flows towards the periphery, and blood pressure is kept relatively close to left ventricular pressure. The dissipated energy attenuates the pulse wave velocity that propagates along the arterial walls as a circumferential distension wave (Fung 1984). In summary, the viscoelastic properties of the arterial wall, together with blood viscosity, prevent the reflected waves from resonating in the arterial network, which would easily happen if the system were perfectly elastic and blood were an ideal non-viscous fluid (Shadwick 1999). The volume of blood discharged by the heart in each beat and the consequent pulsatile regime, together with the reflection phenomena, are buffered by the arterial system. This damping role and the low-resistance conduction ability of the network are the main functions of the arterial system, and depend on the composition and geometry of the vessel walls (O'Rourke 1982).

The arterial wall mainly consists of elastin, collagen and vascular smooth muscle; each of these components contribute to the global mechanical properties of the wall. Elastin is the main protagonist in the damping function of the circulatory system due to its elastic properties: its fibers are easily deformed when a force is exerted on it, and they regain their original length when the force disappears. Large arteries have the highest proportion of elastin, and as such they act as an elastic reservoir. It has been recently stated that the damping function of the arterial walls evolved simultaneously with the heart (Faury 2001), based on the existence of elastin-like proteins in proximal vessels of invertebrates, which confer similar mechanical properties to those found in superior vertebrates. On the other hand, collagen fibers are considered inextensible, and are arranged in such a way that they protect the vessel from tearing by large circumferential strains. At physiological strains, these fibers are not extended enough to oppose intravascular pressure; they are only recruited when deformations exceed physiological limits (Armentano *et al* 1991, Barra *et al* 1993). The configuration of elastin and collagen fibers within the vessel walls make its mechanical behavior nonlinear. This was described over 100 years ago by Charles S Roy. His work, published in 1881, is the first known work on vascular elasticity, and included studies on arteries of humans, rabbits and cats (Roy 1881). It documented the nonlinear elasticity of arteries and that the human aortic distensibility decreases with age (Burton 1954, Dobrin 1978, Shadwick 1999).

Just as elastic properties are determined by elastin and collagen, the viscosity of the wall is attributed to smooth muscle cells. This hypothesis is sustained by the correlation between wall viscosity and: (a) smooth muscle content in segments belonging to different arterial territories (Bauer and Pasch 1971, Bulbring *et al* 1970), and (b) smooth muscle activation (Armentano *et al* 1995a, Bauer and Pasch 1971, Cox 1975). The viscous elements of the arterial wall produce a delay of its dimensional response to changes in parietal stress, with the consequent transformation of kinetic energy into dissipated heat energy. This phenomenon had already observed by Roy in 1881 (Shadwick 1999).

The study of the dynamic behavior of smooth muscle has been inexplicably postponed (Barra *et al* 1993, Armentano *et al* 1995a, 1995b). Since it is a main factor in the pathogenesis of high-prevalence diseases, such as hypertension or arteriosclerosis, smooth muscle is directly or indirectly intensively studied from a metabolic, neuroendocrinological, genetic, biomolecular and pharmacological point of view (Barra *et al* 1997, Armentano *et al* 1998, Berry *et al* 2001, Clark *et al* 2000, Henrion *et al* 2001, Intengan *et al* 1999, Leeson *et al* 2000, Megnien *et al* 2001, Safar *et al* 2000, Van Bortel *et al* 2001). Nonetheless, the mechanical contribution of vascular smooth muscle is being excluded from research in terms of etiology, vascular disease pathogeny, and also circulatory dynamics physiology.

3.1 Biomechanics

Biomechanics is the study of mechanics applied to biological sciences. The term *Mechanics* was coined by Galileo in 1638 to describe forces, movements and deformations to which objects are subjected. This field eventually observed particles and continuum materials, including atoms, quantum, molecules, gases, liquids, solids, structures, stars and galaxies. In a general sense, mechanics is applied to the analysis of any dynamic system (Fung 1981).

Table 3.1 shows the main fields involved in biomechanics. All living tissues in one way or another are included in one or more of these items. The study of stress and strain distribution in biological materials and the determination of mechanical properties through constitutive equations are the main topics of this work.

Table 3.1. Fields of study of biomechanics (Fung 1981).

Stress and strain distribution in materials
Constitutive equations that describe the mechanical properties of materials
Flow of fluids: gas, water, blood, and other tissue fluids
Heat transfer, temperature distribution, thermal stress
Mass transference, diffusion, transport through membranes
Motion of charged particles, plasma, ions in solution
Mechanisms, structures
Stability of mechanical systems
Control of mechanical systems
Shock waves, and waves of finite amplitude

In order to understand the geometric configuration of organisms it is necessary to know about their morphology, the anatomy of the organ or the structure and ultrastructure of tissues. In a similar manner, to completely characterize the material it is necessary to determine the mechanical properties of the observed tissues. When the material is biological, the studies imply a series of challenges: the impossibility of isolating the tissue to test it, or the small size of samples, or the difficulty of keeping the normal conditions of live tissue: the physiological environment, ionic content, pH, pO_2, pCO_2 and temperature have fundamental roles when evaluating the results of an experimental session (Fung 1981, Dobrin, 1984; Milnor 1982). Furthermore, biological tissues are subjected to large deformations, and the stress–strain relationships are generally nonlinear and show hysteresis. The nonlinearity of the constitutive equation makes it difficult to determine it.

In summary, to fully understand the mechanical behavior of living tissues it is necessary to determine their mechanical properties. The best way of doing so is to represent them with a constitutive equation. Fung has pointed out that the most serious frustration to a biomechanics worker is usually the lack of information about the constitutive equations of living tissues, and that without constitutive laws, no analysis can be done (Fung 1981).

3.2 The constitutive equation

The properties of materials can be specified through constitutive equations. There are as many constitutive equations as there are materials. A constitutive equation establishes a mathematical relationship between the stress applied to a material and its consequent strain. This approach may be used for blood vessels, where stress is due to intravascular pressure and strain due to the proportional circumferential deformations of the vessel.

3.2.1 Stress

The force per unit area acting on a surface is known as *stress* (σ). The concept of stress expresses the interaction of the material in one part of the body on another (Fung 1981, Milnor 1982). It is worth mentioning that pressure is also a force per unit area and therefore a stress, but in circular section conduits it implies a radial direction (see section 3.3).

Stress is the value of a force acting on a given plane of a body. If this force is uniformly distributed over a determined area, the stress will be quotient between the two variables (McDonald 1974, Milnor 1982, Nichols and O'Rourke 1998):

$$\sigma = \frac{\text{force}}{\text{erea}} = \frac{\text{mass} \times \text{acceleration}}{\text{area}} = \frac{[\text{mass}]}{[\text{length}] \times [\text{time}]^2}. \tag{3.1}$$

The units of stress are the units of force/area or, in base units, mass $\times$ length^{-1} $\times$ time^{-2}. In the International System of Units (SI), the basic unit for force is the *Newton* (*N*) and the unit for length is the *meter* (m), and the basic unit for stress is *Newtons per square meter* ($N\,\text{m}^{-2}$), or *Pascal* (*P*). Therefore, 1 *N* is the force needed to accelerate 1 kg of mass at the rate of 1 m s^{-2}. Similarly, in the CGS system, 1 dyne is the force needed to accelerate a

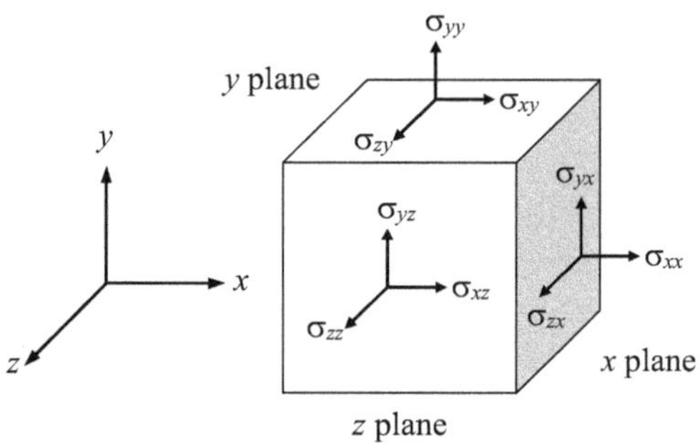

Figure 3.1. Orthogonal coordinate system and stress notation.

mass of 1 g at the rate of 1 cm s^{-2}, therefore the stress can be expressed as dyne cm^{-2} (Fung 1977, 1981)[1].

$$1\frac{N}{m^2} = 10\frac{\text{dynes}}{\text{cm}^2}. \tag{3.2}$$

Strictly speaking, stress at a point is a tensor that combines all the forces that act on the surface of a body, whichever their direction. However, it is analytically more convenient to solve a given tension in three orthogonal directions. Each of these components may be represented as a force vector. This system can be illustrated using a set of orthogonal coordinates x, y, z. (figure 3.1). Stresses are represented using two subscripts: the first one represents its direction and the second one, the plane on which the stress is applied. Each plane is named after its normal axis (Milnor 1982, Fung 1977).

A normal stress tends to lengthen a body (*tensile stress*). It is represented as σ_{xx}, in figure 3.2: a force with direction x acts on the x plane of a body. If the direction of the force were opposite (i.e. if it had a $-x$ direction), the resultant stress would be *compressive stress.*

When a stress parallel to the plane over it is exerted, e.g. σ_{xy} in figure 3.2 (a force with direction x acting on a plane normal to y), it is called *shear stress* (Milnor 1982, Fung 1981).

For the body to maintain a non-rotational state, σ_{ij} and σ_{ji}, $i, j = x, y, z$ must be equal. The tension in any point of the body can be described by six independent stress components (Milnor 1982, Nichols and O'Rourke 1998):

$$\sigma_{xx}, \sigma_{yy}, \sigma_{zz}, \sigma_{xy}, \sigma_{yz}, \sigma_{zx}. \tag{3.3}$$

The first three represent normal stresses (tensile or compressive) and the last three represent shear stress.

---

[1] The conversion from mmHg to dyn·cm^{-2} comes from the hydrostatic pressure formula, $P = h \cdot \rho \cdot g$, where h is the height of a mercury (Hg) column; $\rho = 13.6$ g·cm^{-3} is the density of mercury; $g = 981$ cm·s^{-2} is the gravitational acceleration. A 1 mm high column of Hg exerts a downwards force of 0.1 cm × 1.36 g·cm^{-3} × 981 cm·s^{-2} = 1334 dinas·cm^{-2}.

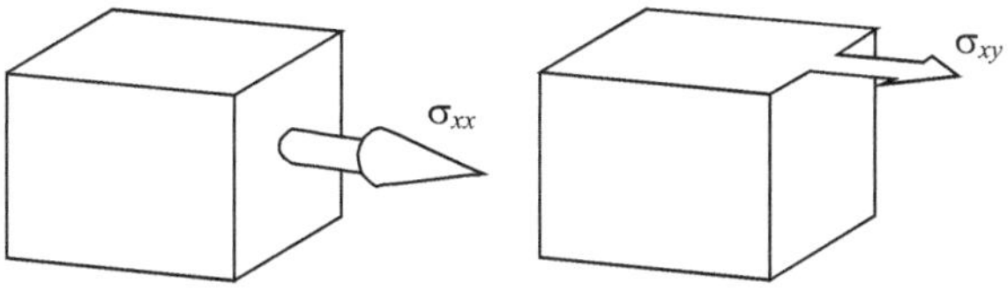

Figure 3.2. Left: normal stress component. Right: shear stress component.

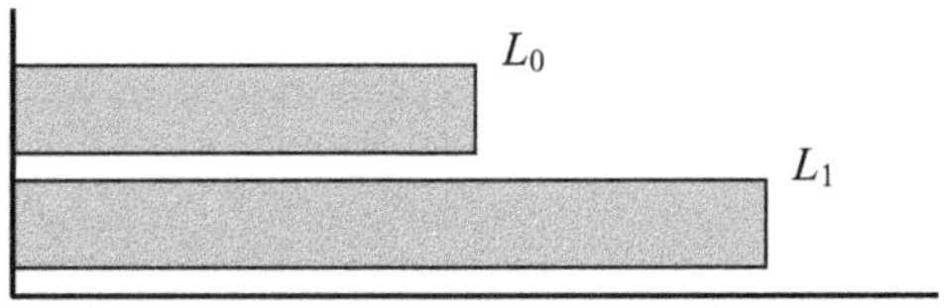

Figure 3.3. Longitudinal deformation.

3.2.2 Strain

Stresses on a body cause a strain (ε). A body of length L_0 is extended to a length L_1, the relative length increment is called *longitudinal* strain, as seen in figure 3.3. Strain is a dimensionless magnitude that is expressed in several ways (Fung 1981, Nichols and O'Rourke 1998, Milnor 1982):

$$\varepsilon = \frac{L_1}{L_0}, \qquad \varepsilon = \frac{L_1 - L_0}{L_0}. \tag{3.4}$$

A tensile stress results in a positive increment in length, a compressive stress in a negative strain.

Strain is therefore a description of the proportional change of the distance between any two points of a body when it is stressed. These two points can be thought of as the adjacent corners of a cube whose faces are normal to a set of coordinates x, y, z. The direction of the strain is described with two subscripts, as stress is. The first subscript indicates the direction and the second one the axis normal to the displaced plane. An infinitesimal cube of the material under study will have nine components of strain: ε_{xx}, ε_{yy}, ε_{zz}, ε_{xy}, ε_{xz}, ε_{yx}, ε_{yz}, ε_{zx}, ε_{zy}. The first three terms are longitudinal strains, the last six of them are shear strains. It can be also demonstrated that strains that share subscripts must be equal, therefore only six independent strains remain:

$$\varepsilon_{xx}, \varepsilon_{yy}, \varepsilon_{zz}, \varepsilon_{xy}, \varepsilon_{yz}, \varepsilon_{zx}. \tag{3.5}$$

The deformation of a body along an axis due to a normal stress generally produces a contraction of the body in the other two axes, i.e. a longitudinal deformation also causes transversal deformations. Figure 3.4 shows that a resting material under a normal stress σ_{xx} produces strains in ε_{xx}, ε_{yy} and ε_{zz}. Each of them are calculated as:

$$\varepsilon_{xx} = \frac{x_1 - x_0}{x_0}, \qquad \varepsilon_{yy} = \frac{y_1 - y_0}{y_0}, \qquad \varepsilon_{zz} = \frac{z_1 - z_0}{z_0}. \tag{3.6}$$

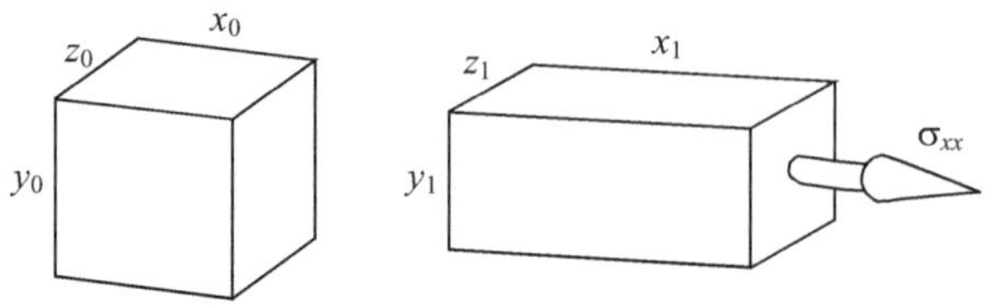

Figure 3.4. An elastic solid of dimensions x_0, y_0, z_0 (left) is deformed by a stress σ_{xx} and has new dimensions x_1, y_1, z_1 (right). x_1 is larger than x_0, whereas y_1 and z_1 become smaller than their initial values.

Transversal strains are proportional to the elongation, and therefore a relationship between these variables can be calculated:

$$-\nu_{yx} = \frac{\varepsilon_{yy}}{\varepsilon_{xx}} \quad \text{and} \quad -\nu_{zx} = \frac{\varepsilon_{zz}}{\varepsilon_{xx}}. \tag{3.7}$$

This proportionality constant is an important characteristic of materials, known as Poisson's ratio. In some applications it can be considered constant (Fung 1977, 1981, 1984).

If the elastic properties of a body are independent of the directions of the stresses, the material is considered *isotropic*, whereas it is *anisotropic* if the elastic properties change according to the direction of the applied stress. Moreover, if the elastic properties remain the same in each point of the body, the material is *homogeneous* (Milnor 1982).

An isotropic material has the same Poisson's ratio for all directions, while anisotropic materials may have several Poisson's ratios. Materials have Poisson's ratios that range between 0 and 1/2. It can be demonstrated mathematically that a Poisson's ratio of 1/2 means the material has a constant volume even if it is deformed (i.e. the volumetric strain is zero). Arterial walls have a Poisson's ratio of approximately 0.5, while most metals have Poisson's values that range between 0.25 and 0.4 (Milnor 1982, Nichols and O'Rourke 1998).

When an angular deformation takes place, i.e. when two points in parallel planes are displaced in a parallel direction, a *shear strain* occurs. Shear strain is expressed as the tangent of the shear angle (figure 3.5).

3.2.3 Hooke's law: the relationship between stress and strain

The properties of materials are determined by their constitutive equations. There are as many constitutive equations as there are materials. It is noteworthy that three simple stress–strain relationships and a system of orthogonal coordinates adequately describe most known materials, i.e. non-viscous fluids, Newtonian viscous fluids and elastic solids. In this way, air, water and many structural materials can be described using these ideal equations. However, most biological materials cannot be described as simply (Fung 1981).

Robert Hooke established, in 1678, that strain is proportional to stress within certain limits. This is known as *Hooke's law*, and as he described, *ut tensio sic vis*, this is *as the extension, so the force*. Any spring-like material subjected to a force suffers an extension proportional to that force (Nichols and O'Rourke 1998, Fung 1981).

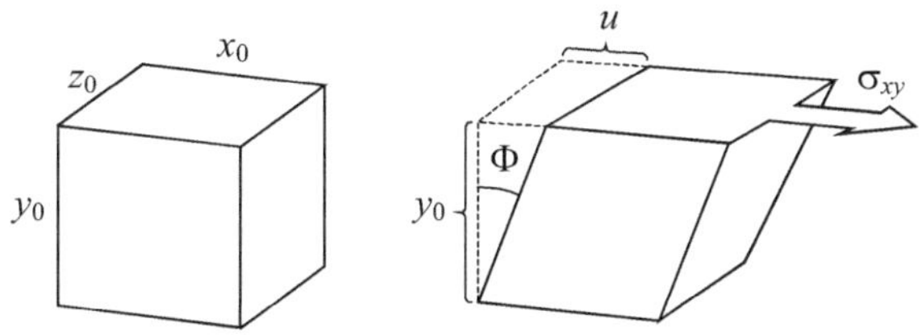

Figure 3.5. Shear strain due to a shear stress σ_{xy}. The shear strain is evaluated through the shear angle (Φ).

The proportionality between stress and strain can explained by the generalized statement of Hooke's law: 'Each of the six components of strain may be expressed as a linear function of the six components of stress, and vice versa'. A complete expression of stress and strain involves 36 constants of proportionality (C_{mn}):

$$\begin{aligned}
\sigma_{xx} &= C_{11}\varepsilon_{xx} + C_{12}\varepsilon_{yy} + C_{13}\varepsilon_{zz} + C_{14}\varepsilon_{yz} + C_{15}\varepsilon_{zx} + C_{16}\varepsilon_{xy} \\
\sigma_{yy} &= C_{21}\varepsilon_{yy} + C_{22}\varepsilon_{zz} + C_{23}\varepsilon_{xx} + C_{24}\varepsilon_{zx} + C_{25}\varepsilon_{yx} + C_{26}\varepsilon_{yz} \\
\sigma_{zz} &= C_{31}\varepsilon_{zz} + C_{32}\varepsilon_{xx} + C_{33}\varepsilon_{yy} + C_{34}\varepsilon_{xy} + C_{35}\varepsilon_{yz} + C_{36}\varepsilon_{zx} \\
\sigma_{yz} &= C_{41}\varepsilon_{xx} + C_{42}\varepsilon_{yy} + C_{43}\varepsilon_{zz} + C_{44}\varepsilon_{yz} + C_{45}\varepsilon_{zx} + C_{46}\varepsilon_{xy} \\
\sigma_{zx} &= C_{51}\varepsilon_{yy} + C_{52}\varepsilon_{zz} + C_{53}\varepsilon_{xx} + C_{54}\varepsilon_{zx} + C_{55}\varepsilon_{xy} + C_{56}\varepsilon_{yz} \\
\sigma_{xy} &= C_{61}\varepsilon_{zz} + C_{62}\varepsilon_{xx} + C_{63}\varepsilon_{yy} + C_{64}\varepsilon_{xy} + C_{65}\varepsilon_{yz} + C_{66}\varepsilon_{zx}.
\end{aligned} \tag{3.8}$$

Fifteen of these constants are redundant, since ($C_{mn} = C_{nm}$), therefore 21 constants remain to be solved when the material is anisotropic. However, if the material is isotropic and incompressible, the number of constants is reduced to two (Milnor 1982, Nichols and O'Rourke 1998, Fung 1981). These constants are known as *Lamé's constants*, G and λ. The constant G is usually identified as the transversal elasticity modulus, or *shear modulus*, and λ as the *longitudinal loading modulus*. Thus, an elastic isotropic solid can be described using only these coefficients or a combination of both:

$$\begin{aligned}
\sigma_{xx} &= \lambda(\varepsilon_{xx} + \varepsilon_{yy} + \varepsilon_{zz}) + 2G\varepsilon_{xx} \\
\sigma_{yy} &= \lambda(\varepsilon_{xx} + \varepsilon_{yy} + \varepsilon_{zz}) + 2G\varepsilon_{yy} \\
\sigma_{zz} &= \lambda(\varepsilon_{xx} + \varepsilon_{yy} + \varepsilon_{zz}) + 2G\varepsilon_{zz} \\
\sigma_{xy} &= 2G\varepsilon_{xy} \\
\sigma_{yz} &= 2G\varepsilon_{yz} \\
\sigma_{zx} &= 2G\varepsilon_{zx}.
\end{aligned} \tag{3.9}$$

Solving for ε:

$$\begin{aligned}
\varepsilon_{xx} &= \frac{1}{E}\left[\sigma_{xx} - \mu(\sigma_{yy} + \sigma_{zz})\right] & \varepsilon_{xy} &= \frac{1+\nu}{E}\sigma_{xy} = \frac{1}{2G}\sigma_{xy} \\
\varepsilon_{yy} &= \frac{1}{E}\left[\sigma_{yy} - \mu(\sigma_{zz} + \sigma_{xx})\right] & \varepsilon_{yz} &= \frac{1+\nu}{E}\sigma_{yz} = \frac{1}{2G}\sigma_{yz} \\
\varepsilon_{zz} &= \frac{1}{E}[\sigma_{zz} - \mu(\sigma_{xx} + \sigma_{zz})] & \varepsilon_{zx} &= \frac{1+\nu}{E}\sigma_{zx} = \frac{1}{2G}\sigma_{zx}.
\end{aligned} \tag{3.10}$$

The constants E and υ are associated with the Lamé constants λ and G. The parameter E is known as *Young's Modulus* and ν as Poisson's ratio. The relationship among these parameters is:

$$\lambda = \frac{2G\nu}{1-2\nu} = \frac{G(E-2G)}{3G-E} = \frac{E\cdot\nu}{(1+\nu)\cdot(1-2\nu)} \tag{3.11}$$

$$G = \frac{\lambda(1-2\nu)}{2\nu} = \frac{E}{2(1+\nu)} \tag{3.12}$$

$$E = \frac{G(3\lambda+2G)}{\lambda+G} = \frac{\lambda(1-\nu)\cdot(1-2\nu)}{\nu} = 2G(1+\nu) \tag{3.13}$$

$$\nu = \frac{3B-2G}{2(3B+G)} = \frac{\lambda}{(3B-\lambda)} = \frac{E}{2G} - 1. \tag{3.14}$$

The compressibility modulus (*bulk modulus*, B) is the relationship between the compressive stress product of a pressure P that is uniform in the three directions ($\sigma_{xx} = \sigma_{yy} = \sigma_{zz} = P$) and the volumetric deformation ($V_0/\Delta V$):

$$B = \frac{P\cdot V_0}{\Delta V}. \tag{3.15}$$

The average stress exerted on a body can be calculated as:

$$-\frac{\sigma_{xx}+\sigma_{yy}+\sigma_{zz}}{3} \tag{3.16}$$

and volumetric deformation is the sum of the strains in all three directions:

$$\frac{\Delta V}{V_0} = \varepsilon_{xx}+\varepsilon_{yy}+\varepsilon_{zz} = (\sigma_{xx}+\sigma_{yy}+\sigma_{zz})\frac{1-2\nu}{E}. \tag{3.17}$$

Therefore, B can be expressed as:

$$B = -\frac{PV_0}{\Delta V} = \frac{(\sigma_{xx}+\sigma_{yy}+\sigma_{zz})V_0}{3(\varepsilon_{xx}+\varepsilon_{yy}+\varepsilon_{zz})} = \frac{E}{3(1-2\nu)}. \tag{3.18}$$

The elastic properties of a material can be expressed as the relationship between stress and strain, or *elastic modulus*. As strain is a proportion, and therefore dimensionless, moduli have the same units as stress.

Young's modulus can also be calculated as the quotient of longitudinal stress and strain:

$$E_{xx} = \frac{\sigma_{xx}}{\varepsilon_{xx}}. \tag{3.19}$$

Shear modulus G can be expressed as the relationship between shear stress and shear strain:

$$G = \frac{\sigma_{xy}}{\varepsilon_{xy}} \tag{3.20}$$

The longitudinal loading modulus, λ, is the relationship between a normal stress and an orthogonal normal strain:

$$\lambda_{xy} = \frac{\sigma_{yy}}{\varepsilon_{xx}}. \tag{3.21}$$

Any of these five constants (E, ν, B, G, and λ) can be calculated from three of them. They all have the same units, except for the dimensionless Poisson's ratio. Table 3.2 shows different ways of calculating these parameters.

The determination of the Young's modulus of an elastic material is a simple procedure, since strain is linearly proportional to stress, according to Hooke's law. If a graph is constructed with strain in the x-axis and stress in the y-axis, the gradient of the linear relationship is the Young's modulus. However, blood vessels and other non-homogeneous materials do not obey Hooke's law, but rather exhibit a curvilinear relationship between stress and strain. Inhomogeneous materials have a variable elasticity modulus that is a function of strain. Under these conditions, the elastic modulus can be defined as the tangent of a certain point in the stress–stress relationship. Krafka, in 1939, studied 10 cm × 1 cm sections of aorta from humans, cows and dogs applying forces equivalent to 25, 50, 100 and 200 g (Krafka 1939). The elastic moduli were calculated as:

$$E = \frac{F \times L \times 980}{A \times \Delta L}, \tag{3.22}$$

where F is the applied force, L is the length of the segment, A is the area and ΔL is the elongation, 980 is a conversion factor. He proposed the comparison of

Table 3.2. Relationship between elastic constants (Milnor 1982).

Constant	Definition expressed as function of stress and strain	Equivalent expression for an isotropic material
Young's modulus	$E_{xx} = \frac{\sigma_{xx}}{\varepsilon_{xx}}$	$E = 2G(1 + \nu)$
Shear modulus	$G = \frac{\sigma_{xy}}{\varepsilon_{xy}}$	$G = \frac{E}{2(1 + \nu)}$
Bulk modulus	$B = \frac{P \cdot V_0}{\Delta V}$	$B = \frac{E}{3(1 + 2\nu)}$
Longitudinal loading modulus	$\lambda_{xy} = \frac{\sigma_{yy}}{\varepsilon_{xx}}$	$\lambda = \frac{E \cdot \nu}{(1 + \nu) \cdot (1 - 2\nu)}$
Poisson's ratio	$\nu_{yx} = -\frac{\varepsilon_{yy}}{\varepsilon_{xx}}$	$\nu = \frac{3B - 2G}{2(3B + G)}$

incremental forces ($E^{200-100}$). As a result of the work of Krafka, Bergel called *incremental elastic modulus* (E_{inc}) the elastic modulus calculated at 20 mmHg pressure increments (Bergel 1961a). In order to calculate the incremental elastic modulus, a stress (σ_1) is applied and the resulting strain (ε_1) is calculated. Then stress is increased (σ_2) and another strain (ε_2) will be observed. The value of E_{inc} corresponds to an average strain $\varepsilon_m = (\varepsilon_1 + \varepsilon_2)/2$ (Milnor 1982):

$$E_{inc} = \frac{(\sigma_2 - \sigma_1) \cdot \varepsilon_m}{(\varepsilon_2 - \varepsilon_1)}. \tag{3.23}$$

The smaller the increment, the more precise the approximation to the real value of the tangent of the curve at the observed strain.

Hooke's law is valid until the *elastic limit*, beyond which a solid suffers a *permanent strain* and is unable to return to its original shape. The classic elasticity theory has been developed to work within elastic limits and is based on two hypotheses: strains are infinitely small, and the structure of the material is continuous, uniform and homogeneous. It is a well-known fact that the arterial wall does not follow any of these premises. Firstly, the vascular wall is easily deformed, comparable to rubber, and the strains to which they are subjected cannot be considered small. Secondly, the main structural components of the elastic nature of the arterial wall are elastin and collagen, which are fibrous and are surrounded by fluids, semifluids, water matrices and mucoproteins (McDonald 1974). From a histological point of view, this is far from homogeneity. However, recent studies have shown that due to the spatial disposition of the elastic laminae, collagen fibers and smooth muscle cells of the tunica media, the arterial wall may be considered a mechanically homogeneous material, even if it is evidently inhomogeneous (Dobrin 1999).

3.3 Physics of the equilibrium of blood vessels

Intravascular pressure is exerted against the vascular wall. The wall is distended in all directions, and an equilibrium of forces is reached. Distensions occur in the circumferential and longitudinal directions, but rotations are negligible and therefore shear stresses are too (see figure 3.5). This allows one to consider the arterial wall as a cylindrical orthotropic body, where strains are aligned with the three main directions. Therefore, the rectangular coordinates (x, y, z) can be replaced by the cylindrical coordinate system: a radial direction ($\breve{r}$), a circumferential or tangential direction ($\breve{\theta}$), and a longitudinal or axial direction ($\breve{z}$) (Burton 1954, Patel and Fry 1969, Dobrin, 1978). Figure 3.6 shows the cylindrical coordinate system.

The two forces that determine a state of equilibrium in the vascular wall are: (a) intravascular pressure, which tends to increase the diameter of the vessel and stretch the wall (radial stress) and (b) the stress within the wall (tangential stress), which opposes the radial stress (Burton 1954, Peterson *et al* 1960). This equilibrium condition has been documented as a special application of Laplace's Law,

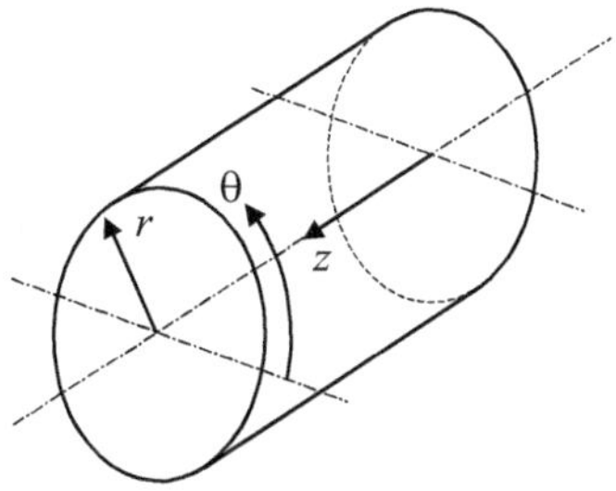

Figure 3.6. Cylindrical coordinate system. The central axis coincides with $r = 0$, whereas $\theta = 0$ and $z = 0$ are arbitrary planes.

formulated in 1841 (Burton 1954): the tangential or circumferential force (T, also called parietal stress) is associated with transmural pressure (P) and radius (R):

$$T = P \cdot R. \tag{3.24}$$

This parietal stress T is different from the classical stress σ, since it is a force per unit length (dyne cm^{-1})

Peterson *et al* (1960) considered this simplified approach inappropriate, since it overlooks the thickness of the wall (h); instead they proposed that the circumferential or tangential stress should be calculated as:

$$\sigma_{\theta\theta} = \frac{P \cdot R}{h}. \tag{3.25}$$

Strictly speaking, $\sigma_{\theta\theta}$ is a simplification of the stresses solved by Love in 1927 (Milnor 1982) in a pressurized isotropic tube of non-negligible wall thickness. The radial ($\breve{r}$), circumferential ($\breve{\theta}$) and longitudinal ($\breve{z}$) components were solved by Love as follows:

$$\begin{aligned} \sigma_{\theta\theta} &= \left(\frac{P_i \cdot r_i^2 - P_e \cdot r_e^2}{r_e^2 - r_i^2}\right) + \left(\frac{P_i - P_e}{r_e^2 - r_i^2} \cdot \frac{r_e^2 \cdot r_i^2}{R^2}\right) \\ \sigma_{rr} &= \left(\frac{P_i \cdot r_i^2 - P_e \cdot r_e^2}{r_e^2 - r_i^2}\right) - \left(\frac{P_i - P_e}{r_e^2 - r_i^2} \cdot \frac{r_e^2 \cdot r_i^2}{R^2}\right) \\ \sigma_{zz} &= \left(\frac{\lambda}{\lambda - G} \cdot \frac{P_i \cdot r_i^2 - P_e \cdot r_e^2}{r_e^2 - r_i^2}\right) + \frac{\varepsilon G(3\lambda + 2G)}{\lambda + G}, \end{aligned} \tag{3.26}$$

where λ is the longitudinal loading modulus and G the shear modulus (see table 3.2), P_i and P_e are the internal and external pressures, respectively, r_i and r_e are the internal and external radii, respectively, and R is the median radius:

$$R = \frac{r_e + r_i}{2}. \tag{3.27}$$

If both the external pressure and ε are null, these equations are simplified:

$$\sigma_{\theta\theta} = P_i\left(\frac{r_i^2}{r_e^2 - r_i^2}\right) + P_i\left(\frac{r_e^2 \cdot r_i^2}{r_e^2 - r_i^2} \cdot \frac{1}{R^2}\right)$$
$$\sigma_{rr} = P_i\left(\frac{r_i^2}{r_e^2 - r_i^2}\right) - P_i\left(\frac{r_e^2 \cdot r_i^2}{r_e^2 - r_i^2} \cdot \frac{1}{R^2}\right) \tag{3.28}$$
$$\sigma_{zz} = \frac{\lambda}{\lambda - G} \cdot P_i \frac{r_i^2}{r_e^2 - r_i^2}.$$

Since equation (3.25) is a well-known equation, it is interesting to demonstrate that it appears in the circumferential component of stress ($\sigma_{\theta\theta}$) of equation (3.28), assuming a thin enough wall to consider $r_e \approx R$.

Since $r_e - r_i = h$ and $r_e^2 - r_i^2 = (r_e - r_i) \cdot (r_e + r_i) = (r_e + r_i) \cdot h = 2 \cdot r_i \cdot h + h^2$, h^2 is negligible against $2 \cdot r_i \cdot h$. Therefore, circumferential stress ($\sigma_{\theta\theta}$) can be expressed as:

$$\sigma_{\theta\theta} = P_i\left(\frac{r_i^2}{2 \cdot r_i \cdot h}\right) + P_i\left(\frac{r_e^2 \cdot R^2}{2 \cdot r_i \cdot h} \cdot \frac{1}{R^2}\right)$$
$$\sigma_{\theta\theta} = \frac{P_i \cdot r_i}{2 \cdot h} + \frac{P_i \cdot r_i}{2 \cdot h} = \frac{2 \cdot P_i \cdot r_i}{2 \cdot h} \tag{3.29}$$
$$\sigma_{\theta\theta} = \frac{P \cdot R}{h}.$$

3.4 Viscoelasticity

Until now, materials have been considered as purely elastic, i.e. a strain disappears as soon as the stress disappears and the frequency at which stress is applied is not taken into account. Some materials, blood vessels included, need a certain amount of time to reach a degree of strain, and in a similar manner do not return to their original shape immediately, when a force is applied and removed. Thus, the time factor is important and materials that exhibit this behavior are called *viscoelastic* (McDonald 1974, Milnor 1982).

A way of expressing the hypotheses of the mechanical behavior of these materials is through *models*. These models are represented with elemental mechanical components and allow one to carry out purely elastic, purely viscous, or viscoelastic approaches. The vascular wall has been represented with conventional mechanical models, but none of them has adequately represented its true behavior. These models combine springs (purely elastic element) and dampers (a stiff cylinder suspended in a viscous fluid) (Milnor 1982, Fung 1981).

A spring is assumed to have linear behavior (figure 3.7) that strains proportionally to the applied force. This proportionality constant obeys Hooke's law:

$$\sigma_{\text{elastic}} = E \cdot \varepsilon. \tag{3.30}$$

Likewise, a damper is assumed to move at a velocity that is proportional to the applied load (figure 3.8). As velocity is the first time derivative of strain, the viscous stress is:

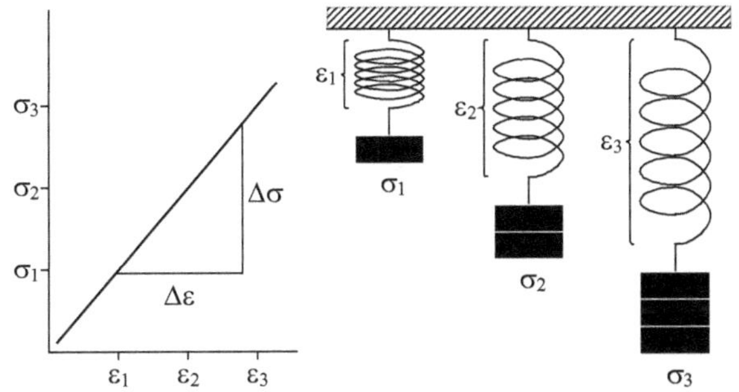

Figure 3.7. Left panel: stress–strain relationship of a linear spring. Its gradient is the elastic modulus $E = \Delta\sigma/\Delta\varepsilon$. Right panel: the length reached by the spring is proportional to the load.

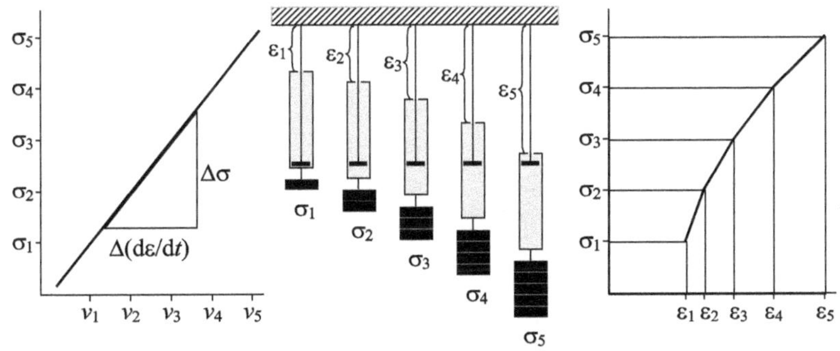

Figure 3.8. Left panel: stress–velocity (σ–v) relationship of a damper, where $v = d\varepsilon/dt$. The gradient of the relationship is the viscous modulus $\eta = \Delta\sigma/\Delta(d\varepsilon/dt)$. Central panel: dampers in five stages of equal time interval. Right panel: even though the displacement velocity is constant, the strain is not linear with load.

$$\sigma_{\text{viscous}} = \eta \cdot \frac{d\varepsilon}{dt}. \tag{3.31}$$

After the behavior of the purely elastic and viscous components has been described, a model that combines both, i.e. a viscoelastic model, can be elaborated. Figure 3.9 shows the most conventional models used to describe the mechanical properties of blood vessels. The Maxwell model has an elastic and a viscous element connected in series, the Voigt model has the same elements but in parallel. The Saint Venant model has an elastic element connected in series to a Voigt model, and the Kelvin model has an elastic element in parallel with a Maxwell model.

In the Maxwell model (figure 3.9(a)) a spring instantaneously deforms when a force is applied, while the damper progressively stretches. In the Voigt model (figure 3.9(b)), the spring is held back by the damper and their deformation is simultaneous until they reach equilibrium.

Three-element models best describe the mechanical behavior of the vascular wall. Although it is not entirely true, the Kelvin model is frequently called modified Maxwell model or Hill model, and the Saint Venant model is called Voigt model in literature on physiology.

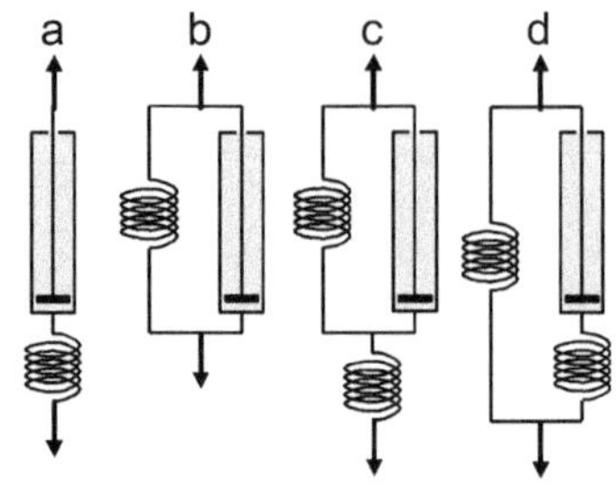

Figure 3.9. Configuration of the models used to characterize viscoelastic materials: (a) Maxwell, (b) Voigt, (c) Saint Venant, (d) Kelvin (or Hill) models.

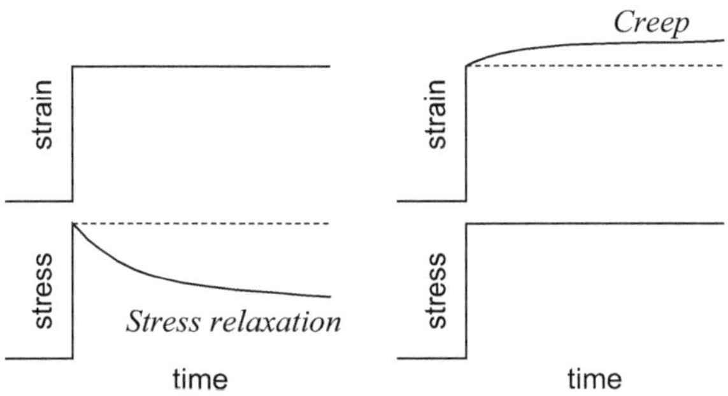

Figure 3.10. *Stress relaxation* (left panel), the decay of stress while strain remains constant. *Creep* (right panel), the slow and prolonged strain when the material is constantly stressed.

3.4.1 Stress relaxation, creep and hysteresis

When a viscoelastic material is suddenly deformed, a stress is immediately formed to oppose this deformation; but even though this deformation is kept constant, the stress decreases with time. This phenomenon of the decay of stress in the viscoelastic material while strain is constant is known as *stress relaxation* (table 3.1, equation (3.19)).

On the other hand, if a stress is suddenly applied to a viscoelastic material and kept constant, the material suffers an immediate strain, followed by a slow and prolonged deformation(figure 3.10). This phenomenon of slow and prolonged strain of a viscoelastic material subjected to a constant stress is called *creep* (table 3.1, equation (3.19)).

It is precisely due to creep and stress relaxation that during cyclical stress and strain conditions (e.g. blood vessels in each cardiac cycle), the combined effects of elasticity and viscosity determine a delay between the applied stress and the resulting strain. This delay is known as *hysteresis* (Gow and Taylor 1968, Dobrin 1978, Fung 1981, Bauer *et al* 1982). The periodic behavior allows one to study stress and stress as a function of time and with a simple harmonic motion approach. As it has become clear, a cycle is completed by covering the 360° or 2π radians of a circumference, independently of the time it takes.

3.5 Frequency dependence of the elastic modulus $E_{(\omega)}$

In 1952, Hardung described the viscoelasticity of vessels through a complex elastic modulus E':

$$E' = E_{dyn} + j\eta\omega. \tag{3.32}$$

The real part of E', its first term, is the dynamic modulus (E_{dyn}), which describes the purely elastic properties of the wall. The second and complex term of E' describes the purely viscous properties, and is called loss modulus, where ω is the angular velocity and η is the viscosity of the wall. The complex operator j is the imaginary unit, defined as the square root of -1 ($\sqrt{-1} = j$).

The complex modulus of the Hardung equation (3.32), E', is a complex number that can be decomposed into its modulus $|E'|$ and its argument φ, also called the phase angle:

$$|E'| = \sqrt{E_{dyn}{}^2 + (\eta\omega)^2} \tag{3.33}$$

$$\varphi = \text{arctg}\left(\frac{\eta\omega}{E_{dyn}}\right). \tag{3.34}$$

In practice, it is usual to separate the real and complex components with respect to the phase angle:

$$E_{dyn} = |E'| \cdot \cos\varphi$$
$$\eta\omega = |E'| \cdot \text{sen}\ \varphi.$$

The argument φ is the phase angle between the stress and the resulting strain, and is responsible for hysteresis. Hysteresis is evidenced when representing both signals in an X–Y graph (Lissajou figure; figure 3.11). Two sinusoidal signals with the same amplitude and frequency may or may not have the same phase. If they do, an X–Y

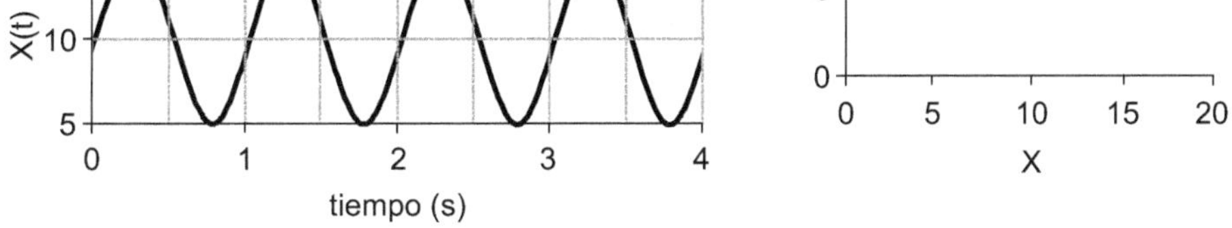

Figure 3.11. Lissajou figure (right panel) for the two sinusoidal signals in the left panel. As both signals are phased with respect to time, the X–Y composition shows a straight line. Viscosity is null ($\eta = 0$).

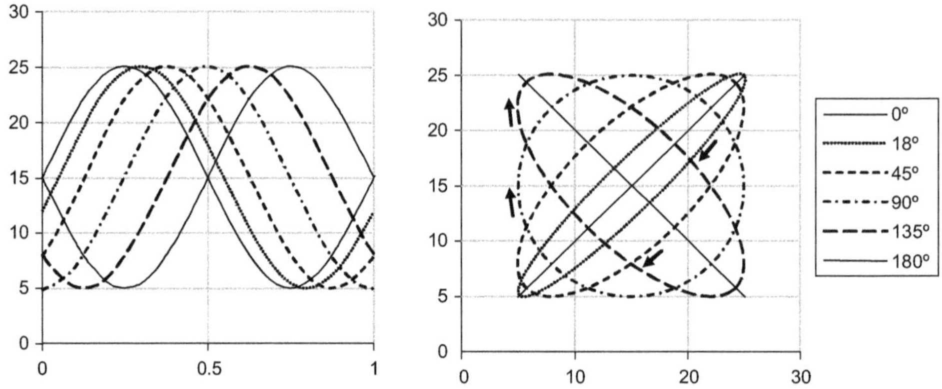

Figure 3.12. Hysteresis loop with respect to the phase angle between two signals of equal amplitude and frequency. Left panel: signals and phase difference angles with respect to the original signal (0°). Right panel: Lissajou figure for one *Y* signal but several *X* signals. The arrows indicate the direction of rotation.

composition will show a straight line. This is the case of a purely elastic material, which shows no hysteresis in the Lissajou figure. Viscosity is null ($\eta = 0$).

However, if signals are temporarily out of phase, their *X–Y* composition will show a hysteresis loop encircling a certain area, which increases with phase difference. Figure 3.12 shows the effects of delaying a signal *X* with respect to *Y*. The straight line becomes elliptical, and finally a circle as the phase is 90°. The phase difference between two signals can be expressed in terms of time (e.g. in milliseconds), but also as the phase angle difference. As each cycle can be represented as a 360° quadrant, the maximum achievable phase difference is 90°, a circle in the *X–Y* composition and the largest possible enclosed area. Phase differences larger than 90° do not increase the hysteresis area, but change the gradient of the *X–Y* relationship until it reaches 180° and a straight line (figure 3.12). Loops at phases of 0° and 180° are the same as 180° and 360° but with an opposite direction of rotation.

There exists a relationship between the time delay (t) and the phase angle (φ), expressed as:

$$\frac{t}{T} = \frac{\varphi(\text{degrees})}{360} = \frac{\varphi(\text{radians})}{2\pi}. \tag{3.35}$$

There is a temporal dependence of the stress and the resulting strain. This behavior is typical of blood vessels, and the time lag is a way of measuring wall viscosity (Milnor 1982).

The elastic modulus is calculated as the quotient between stress and strain, $\sigma = E \cdot \varepsilon$. However, the elastic modulus is frequency dependent ($E_{(\omega)}$):

$$\begin{aligned} E' &= E_{dyn} + j\eta\omega \\ E_{(\omega)} &= E_{real} + jE_{imag}, \end{aligned} \tag{3.36}$$

where E_{real}, the real part, is also called the *storage modulus*, and E_{imag} is the complex part also called *loss storage*. $E_{(\omega)}$ has a modulus $|E_{(\omega)}|$ and an argument $\varphi = \omega t$:

$$\begin{aligned} \left|E_{(\omega)}\right| &= \sqrt{E_{real}^2 + jE_{imag}^2} \\ \omega t &= \text{arctg}\left(\frac{E_{imag}}{E_{real}}\right) \\ E_{real} &= E_{(\omega)}\cos\,\omega t \\ E_{imag} &= E_{(\omega)}\text{sen}\,\omega t. \end{aligned} \tag{3.37}$$

The frequency dependence between stress and strain can be studied by means of a sinusoidal stress at a given frequency, and measuring strains and the consequent phase difference. Then, the frequency is modified and measurements are repeated, and so on. These studies have been carried out in arteries *in vitro*, and have provided important information regarding the behavior or the vascular wall facing frequency changes (Bergel 1961b), however these techniques cannot be reproduced *in vivo*.

The dynamic elastic modulus can also be calculated as:

$$\begin{aligned} E_{(\omega)} &= \frac{\sigma_{(\omega)}}{\varepsilon_{(\omega)}} = \frac{\sigma_0 e^{j\omega t}}{\varepsilon_0 e^{j\omega t}} \\ \sigma_{(\omega)} &= E_{(\omega)} \cdot \varepsilon_{(\omega)}, \end{aligned} \tag{3.38}$$

where σ_0 and ε_0 are stress and strain at zero frequency, and $e^{j\omega t}$ is the exponential representation of $e^{j\omega t} = \cos\,\omega t + j\,\sin\,\omega t$. Then,

$$\begin{aligned} \sigma_{(\omega)} &= (E + j\omega\eta) \cdot \varepsilon_{(\omega)} \\ \sigma_{(\omega)} &= E \cdot \varepsilon_{(\omega)} + j\omega\eta \cdot \varepsilon_{(\omega)} \\ \sigma_0 e^{j\omega t} &= E \cdot \varepsilon_0 e^{j\omega t} + j\omega\eta \cdot \varepsilon_0 e^{j\omega t}. \end{aligned} \tag{3.39}$$

Periodic waves can be numerically represented by decomposing them into their oscillatory components. This *harmonic analysis* was developed by French mathematician Jean Baptiste Joseph Fourier (1768–1830), in 1807.

Fourier analysis establishes that any function $f(t)$ is equivalent to the infinite sum of sinusoidal waves:

$$f_{(t)} = m_0 + \sum_{k=1}^{\infty}[2A_k \cos\,(k\omega t - \varphi_k)], \tag{3.40}$$

where m_0 is the mean value of the function, and the summation term encloses a sinusoidal function $s_{(t)} = m\,\cos\,(\omega t - \varphi)$. $k = 1, 2, 3, \ldots, \infty$, and $k\omega$ is the sinusoidal frequency. The first sinusoidal wave ($k = 1$) is called *first harmonic*, or *fundamental harmonic*. In the aortic pressure, the frequency of the first harmonic is equal to the heart rate. The second harmonic, $k = 2$, has a frequency that is two times the fundamental frequency and so on. Each wave has its own modulus m_k and phase φ_k.

The fast Fourier transform (FFT) is an efficient algorithm to decompose a complex signal. Figure 3.13 shows a wave and its sinusoidal harmonic components.

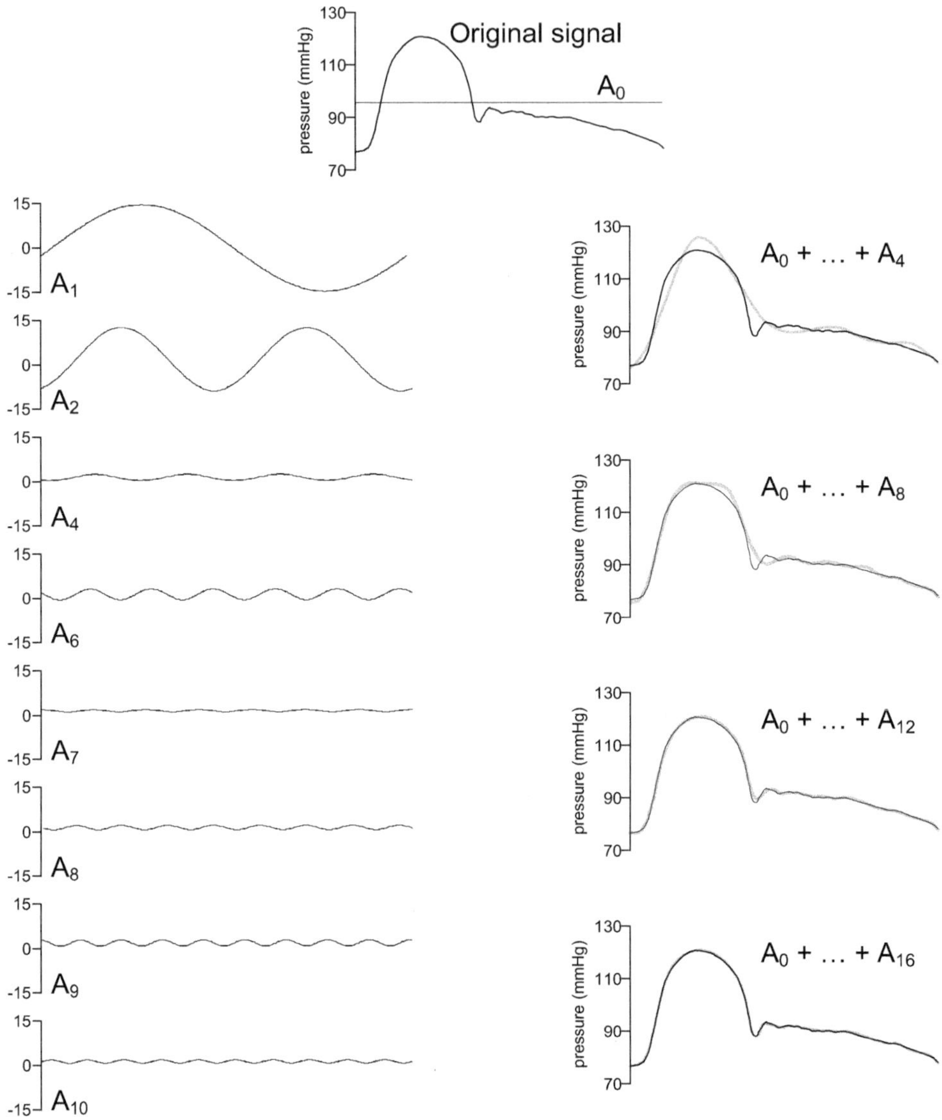

Figure 3.13. Example of the decomposition and synthetization of an aortic pressure signal of a dog through Fourier analysis. The original signal is decomposed into sinusoidal wakes of increasing frequency, called harmonics. The first ten harmonics are represented ($A_1,\dots A_{10}$). Each harmonic has its own amplitude and phase difference with respect to the fundamental harmonic. The mean value of the original signal is the 0 harmonic (A_0). The reconstruction of the signal is done by adding the different harmonics ($A_0 + A_1 + A_2 + \dots + A_n$). It is noteworthy that the more harmonics are considered, the better the representation of the original wave.

The decomposition of the signal into its respective harmonics was done using a FFT, an application present in most programming languages. Generally, a signal is input and the output is a series of data that correspond to the moduli and phase of each harmonic (see figure 3.14).

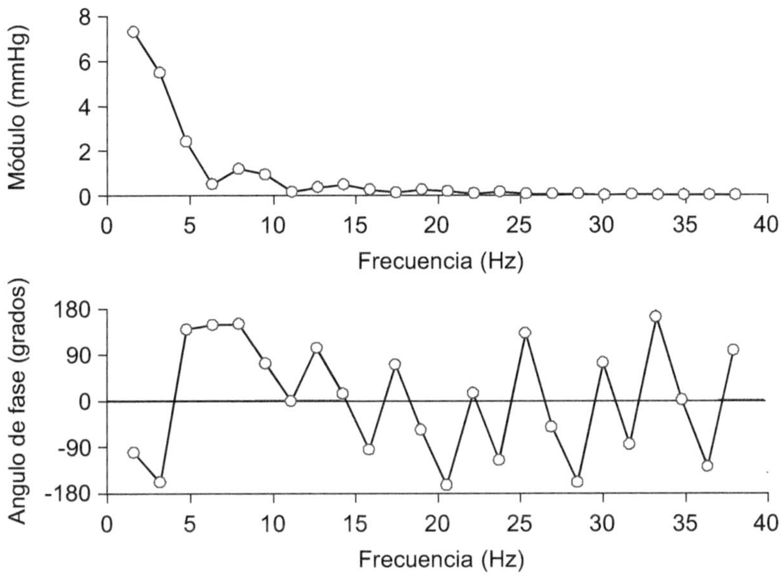

Figure 3.14. Modulus and phase calculated for the pressure wave of figure 3.13. The x-axis has the frequencies that correspond to the harmonics A_1 to A_{24}.

Equation (3.40) defines the model that responds to the dynamic behavior of a viscoelastic material. This model can be further developed to include an inertial component (M). Thus, a model that includes an elastic, viscous and inertial component is expressed as:

$$\begin{aligned} \sigma_0 e^{j\omega t} &= E \cdot \varepsilon_0 e^{j\omega t} + j\omega\eta \cdot \varepsilon_0 e^{j\omega t} + j^2\omega^2 M \cdot \varepsilon_0 e^{j\omega t} \\ \sigma_{(\omega)} &= E \cdot \varepsilon_{(\omega)} + j\omega\eta \cdot \varepsilon_{(\omega)} + j^2\omega^2 M \cdot \varepsilon_{(\omega)}. \end{aligned} \tag{3.41}$$

Since $\frac{d(e^{at})}{dt} = ae^{at}$, equations (3.40) and (3.42) can be rewritten as:

$$\begin{aligned} \sigma_0 e^{j\omega t} &= E \cdot \varepsilon_0 e^{j\omega t} + \eta \frac{d(\varepsilon_0 e^{j\omega t})}{dt} \\ \sigma_{(\omega)} &= E \cdot \varepsilon_{(\omega)} + \eta \frac{d\varepsilon_{(\omega)}}{dt} \end{aligned} \tag{3.42}$$

$$\begin{aligned} \sigma_0 e^{j\omega t} &= E \cdot \varepsilon_0 e^{j\omega t} + \eta \frac{d(\varepsilon_0 e^{j\omega t})}{dt} + M \frac{d^2(\varepsilon_0 e^{j\omega t})}{dt^2} \\ \sigma_{(\omega)} &= E \cdot \varepsilon_{(\omega)} + \eta \frac{d\varepsilon_{(\omega)}}{dt} + M \frac{d^2\varepsilon_{(\omega)}}{dt^2}. \end{aligned} \tag{3.43}$$

Equations (3.43) and (3.44) can be rewritten in the time domain using first and second order differential equations:

$$\sigma_{(t)} = E \cdot \varepsilon_{(t)} + \eta \frac{d\varepsilon_{(t)}}{dt} \tag{3.44}$$

$$\sigma_{(t)} = E \cdot \varepsilon_{(t)} + \eta \frac{d\varepsilon_{(t)}}{dt} + M \frac{d^2\varepsilon_{(t)}}{dt^2}. \tag{3.45}$$

These last equations are the expression of the mathematical relationship between stress and strain in the time domain equation (3.45) and the frequency domain equation (3.42), i.e. they are constitutive equations that respond to the chosen model to mathematically represent the arterial wall.

References

Alexander R M 1983 *Animal Mechanics* 2nd edn (Chichester: Packard Publishing Ltd)

Armentano R L, Levenson J, Barra J G, Cabrera Fischer E I, Breitbart G J, Pichel R H and Simon A C 1991 Assessment of elastin and collagen contribution to aortic elasticity in conscious dogs *Am. J. Physiol.* **260** H1870–7

Armentano R L, Barra J G, Levenson J, Simon A and Pichel R H 1995a Arterial wall mechanics in conscious dogs: assessment of viscous, inertial, and elastic moduli to characterize the aortic wall behavior *Circ. Res.* **76** 468–78

Armentano R L, Megnien J L, Simon A, Bellenfant F, Barra J G and Levenson J 1995b Effects of hypertension on visco-elastic properties of common carotid and femoral arteries in humans *Hypertension* **26** 48–54

Armentano R L, Graf S, Barra J G, Velikovsky G, Baglivo H, Sanchez R, Simon A, Pichel R H and Levenson J 1998 Carotid wall viscosity increase is related to intima-media thickening in hypertensive patients *Hypertension* **31** 534–9

Barra J G, Armentano R L, Levenson J, Cabrera Fischer E I, Pichel R H and Simon A 1993 Assessment of smooth muscle contribution to descending thoracic elastic mechanics in conscious dogs *Circ. Res.* **73** 1040–50

Barra J G, Levenson J, Armentano R L, Cabrera Fischer E I, Pichel R H and Simon A 1997 *In vivo* angiotensin II receptor blockade and enzyme inhibition on canine aortic viscoelasticity *Am. J. Physiol.* **272** H859–68

Bauer R D and Pasch T 1971 The quasi-static and dynamic circumferential elastic modulus of the rat tail artery studied at various wall stresses and tones of the vascular smooth muscle *Pflügers Arch.* **330** 335–46

Bauer R D, Büsse R and Schabert A 1982 Mechanical properties of arteries *Biorheology* **19** 409–24

Bergel D H 1961a The static elastic properties of the arterial wall *J. Physiol.* **156** 445–57

Bergel D H 1961b The dynamic elastic properties of the arterial wall *J. Physiol.* **156** 458–69

Berry C, Touyz R, Dominiczak A F, Webb R C and Johns D G 2001 Angiotensin receptors: signaling, vascular pathophysiology, and interactions with ceramide *Am. J. Physiol.* **281** H2337–65

Bulbring E, Brading A F, Jones A W and Tomita T (ed) 1970 *Smooth Muscle* (Baltimore, MD: Williams & Wilkins)

Burton A C 1954 Relation of structure to function of the tissues of the wall of blood vessels *Physiol. Rev.* **34** 619–42

Clark C J, Davies E, Anderson N H, Farmer R, Friel E C, Fraser R and Connell J M C 2000 α-adducin and angiotensin I-converting enzyme polymorphisms in essential hypertension *Hypertension* **36** 990–4

Cox R H 1975 Arterial wall mechanics and composition and the effects of smooth muscle activation *Am. J. Physiol.* **229** 807–12

Dawkins R 1985 *The Selfish Gene* (Oxford: Academic)
Traducido por ed Suárez J R 1985 *El Gen Egoísta, Las Bases Biológicas de Nuestra Conducta* (Barcelona, España: Salvat Editores)

Dobrin P B 1978 Mechanical properties of arteries *Physiol. Rev.* **58** 397–460

Dobrin P B 1984 Mechanical behaviour of vascular smooth muscle in cylindrical segments of arteries *in vitro Ann. Biomed. Eng.* **12** 497–510

Dobrin P B 1999 Distribution of lamellar deformations. Implications for properties of arterial media *Hypertension* **33** 806–10

Faury G 2001 Function-structure relationship of elastic arteries in evolution: from microfibrils to elastin end elastic fibres *Pathol. Biol.* **49** 310–25

Fung Y C 1977 *A First Course in Continuum Mechanics* (Upper Saddle River, NJ: Prentice-Hall)

Fung Y C 1981 Biomechanics *Mechanical Properties of Living Tissues* (New York: Springer)

Fung Y C 1984 Biodynamics *Circulation* (New York: Springer)

Gow B S and Taylor M G 1968 Measurements of viscoelastic properties of arteries in the living dog *Circ. Res.* **23** 111–22

Henrion D, Kubis N and Lévy B I 2001 Physiological and pathophysiological function of the AT2 subtype receptor of angiotensin II. From large arteries to the microcirculation *Hypertension* **38** 1150–7

Intengan H D, Deng L Y, Li J S and Schiffrin E L 1999 Mechanics and composition of human subcutaneous resistance arteries in essential hypertension *Hypertension* **33** 569–74

Johansen K and Martin A W 1965 *Handbook of Physiology* Section 2: Circulation ed W F Hamilton and P Dow vol III (Washington, DC: American Physiological Society) ch 73, pp 2583–614

Krafka J 1939 Comparative study of the histo–physics of the aorta *Am. J. Physiol.* **125** 1–14

Leeson C P, Whincup P H, Cook D G, Mullen M J, Donald A E, Seymour C A and Deanfield J E 2000 Cholesterol and arterial distensibility in the first decade of life: a population-based study *Circulation* **101** 1533–8

Martin A W and Johansen K 1965 *Handbook of Physiology* Section 2: Circulation ed W F Hamilton and P Dow vol III (Washington, DC: American Physiological Society) ch 72, pp 2545–81

McDonald D A 1974 *Blood Flow in Arteries* 2nd edn (London: Edward Arnold)

Megnien J L, Simon A, Mikaberidze E, Denarie N, Chironi G, Barra J G, Armentano R L and Levenson J 2001 Do arterial effects of antihypertensive drugs depend on subject's serum cholesterol? *J. Cardiovasc. Pharmacol.* **38** 520–8

Milnor W K 1982 *Hemodynamics* (Baltimore, MD: Williams & Wilkins)

Nichols W W and O'Rourke M F 1998 McDonald's blood flow in arteries *Theoretical, Experimental and Clinical Principles* 4th edn (London: Edward Arnold)

O'Rourke M F 1982 *Arterial Function in Health and Disease* (New York: Churchill Livingstone) pp 153–69

Patel D J, Mallos A J and Fry D L 1961 Aortic mechanics in the living dog *J. Appl. Physiol.* **16** 293–9

Patel D J and Fry D L 1969 The elastic symmetry of arterial segments in dogs *Circ. Res.* **24** 1–8

Peterson L H, Jensen R E and Parnell J 1960 Mechanical properties of arteries *in vivo Circ. Res.* **8** 622–39

Roy C S 1881 The elastic properties of the arterial wall *J. Physiol. Lond.* **3** 25–162

Safar M E, Blacher J, Mourad J J and London G M 2000 Stiffness of carotid artery wall material and blood pressure in humans: application to antihypertensive therapy and stroke prevention *Stroke* **31** 782–90

Scher A M 1974 *Physiology and Biophysics* In: ed T C Ruch and H D Patton vol II (Philadelphia, PA: WB Saunders Company) ch 1, pp 1–9

Shadwick R E 1999 Mechanical design in arteries *J. Exp. Biol.* **202** 3305–13

Van Bortel L M, Struijker-Boudier H A and Safar M E 2001 Pulse pressure, arterial stiffness, and drug treatment of hypertension *Hypertension* **38** 914–21

Chapter 4

Modeling of the cardiovascular function

Edmundo I Cabrera Fischer

In this chapter both a hydraulic *in vitro* model of the cardiovascular function and animal models that mimic the function of the heart and vessels in a healthy state will be analyzed. Firstly, small vascular structures that are studied *in vitro* will be described, followed by animal models.

4.1 *In vitro* models

The Latin denomination '*in vitro*' refers to a condition in which the biological material under research is extracted from the body and placed in a controlled external environment. Cells and tissues of the specimen under study receive all the elements that allow one to maintain biological parameters within physiological ranges. Once the *in vitro* preparation is equilibrated, a biological study can be carried out in organs or tissues in which the physiological variables are similar to those found in unrestrained conscious experimental animals.

This type of research allows one to obtain results that could be extrapolated to humans, and is sometimes done directly in tissues obtained during surgical procedures. For example, human arteries are maintained in physiological conditions using an *in vitro* set-up. On the other hand, an *in vitro* preparation allows for important hemodynamic changes to occur, which in humans or animals determines homeostatic responses for a long period of time. This is the case for increases of arterial pressure higher than 100 mmHg, where uncontrolled changes of multiple biologic variables preclude any data analysis. In general terms, *in vitro* research allows one to control the physiological variables better than *in vivo* research, where a change in an organ or tissue may have an effect elsewhere.

In cardiovascular research, the use of hydraulic models of the cardiovascular system using elastic tubes has been reported for over 100 years (Von Frey 1911). A basic cardiovascular model should mimic at least the following structures:

(a) a pressure pump to model the left ventricle, with a one-way inlet and outlet valves.

doi:10.1088/2053-2563/aafb0dch4

(b) an elastic tube to represent the arterial system, connected to the pump on one end and to a resistance modulator on the other end.
(c) a wide tubular structure to connect the pump to a reservoir to represent the venous system and the left atrium.

The authors of this book have used, for the past 20 years, a perfusion line made up by a pneumatic pump that was part of an analogic artificial heart (Jarvik model 5, Kolff Medical; Salt Lake City, Utah; Colorado, USA). This device was developed to produce fluid streams at physiological pressure and flow values of the systemic territory. Moreover, adjustments were so wide that they could be used in experimental animal models using small specimens and cows weighing 200 kg (Fischer *et al* 2002) (see figure 4.1).

The outlet of the pump is connected to a perfusion line made up of polyethylene tubing and a Windkessel chamber. Since tubes are not compliant, the Windkessel chamber represents compliance in the model by increasing or decreasing the volume of air in the reservoir.

The control system of this device allows one to set the fluid flow, pressure and heart rate, and to make fine adjustments of the length of the systolic and diastolic periods of each cycle. Once the circulation begins, a stabilization period of at least 15 min is needed. Stretching rate, fluid pressure and flow levels are adjusted to best fit the values found in the observed subject. This set-up can generate transit changes that allow one to analyze dynamic adaptations of the biological structures under research, e.g. an artery segment.

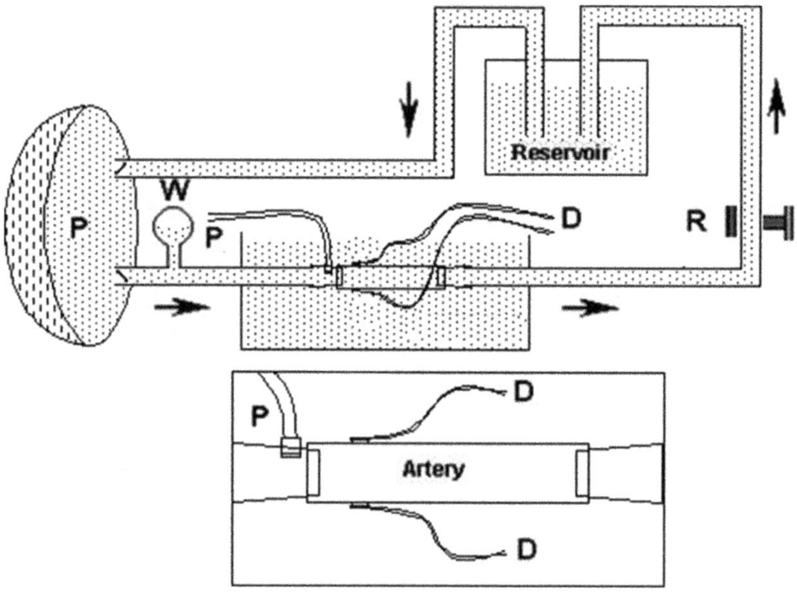

Figure 4.1. Experimental set-up to study tubular structures (vessels and prostheses). P: pneumatic pump, W: Windkessel, R: resistance regulator, D: diameter sensors, P: pressure sensor. Arrows indicate the direction of flow.

The most important attribute of the circulating loop is the ability to keep the experimental animal tissues alive. Figure 4.1 shows an artery segment that is mounted in the perfusion line. The vessel is immersed in a Tyrode's solution contained in a reservoir. The solution is kept at 37 °C with a pH of 7.4.

During an experimental session, an artery is instrumented with two ultrasonic crystals (5 MHz) that are sutured to the arterial wall in order to measure the external diameter. A solid pressure microtransducer (1200 Hz frequency response) is implanted in the vessel lumen through a collateral branch and positioned in the proximity of diameter sensors.

The ultrasonic crystals are connected to a sonomicrometer (Triton Technology Inc.) that converts the transit time of the ultrasonic signal (1580 m s^{-1}) into distance. The diameter and intraluminal pressure instantaneous signals are monitored on the screen of a computer and digitized using specific software (Fischer *et al* 2005).

The solid state pressure microtransducer (Königsberg Instruments, Inc. Pasadena, CA) is calibrated *in vitro* in saline solution at 37 °C against a pressure caliper (Xcaliber, Viggo-Spectramed, Oxnard, CA). The diameter signals are calibrated using the step calibration facility of the sonomicrometer (Triton Technology Inc., San Diego, CA).

When an artery or vein is analyzed, the biological parameters of the donor animal and the physiological state at the moment of harvesting should be considered e.g. blood pressure, flow and length of the vessel. As the isolation of an arterial segment immediately shortens it, the preservation of *in vivo* length should be respected when the specimen is mounted in the circulating loop.

When a potential artery graft (a synthetic arterial prosthesis or a preserved vein) is observed, the biomechanical properties can be analyzed using an *in vitro* set-up. In these cases, several variables should be considered besides those that characterize a healthy state. Moreover, when an arterial prosthesis is investigated, the pathological state of the receptor should be taken into account. The recipients of arterial prostheses are hardely in a healthy condition, and it is important to take into account the alterations (atherosclerosis, systemic hypertension, etc) that change both the structure and the function of the vessel.

In an experimental set-up, pressure and diameter signals can be controlled using a Utah driver control and performing fine adjustments of the resistance simulator (figure 4.1). Furthermore, any solution can be used as a working fluid in the *in vitro* set-up thus controlling variables such as osmolality, hematocrit, oxygen concentration and pharmacological dosages in order to produce changes in the active constituents of the vessel under analysis.

Data acquisition is possible for further offline processing while the physiological steady state of the vessel under study is maintained and the device ensures stability within the previously set parameters. In figure 4.2, instantaneous pressure and diameter signals are shown. In these signals, both the quantitative parameters and the waveforms are similar to those recorded during *in vivo* experimental procedures in animals.

The simultaneous *in vitro* recording of pressure and diameter signals of an artery allows the study of the relationship between these variables, both during a steady

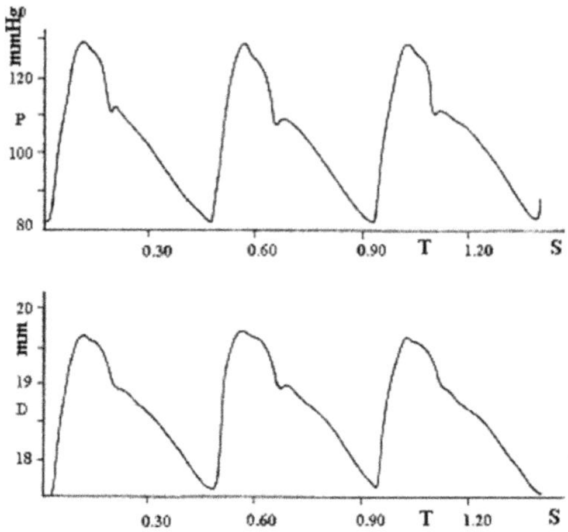

Figure 4.2. Instantaneous pressure (P) and diameter (D) signals obtained in *in vitro* conditions using a circulating loop. The vessel under study is an ovine iliac artery.

state and after changes introduced during the experimental session. The waveforms of these signals depend on the structural constituents of the vessel wall and the parameters of the intraluminal fluid. A proper analysis could distinguish between the contributions of each arterial constituent to the vessel wall dynamics. The quantification of elastic, viscous and inertial effects allows one to understand the arterial mechanical behavior.

The dynamic behavior of an artery wall can be analyzed using pressure–diameter loops, equivalent to stress–strain relationships, which allow one to detect physiological and pathological changes, as previously reported by our team (Armentano *et al* 1991, Fischer *et al* 1991a).

The pressure–diameter loop observed in figure 4.3 was obtained in an arterial segment with the following adjustments in the *in vitro* set-up: stretching rate of 100 cycles/min intravascular mean pressure of 100 mmHg and pulse pressure of 45 mmHg. Both the Utah driver machine and the resistance regulator were used to cause changes in the circuit.

The clockwise rotation of the pressure–diameter loop encloses an area of hysteresis that represents the viscous component of the arterial wall dynamics. The preservation of the hemodynamic parameters introduced in the set-up ensures an isobaric and isofrequency analysis of all possible tubular segments under research.

Furthermore, this circuit allows one to study the effects of substances such as toxins or new drugs with vascular effects.

The circulating loop described is used to evaluate the viscoelastic characteristics of vessels harvested from experimental animals or obtained during surgery in revascularization procedures (i.e. vessel replacement). Moreover, it is capable of simulating heart failure states and allows one to analyze the performance of circulatory assistance by cardiac assist devices under research (i.e. prototypes).

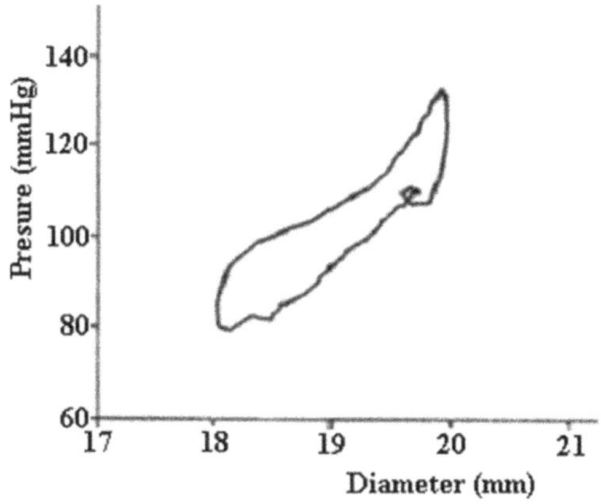

Figure 4.3. Pressure–diameter clockwise loop obtained in an *in vitro* condition using a circulation loop. The vessel under study was an ovine iliac artery.

The *in vitro* circulating loop described is usually used to study fresh human arteries of cadaveric donors. In this case, the protocol is similar to the one used for synthetic vascular prostheses.

4.2 Isolated perfused animal heart

The first arterial pressure wave recording was done in a dog in the Karl Ludwig Institute, in 1847 (Zimmer 1999). The *in vitro* study of cardiac physiology began at the end of the nineteenth century. Otto Frank and Oskar Langendorff (Frank 1895, Langendorff 1895) developed *in vitro* models in which hearts obtained from a frog and rabbits were used with specific purposes.

The Langendorff preparation is still used today as a commercial device, including several modifications. Nowadays, this technology is used to study cardiac function in mice, rats, guinea pigs and rabbits. From a technical point of view, the most important organ in the Langendorff preparation is the aorta, which is perfused to maintain a coronary flow able to provide the myocardium with the basic nutrients and oxygen, and ensuring the scavenger function that removes metabolic waste.

A basic Langendorff *in vitro* preparation has a reservoir that provides fluid to the left atrium through an inflow cannula. Once this fluid goes through the mitral valve and completes ventricular filling, a myocardial contraction takes place. In modified versions, heart rate is modulated using a pacemaker. The inflow cannula has a roller pump that allows quick changes in pressure and flow of the fluid that enters the left atrium. A physiological myocardial perfusion is achieved through an adequate fluid pressure at the aortic root; moreover, a coronary vein flow is recirculated by using a roller pump that fills the reservoir through an outflow cannula. The circuit also includes an oxygenator and a heater.

In summary, this modified version of the Langendorff preparation allows one to perform changes in preload and afterload, heart rate and characteristics of the circulating fluid. Moreover, pressure and flow sensors allow one to measure hemodynamic variables and calculate parameters such as vascular resistance, stroke work, stroke volume, among others.

4.3 *In vivo* animal model

In vivo research provides physiologic conditions to study the cardiovascular system that are closer to reality than those provided by *in vitro* investigations. On the other hand, biological variables are not usually controlled and a biological equilibrium is reached after a certain period of time during experimental sessions.

In cardiovascular research, several models have been validated in *in vivo* conditions. The next section summarizes a description of (a) open-chest surgeries in different experimental animals, (b) anesthetized intact animals, (c) chronically instrumented conscious animals, and (d) blood pressure studies in intact unanesthetized animals.

4.3.1 Cardiovascular function research during open-chest surgeries in animals

There are several techniques that allow a dynamic analysis of left ventricular function. The use of laboratory animals, under international accepted guidelines, provides scientific information of both physiological and pathological states in conscious and anesthetized animals.

Cardiac function can be evaluated using similar techniques to those described for *in vitro* research. As seen in figure 4.4, ultrasonic crystals are placed to measure left ventricular diameter and thickness of the ventricle. A balloon catheter increases left ventricular afterload and a coronary occluder decreases coronary blood flow. Pressure sensors inside the left ventricle and the aorta are able to detect changes synchronically with an ultrasonic flow sensor, and the diameter variations measured by ultrasonic crystals. Ultrasonic non-constricting perivascular flow probes can be placed around the aorta and femoral, carotid and coronary arteries (Transonic Systems Inc. Model T206, Ithaca, New York, USA).

This type of experimental research is usually done with Corriedale sheep, weighing 25–35 kg and aged 25–45 months. All animals are properly immunized and treated against intestinal parasites and skin diseases. All animals are kept for 20 days prior to surgery in a stable environment, eating a balanced diet and clinically controlled by specialized personnel. Animal care is in compliance with international regulations for laboratory animals.

All sensors are placed with the animal under general anesthesia, induced by sodium thiopental (20 mg kg^{-1}, IV), followed by endotracheal intubation and a 1% halothane as maintenance dose through a Bain tube connected to a respirator (Mark VIII, Bird Electronic Corp., Cleveland, Ohio, USA).

The above-described animal instrumentation needed to obtain biological signals is only part of the animal model. In figure 4.5, a graphic description of the elements ordinarily used in an experimental session is shown.

Cardiovascular catheterization is a useful tool that, without significant modification of systemic parameters, allows one to obtain data that are easily extrapolated to human physiology. Different techniques that use catheters have been introduced to assess hemodynamic parameters for almost a century. For example, the use of an

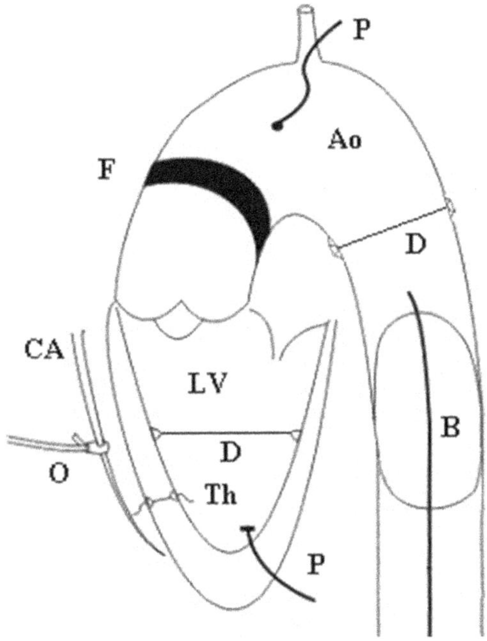

Figure 4.4. Instrumentation in an animal model to analyze left ventricle and arterial functions. Different instruments are placed in the aorta (Ao): solid pressure catheter (P), aortic diameter sensors (D), a flow sensor (F), and a balloon catheter (B), introduced through the left femoral artery. In the left ventricle (LV), blood pressure (P), internal diameter (D) and myocardial wall thickness (Th) are also measured. A pneumatic coronary occluder (O) is placed around a coronary artery (CA).

admittance catheter allows one to measure left ventricular volume and changes during systolic and diastolic periods. The admittance catheter is placed in the left ventricle along the longitudinal axis. The electrodes are in the distal 10 cm of the catheter, and allow not only left ventricular measurements but also the relative regional changes during myocardial contraction (Fischer *et al* 1988).

The Swan–Ganz catheter is another type of instrument that is used in the pulmonary circuit. This technique is done with fluoroscopy control and provides the values of right ventricular and pulmonary pressures. Furthermore, a thermistor situated in the distal portion of the catheter can generate a temporal thermic curve used to measure cardiac output (Fischer *et al* 2009).

Periodic instantaneous signals allow on-line monitoring of the cardiac cycle in steady and transient states: in healthy animals, after the induction of a pathological change and during therapeutic interventions. In figure 4.6, five calibrated signals are displayed on the screen of a computer. Signal monitoring allows the operator to select the appropriate time to initiate mechanical maneuvers allowing accurate records and repetition if required.

Data acquisition allows one to record not only static or dynamic signals from an animal model, but also those originated in experimental devices. That is the case of electrical stimuli that contract skeletal muscle. In figure 4.7, the effect of the electrostimulation of skeletal muscle using an external device is shown. In this

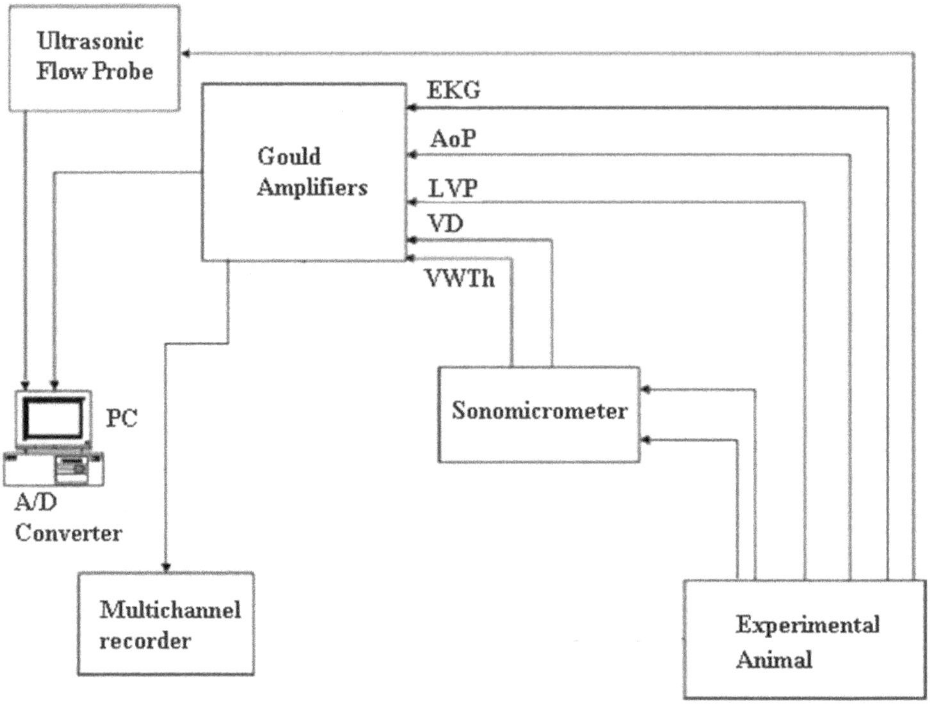

Figure 4.5. Block diagram showing the recorded biological signals. The analogic signal of the experimental animal end as digitized data in the hard disc of a computer (PC). EKG: electrocardiogram, AoP: aortic pressure, LVP: left ventricular pressure, VD: ventricular diameter, VWTh: ventricular wall thickness.

experimental session, the heart was wrapped with a muscle that was stimulated using a pulse amplitude of 5 V, pulse width of 210 μs, burst rate of 30 Hz and burst duration 185 ms (depending on heart rate). This stimulus was synchronized with the cardiac cycle to reproduce the contraction during the natural systole and avoiding the diastolic period. The consequence of this skeletal muscle stimulation during myocardial contraction is an increase of left intraventricular systolic pressure and a decrease of pressure during the early filling period.

The origin of the negative pressure developed in the early diastolic period in the assisted left ventricle has been explained in chapter 2, and is observed when the remaining blood volume after myocardial contraction is further decreased. Thus, increases in the left ventricular emptying, usually determined by the augmentation of myocardial contractility, determine negative pressures during the left ventricular relaxation period (Fischer *et al* 1991b, 2005). Negative left ventricular pressure is an interesting subject that was extensively studied many years ago by Brecher, Bloom, Nikolic and Fowler. These authors investigated the diastolic left ventricular function using *in vitro* and *in vivo* experimental animal models (Brecher 1956, Bloom and Ferris 1956, Fowler *et al* 1957).

The intrinsic mechanism that determines these negative pressures in the left ventricle during the early diastolic period are related to the passive elastic properties

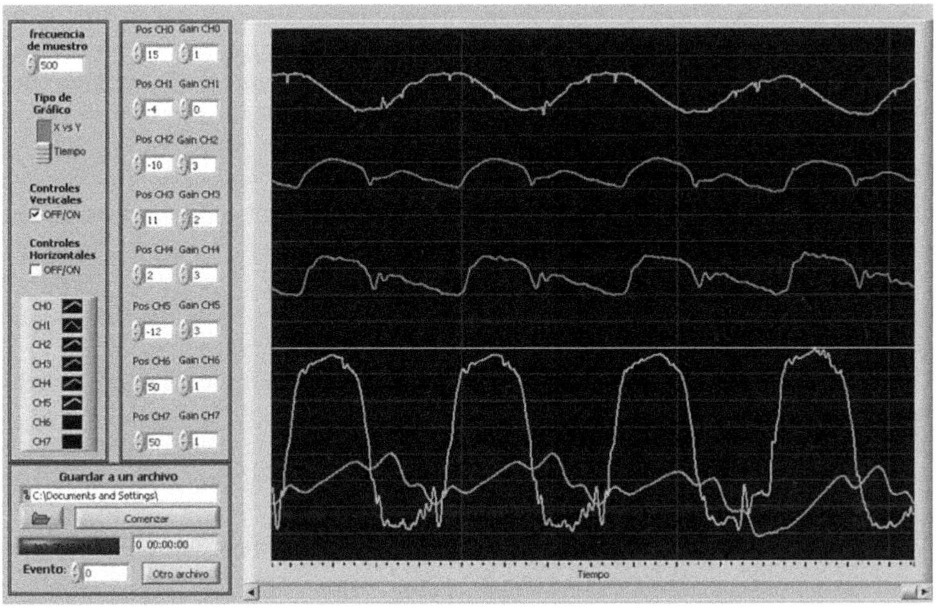

Figure 4.6. Simultaneous monitoring of cardiovascular signals. From top to bottom: ventricular diameter, aortic diameter, aortic pressure measured using a fluid-filled catheter, left ventricular pressure and left ventricular wall thickness.

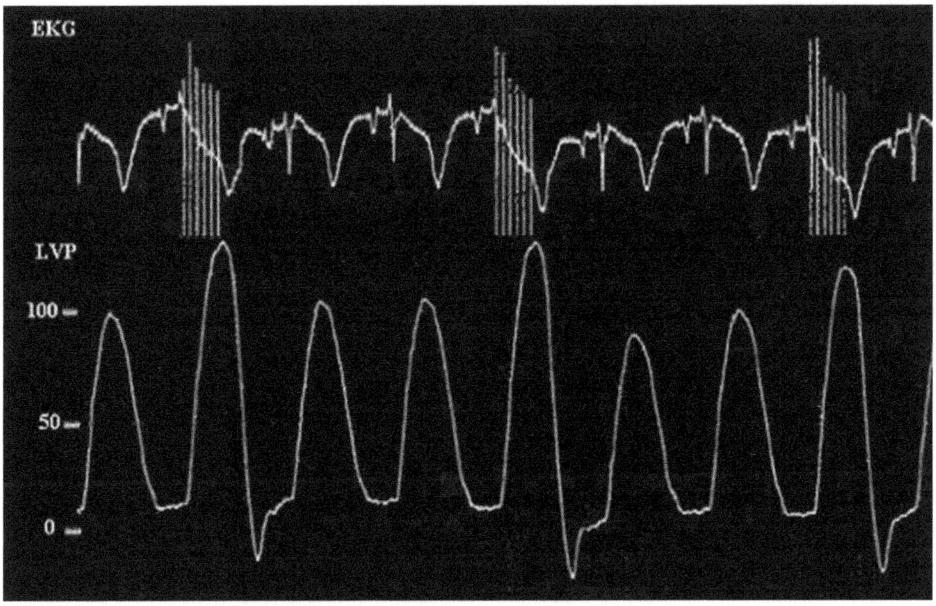

Figure 4.7. Effects of the stimulation of the latissimus dorsi muscle flaps wrapping the heart, obtained in an experimental animal. Upper panel: electrical stimulation obtained with pulse trains 1:3 on the electrocardiogram signal (EKG). Lower panel: left ventricular pressure (LVP) showing negative values simultaneously with the electrical stimulation.

of the ventricular wall and this particular phenomenon was observed for the first time in 1930 (Katz 1930). Detection of left ventricular negative pressures during experimental sessions using an animal model is usually surprising. Frequently, these unusual findings are attributed to operator failure, due to calibration mistakes. In this case, a new calibration of pressure sensor is obligatory to analyze the physiological condition of left ventricular filling.

Sometimes, the use of left ventricular assistance devices, also determines undesirable negative pressures during the diastolic period. Moreover, in pathological states such as mitral stenosis, failure in left ventricular filling determines significant decreases in diastolic left ventricular pressure. In these cases, negative end diastolic left ventricular pressures have been reported (Sabbah *et al* 1980).

The open-chest animal model is useful when there are many biological variables to record, several of which must be modified to emulate physiological or pathological states. Currently, records are performed before and after induced changes allowing one to compare an initial state (control state) with those obtained afterwards during the experimental session.

All of the above-described experiments were in agreement with the National Institute of Health Guidelines for the care and use of laboratory animals (NIH Publication No. 85-23, revised 1996).

4.3.2 Cardiovascular function research in intact anesthetized animals

Sometimes experimental research is carried out in chronically instrumented anesthetized animals. For example, when pressure, flow and/or diameter sensors are implanted in an experimental animal and a catheter must be introduced in the circulatory system during the experimental session.

Figure 4.8 shows a change in arterial pressure in an anesthetized chronically instrumented animal. This change is produced by the inflation of a balloon catheter introduced in the descending aorta through the left femoral artery. Due to ethical recommendations, this procedure is not done in conscious laboratory animals. This

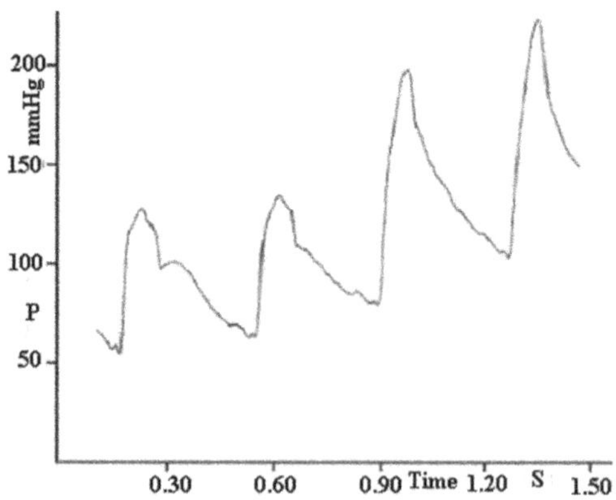

Figure 4.8. Aortic pressure signal (P) recorded along four cardiac cycles in an experimental animal in which the first beat is obtained in basal state and the following during continuous afterload increases obtained by inflating a catheter balloon in the descending aorta.

animal model is useful when there are many biological variables to record and maneuvers that involve the use of acute invasive techniques are carried out.

4.3.3 Chronically instrumented conscious animals

In experimental research that involves the recording of multiple signals in conscious animals weighing 30 kg, it is necessary to consider several aspects that are described as follows.

Firstly, signal sensors should be implanted and tunneled to emerge from the interscapular space of the animal. This is the case of pressure, diameter and flow sensors. As these sensors may become uncomfortable for the animal it is important to maintain cables and wires far from any possible external contact. Similar criteria are considered for catheters, electrodes and maneuver devices.

Secondly, during animal instrumentation surgery, anesthesia is similar to acute experimentation, but it is performed under strict sterile conditions. Furthermore, all surgical procedures must guarantee a complete recovery of vital functions. In the case of the closure of a thoracotomy, the negative intrapleural pressures and the complete closure of the thoracic cage must be ensured.

Thirdly, during the recovery period, which usually takes several days, antibiotic preventive administration is indicated under veterinary supervision. Moreover, all catheters must be flushed daily using heparinized saline solutions. Basically, implanted signal sensors are the same as those used in open-chest animal models.

Animal experimentation is performed after a recovery period, usually one week after surgery, ensuring the animal is active, eating well and free of any apparent signs of disease. The animal is conscious and free of sedative drugs, lying quietly on one side during the experimental session.

In figure 4.9, pressure and diameter signals show a hypertensive, progressive state obtained through administration of angiotensin. Drugs are continuously

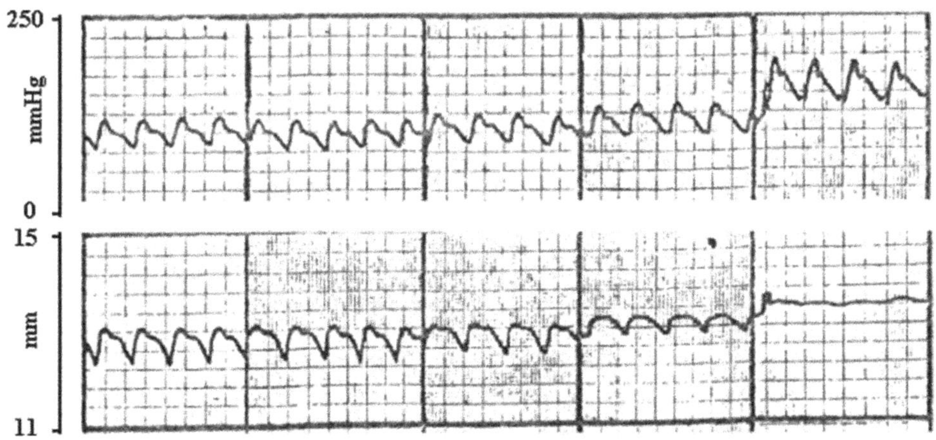

Figure 4.9. Aortic pressure (upper panel) and diameter (lower panel) signals recorded in basal state (left) and during angiotensin administration i.v. in four incremental steps of 1.25, 2.50, 5 and 10 μg min^{-1}. As seen, there is a hypertensive response, while diameter augmentation is accompanied by a loss of pulsatility.

administered using an intravenous catheter placed in a central vein during the instrumentation surgery, which is daily flushed.

As only one chemical substance is administered each time, the pure effect of the drug (e.g. Angiotensin) is ensured.

4.3.4 Blood pressure research in intact unanesthetized animals

The body has several mechanisms to increase or decrease systemic arterial pressure keeping physiological values according to daily activities. One of these mechanisms belongs to the nervous system and includes arterial baroreceptors located in specific areas of the arterial tree.

Arterial baroreceptors and neural circuits provide a quick control of arterial pressure, which is modulated continuously along human life. Baroreceptor denervation is a method to study the physiological role of this important control system. The mentioned denervation is performed through an *in vivo* section of the carotid sinus and aortic nerves, which is usually followed by an arterial pressure increase.

Since changes in arterial pressure post baroreceptor denervation should be monitored for periods of 12 h an appropriate animal instrumentation is needed. Next, an animal model using cats will be described.

Under general anesthesia (ketamine 50 mg^{-1} kg^{-1} i.m.) the sino-aortic nerves are sectioned after a midline neck incision. A fine dissection is performed and tissues situated between the internal and external carotid arteries are eliminated. Then, common carotid arteries are dissected and all sympathetic and parasympathetic nerves are cut.

Blood pressure is measured in this animal model through a catheter positioned in the abdominal aorta through a femoral artery. This catheter is tunneled subcutaneously to emerge at the back of the animal in the inter scapulae space, and secured with sutures.

Continuous recordings of arterial blood pressure are repeated for periods of 12 h while the animal remains conscious, unsedated and lying quietly in a plexiglass box (Ramirez *et al* 1985).

4.4 *Ex vivo* animal model

In some experimental sessions that use animal models it is necessary to maintain certain hemodynamic parameters within basal ranges but also carry out maneuvers that produce great change in other physiological variables. This is the case of changes of arterial blood pressure higher than 100 mmHg. This produces a hemodynamic compensation that reaches an equilibrium after a certain period of time. Moreover, once the mentioned hypertensive maneuver is over, recovering the basal state can take up to an hour. Certain studies may involve cyclical maneuvers that may interrupt the recovery periods.

All of the above-described difficulties can be solved using *ex vivo* animal models, in which abrupt changes of a certain variable determine only slight biologic compensations. In the following paragraphs an *ex vivo* experimental procedure used in our animal laboratory will be described.

As the arterial wall dynamic responds to abrupt increases of intraluminal blood pressure by changing its viscoelastic properties, we developed an animal model in which the right femoral artery was gently dissected. An arterial segment of 10 cm and its collateral branches were dissected in anesthetized Corriedale sheep. The experiments were performed in accordance with the National Institutes of Health Guidelines for the care and use of laboratory animals (NIH Publication No. 85-23, revised 1996).

Two tourniquets were placed at both ends of the arterial segment and a pressure transducer was inserted in the intraluminal space through a collateral branch using a cannula. A polyvinyl catheter was inserted in the artery using a similar technique to inject or withdraw fluids into or from the vessel under analysis. The instrumentation was completed by fixing two ultrasonic micro-crystals that measure the external arterial diameter. During the experimental session, pressure and diameter were measured using similar techniques to *in vitro* and *in vivo* animal models (see figure 4.10).

Using the described instrumentation and keeping the animal anesthetized, changes in intraluminal pressure were obtained after isolation of the arterial segment using the vascular tourniquets, inflating the vessel with a physiologic solution. The arterial segment had been previously emptied of blood.

After each transient change in the isolated arterial segments, blood flow was recovered in order to establish a normal perfusion of the vessel wall.

This technique allows one to perform changes in biological parameters similar to those obtained in *in vitro* conditions while preserving the natural *in vivo* environment (Chau *et al* 1992).

4.5 Steady and transient states

Cardiovascular signals can be monitored on the screen of a computer, before and after data digitalization. Biological signals recorded in a cardiovascular system free of mechanical and/or pharmacological maneuvers show the real state of physiologic variables. During this condition the hemodynamic parameters remain unchanged.

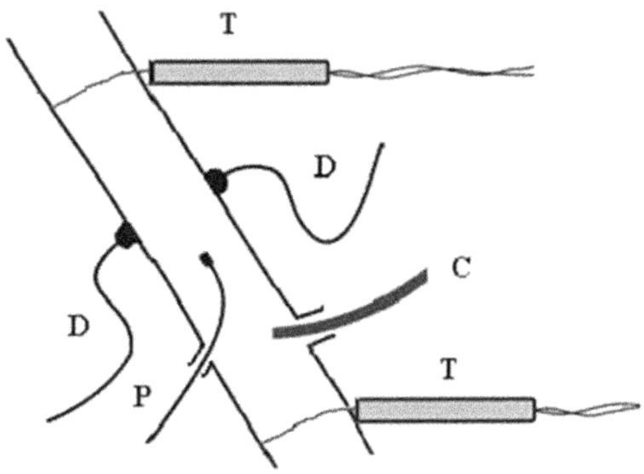

Figure 4.10. Arterial pressure (P) and diameter (D) signals are recorded using sensors after isolating the vessels using tourniquets (T). Changes are produced by fluid infusion through a catheter (C) placed in an arterial branch.

An equilibrium state can also be reached during a continuous infusion of a certain drug with vascular smooth muscle effects. This state is also called 'steady state', and equilibrium is reached after the complete pharmacological effect is obtained, and remains while the drug is infused.

In the above-described situations, a biological signal in steady state remains unchangeable in a range that expresses the equilibrium that exists in both structures and the recorded variables. An example is the aortic pressure shown in figure 4.11, where a low speed recording shows only respiratory modulation along the analyzed period.

In the same experimental animal, the basal state is recorded and then compared to transient states after induced changes. When transient states stabilize, another steady condition is reached; even after an induced variation of the signals. Therefore, several 'steady states' can be recorded: in a basal condition and after induced changes (see figure 4.12).

Instantaneous pressure–diameter loops can be obtained in steady state from the data shown in figure 4.12. In figure 4.13, a clockwise hysteresis loop obtained from an experimental animal is shown.

Some studies require rapid changes of cardiovascular variables in order to study the physiological response to stimuli. In this case, changes correspond to physiological adaptation of the cardiovascular system and not necessarily to pathological variations due to structural damage.

This type of signal analysis is currently employed in studies of the smooth muscle response to quick changes that determined electrochemical adaptation along a time that should be measured in milliseconds. Here, it is important to remember that a cardiac cycle is completed in 1000 ms in a human under study that is in the inferior limit of normality: 60 beats/minute.

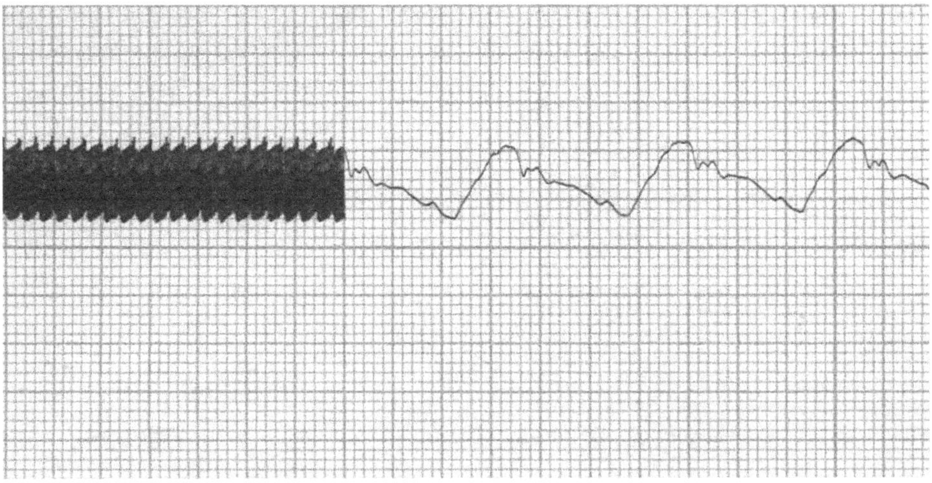

Figure 4.11. Aortic pressure temporal signal at a low recording speed (left) and at a high recording speed (right). The high-speed recording allows one to see the pressure waveform, whereas at a low speed only the respiratory modulation is observed as a periodic variation.

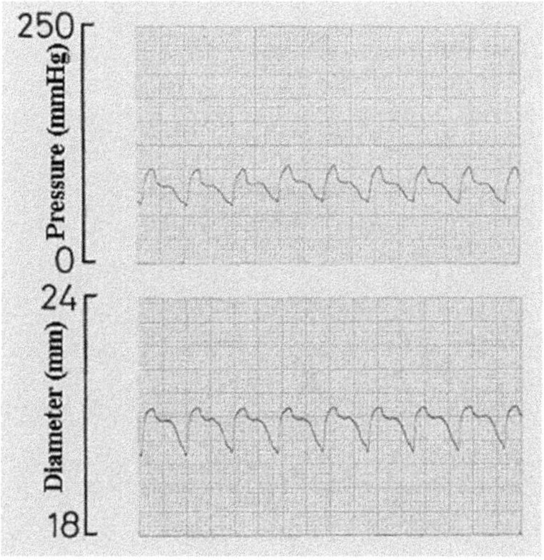

Figure 4.12. Aortic pressure and diameter signals obtained in steady state in an experimental animal. Note the similarity of signals among cardiac cycles along the time recording.

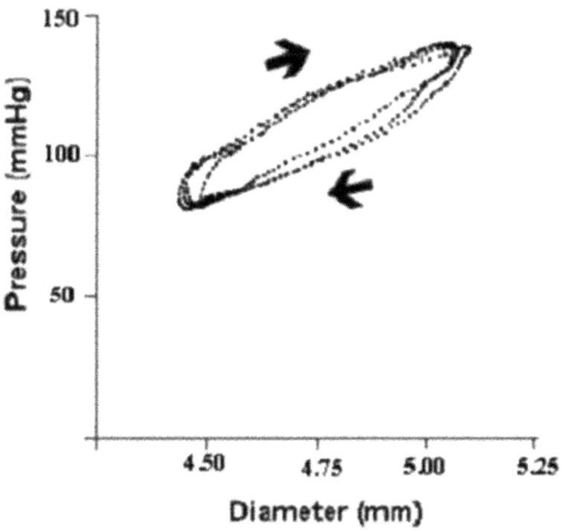

Figure 4.13. Aortic pressure and a diameter hysteresis loop obtained in steady state from an experimental animal.

The signal acquisitions in transient states are fundamental in specific physiological studies. In figure 4.14, changes in aortic pressure and diameter relationship are produced in an experimental animal. As seen, there is a pressure–diameter loop in a basal position (bold line) and two types of changes are induced: (a) decreases in terms of arterial pressure and diameter through inflation of a cuff in the inferior cava vein, and (b) arterial pressure and diameter increases through the injection of an angiotensin bolus of 0.1 μg kg^{-1}.

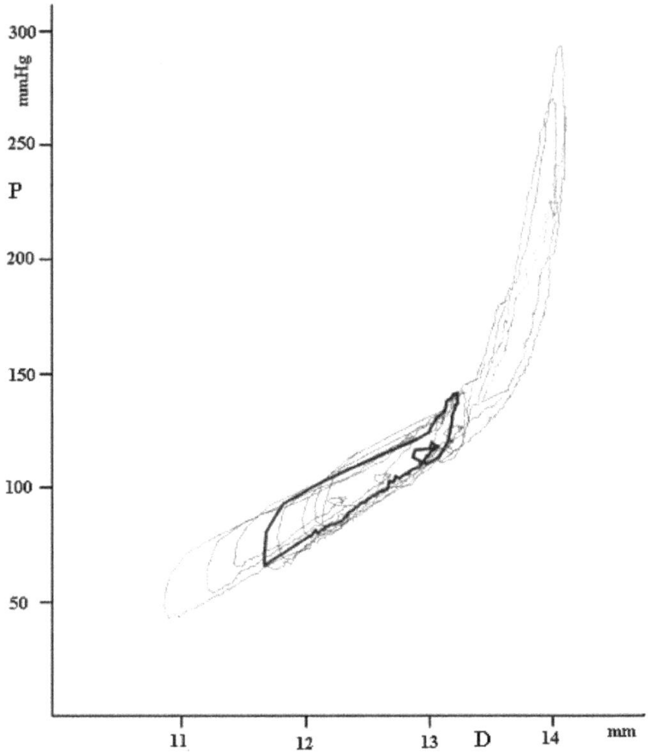

Figure 4.14. Pressure (P) and diameter (D) values allow one to obtain a continuous loop in basal state (bold line) and after maneuvers, done to characterize the arterial wall dynamic behavior along a wide range of changes.

A continuous loop can be observed in figure 4.14, since arterial pressure and diameter change continuously due to the maneuvers: towards lower values during physical occlusions and towards higher values during drug administration (Fischer *et al* 1991a).

4.6 Final comments

The use of *in vitro* studies and animal models contributes to human medicine given the experimental basis to clinical research and contributing to the safety of new technologies used to correct changes provoked by diseases that frequently affect large populations (Bianco *et al* 2013).

In the following chapter, animal models similar to those summarized above are described in research aimed to characterize pathological states.

References

Armentano R L, Levenson J, Barra J G, Fischer E I, Breitbart G J, Pichel R H and Simon A 1991 Assessment of elastin and collagen contribution to aortic elasticity in conscious dogs *Am. J. Physiol.* **260** H1870–7

Bianco R W, Wasiluk K R, Voight J M, Lahti M T, Rivard A L and Gallegos R P 2013 Large animal models in cardiac and vascular biomaterials research and assessment Chapter II.3.7 *Biomaterial Science* 3rd edn (Canada: Academic)

Bloom W L and Ferris E B 1956 Negative ventricular diastolic pressure in beating heart studied *in vitro* and *in vivo Proc. Soc. Med. Biol.* **93** 451–4

Brecher G A 1956 Experimental evidence of ventricular diastolic suction *Circ. Res.* **4** 513–8

Chau N P, Simon A, Vilar J, Fischer E I C, Pithois-Merli I and Levenson J 1992 Active and passive effects of antihypertensive drugs on large artery diameter and elasticity in human essential hypertension *J. Cardiovascular Pharmacol.* **19** 78–85

Fischer E I, Bia D, Zócalo Y and Armentano R L 2009 Smooth muscle-dependent changes in aortic wall dynamics during intra-aortic counterpulsation in an animal model of acute heart failure *Int. J. Artif. Organs* **32** 354–61

Fischer E I, Spinelli J C, Willshaw P, Crottogini A J, de Forteza E, Clavin O E, Valentinuzzi M E and Pichel R H 1988 Detection of left ventricular regional myocardial ischaemia in dogs by intraventricular conductance catheter *Cardiovasc. Res.* **22** 185–92

Fischer E I C, Armentano R L, Levenson J, Barra J, Morales M C, Breitbart G, Pichel R and Simon A 1991a Paradoxically decreased aortic wall stiffness in response to Vitamin D3-induced calcinosis. A biphasic analysis of segmental elastic properties in conscious dogs *Circ. Res.* **68** 1549–59

Fischer E I C, Armentano R L, Pessana F M, Graf S, Romero L, Christen A I, Simon A and Levenson J 2002 Endothelium-dependent arterial wall tone elasticity modulated by blood viscosity *Am. J. Physiol. Heart. Circ. Physiol.* **282** H389–94

Fischer E I C, Bia D, Cassanello G L, Zócalo Y, Crawford E V, Casas R F and Armentano R L 2005 Reduced elastic mismatch achieved by interposing vein cuff in expanded polytetrafluoroethylene femoral bypass decreases intimal hyperplasia *Artif. Organs* **29** 122–30

Fischer E I C, Chachques J C, Garcia A, de Fortezza E, Haab F, Cron C and Carpentier A 1991b Effect of cardiomyoplasty on left ventricular diastolic function *BAM* **1** 253–8

Fowler N O, Bloom W L and Ferris E B 1957 Systolic and diastolic pressure relationships in the isolated rat heart *Circ. Res.* **5** 485–8

Frank O 1895 Zur Dynamik des Herzmuskels *Z. Biol.* **32** 370–437

Katz L N 1930 The role played by the ventricular relaxation process in filling the ventricle *Am. J. Physiol.* **95** 542–53

Langendorff O 1895 Untersuchungen am Überlebenden Saugetierherzen *Pflügers Arch. Ges. Physiol. Mensch. Tiere.* **61** 291–332

Ramirez A J, Bertinieri G, Belli L, Cavallazzi A, Di Rienzo M, Pedotti A and Mancia G 1985 Reflex control of blood pressure and heart rate by arterial baroreceptors and by cardiopulmonary receptors in the unanaesthetized cat *J. Hypertens.* **3** 327–35

Sabbah H N, Anbe D T and Stein P D 1980 Negative intraventricular diastolic pressure in patients with mitral stenosis: evidence of left ventricular diastolic suction *Am. J. Cardiol.* **45** 562–6

Von Frey M 1911 Die Arbeit des Herzens *Vorlesungen über Physiologie* ed M von Frey (Berlin, Germany: Springer)

Zimmer H G 1999 The contribution of Carl Ludwig to cardiology *Can. J. Cardiol.* **15** 323–9

Chapter 5

Modeling of cardiovascular dysfunction

Edmundo I Cabrera Fischer

The study of physiology in healthy animals provides data that allows one to understand the normal mechanisms involved in the biological activities of humans in the basal state and during physiological changes induced by stimulus, such as muscular exercise, infusion of human hormones or changes in environmental parameters (e.g. oxygen concentration, temperature, etc). However, human medicine aims to restore a lost function and to control pathologies that modify physiologic parameters. Consequently, in cardiology, it is necessary to demonstrate the effectiveness of a drug or device using animal models with cardiovascular alterations like those observed in human beings in heart failure. In this chapter, animal models of heart dysfunction and changes produced by abnormalities determined by vessel disease will be described.

5.1 Characteristics of human cardiovascular failure

In humans, heart failure is a syndrome that is characterized by structural and functional changes that involve cardiac and vascular tissues, accompanied by neurohormonal compensatory mechanisms. Cardiac failure has been defined as the last stage of most cardiac diseases. However, some cardiac diseases are successfully treated. On the other hand, there are some changes, such as myocardial hypertrophy, that may be found in healthy and in pathological states. Consequently, it is necessary to model a considerable number of diseases that are currently observed in clinical practice, including minor alterations of the cardiovascular system and heart failure refractory to medical treatment (see table 5.1).

Patients in the end-stage of heart failure have an increased end-diastolic left ventricular pressure, decreased systemic blood pressure, low cardiac output, increased peripheral vascular resistance, elevated right atrial pressure and increased pulmonary vascular resistance. Regardless of the cause of the cardiac failure, most of the above-mentioned characteristics are the response of the control system of cardiovascular structures. In fact, neurohormonal changes are triggered by the hemodynamic decline

doi:10.1088/2053-2563/aafb0dch5

Table 5.1. Types of cardiovascular diseases.

Heart	Vessels
Coronary disease	Atherosclerosis
Cardiac arrhythmias	Arteriosclerosis
Cardiomyopathies	Aortic dissection
Congenital defects	Arteritis
Heart valve disease	Arterial embolism
Hypertensive heart disease	Venous thrombosis
Inflammatory cardiac disease	
Pericardial disease	
Rheumatic cardiac disease	

and are characterized by the increase of sympathetic activity, the activation of the renin–angiotensin system and the stimulation of the antidiuretic hormone. Unfortunately, the increase of the systemic vascular resistance and the decrease of diuresis help to maintain the initial heart failure condition (Hasenfuss 1998).

As mentioned above, the initial heart failure involves changes that modify both the control system and the cardiovascular structures. As the circulatory system is, in fact, a circle in which elements are connected in series, damage in one of them determines changes in elements up or downstream. For example, left ventricular failure produces changes in the pressure in the pulmonary vein and the resistance in systemic arteries. These changes, if not treated, end in right ventricular failure.

Damage in cardiac structures is the main factor that leads to heart failure, and is accompanied by changes in the vessels of the systemic and pulmonary circuits. However, some vascular diseases lead to heart failure, e.g. non-controlled systemic hypertension. The main characteristics of isolated vascular dysfunction are the ischemic involvement of the organs which perfuse the damaged artery.

Blood perfusion to a specific territory depends on arterial flow that is determined by the integrity of the arterial wall. Arterial stenosis higher than 70% of vessel diameter determines significant changes in organ blood perfusion and, consequently, in the functioning of the compromised tissues. The etiology of lumen decrease is mainly due to atherosclerosis and other pathologies such as arterial wall dissection, arteritis and embolic episodes, among others (see table 5.1).

Successful circulatory left ventricular assistance (i.e. using support devices) may uncover right cardiac failure symptoms due to myocardial damage that were previously hidden by the low cardiac output syndrome.

5.2 Anatomy and physiology of animals used to model human cardiovascular diseases

There are many animal models of cardiovascular dysfunction that are currently used in cardiovascular disease research. Specialized literature has classified them according to animal size. Usually, two sizes are considered: small (rats, hamsters, rabbits) and large (ovine, bovine and porcine species). Many animal species are used to model the cardiovascular system, producing cardiac function changes and/or vascular dysfunction (Yarbrough and Spinale 2003). Some species, such as dogs, were largely used in cardiovascular research and mentioned frequently in specialized literature. However, this animal model has been discontinued after significant contributions to medicine (Bianco *et al* 2013).

As in many areas of medicine, the ideal animal model is unachievable. Some important factors should be considered when selecting an animal species for research purposes. An animal to be used in experimental research must be easy to obtain, inexpensive, docile, its food easily available, and the extrapolation of results to humans should be previously validated. Furthermore, the time necessary to develop the cardiovascular dysfunction that mimics the natural disease should not be extremely long. There are many currently validated animal models to choose from, depending on the above-mentioned factors (see table 5.2).

The extrapolation of results obtained in animal models has certain limitations, and it is important to know the anatomic and physiological differences. For example, a well-known animal model of myocardial ischemia is the coronary ligation in dogs. This model has been previously validated, but it is important to consider that dogs have coronary collateral circulation that limits the infarct size and the heart failure relevance (Hongo *et al* 1997).

The rat is an animal model that is widely used to study cardiovascular diseases. The availability of subjects is usually ensured; however, an initial mortality of 50% is observed when studying myocardial infarction. This undesirable characteristic should be considered in the research project (Muders and Elsner 2000).

For technical reasons, the anatomic differences between animals and humans must be considered. For example, humans have three aortic-arch branches: the brachiocephalic trunk, the left common carotid artery and the subclavian arteries. These arteries perfuse the upper limbs, neck and head. In dogs, the aortic arch only has two branches, and sheep only have one branch that bifurcates downstream into the subclavian and common carotid arteries.

Table 5.2. Animals used in cardiovascular research.

Large	Small
Baboon	Chicken
Bovine	Ferret
Cat	Frog
Dog	Guinea pig
Goat	Hamster
Ovine species	Mouse
Swine species	Rabbit
	Rat
	Turkey

Mathematical modeling of cardiac dysfunction is a modality in which a validation process is required. For example, there are mathematical models that have analyzed the impact of heart failure on experimentally identified myocyte components, but their integration into a ventricular model that is part of a multiscale circulatory approach has not been properly attempted. In this case, experimental research has been carried out to demonstrate that a new model may be useful to predict the contractile and hemodynamic response to myocardial cell changes (Lascano *et al* 2018).

Small animals, such as rats and mice have been useful to understand molecular and cellular mechanisms of cardiovascular physiology; however, there are major differences with human beings. These are particularly significant when heart rate, myocardial oxygen consumption or stem cells' characteristics are analyzed. Consequently, the use of large animals is an alternative to develop new therapies, including surgical and endoluminal procedures (Dixon and Spinale 2009).

5.3 Models of cardiac disease

The most considerable heart diseases involve left ventricular function. They may originate in extra-cardiac territories (e.g. endotoxic shock) or in constitutive structures (e.g. valves, interventricular septum, ventricles, auricles, conduction system, coronary arteries and congenital heart defects). A very simple classification takes into account the timing in the developing process that, after acute cardiac damage, progresses to cure, death or chronicity.

5.3.1 Myocardial ischemia

One of the oldest animal models of myocardial injury is the complete ligation of the coronary arteries. This modality has been used in multiple animal models. Initially used to examine the evolution of acute myocardial infarction, it was later used as an experimental model to study the progression of left ventricular dysfunction (Abarbanell *et al* 2010).

A canine model of 'regional' and 'global' coronary ischemia has been used to analyze the ability of a conductance catheter to detect acute left ventricular dysfunction (Fischer *et al* 1988). This animal model of reversible myocardial ischemia used a pneumatic cuff occluder placed in the left anterior descending coronary artery to obtain a small ischemic area. Another cuff occluder was placed in the origin of the circumflex coronary artery to obtain a larger ischemic myocardial mass. In both cases, reversible ischemia was attained through the inflation of occluders.

Although several of the findings regarding ischemia and myocardial infarction have been achieved using dogs, this animal has a remarkable collateral coronary circulation. Consequently, this type of animal experimentation is currently mostly done in small animals like rats (Hodsman *et al* 1988), pigs (Barandon *et al* 2010) and sheep (Rademaker *et al* 2002). Large animal models are closer to the ideal to evaluate myocardial ischemia because of their similarities to human anatomy and physiology. Pig models are similar to humans not only in the gross anatomy of the heart, but also in the distribution of coronary arteries and the poor collateral circulation. Thus, the ability to develop a predictable ischemic necrotic area in size and location, has made pig models the most suitable to study ischemia, infarction and ventricular remodeling. Limitations of the myocardial ischemia pig model are: its high predisposition to arrhythmias, the need for careful control of the airway and ventilation, strict control of electrolyte imbalances and the recommendation to administrate antiarrhythmic drugs (Mukherjee *et al* 2003).

Because of their similarity with human coronary irrigation, sheep are the second species of choice to study congestive heart failure of ischemic etiology (Yarbrough and Spinale 2003, Monnet and Chachques 2005). The model of coronary artery ligation in sheep has enabled the study of ventricular remodeling after infarction, necrotic quantification of the involved territory and the sequence of development of mitral regurgitation in the context of infarction. It has been estimated that the necrotic myocardial mass in a sheep model, with ligation of the first and second diagonal branch of the left anterior descending artery, induced 23.9% of necrotic tissues (Moainie *et al* 2002). The sheep model of myocardial ischemia is also very useful for studying the relationship between neurohormonal activation and left ventricular dysfunction; furthermore, studies using endovascular devices found this animal to be an appropriate model (Yarbrough and Spinale 2003, Monnet and Chachques 2005, Bianco *et al* 2013).

In figure 5.1, a model of right ventricular ischemia used in the laboratory of the authors is reproduced. In this model, myocardial injury and right ventricular enlargement is obtained through a complete ligation of the right coronary artery.

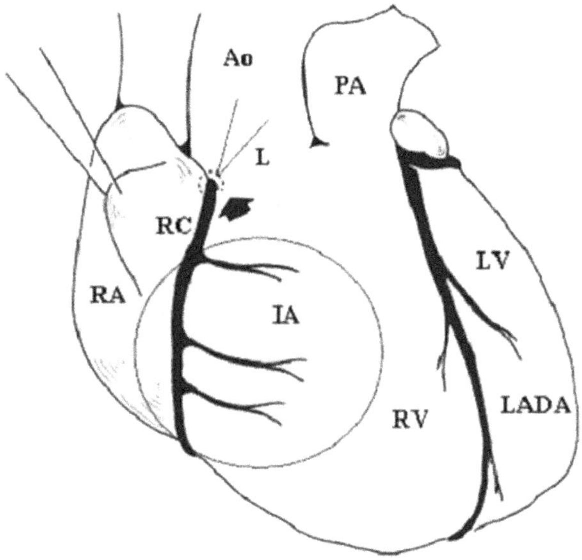

Figure 5.1. Ligation (L) of the right coronary artery (RC) at its origin (arrow). The ischemic risk area (IA) is encircled and involves the free wall of the right ventricle (RV). Ao: aorta, LV: left ventricle, LADA: left anterior descending coronary artery, RA: right atrium and PA: pulmonary artery.

5.3.2 Interventricular communication

Interventricular communication is a cardiac disease in which there exists a passage of blood from the left to the right ventricle, usually due to a congenital defect and seldom to interventricular septum myocardial infarct. In figure 5.2, a model used in the laboratory of the authors is reproduced.

This surgical alternative to generate heart disease is characterized by volume overload in the right cavities, as previously reported (Matsuoka *et al* 1986). The technique described in figure 5.2 is a modification of that reported by Matsuoka *et al* and used in the laboratory of the authors. The surgical technique is as follows: after a left lateral thoracotomy of an experimental animal (dog, sheep or swine), a purse-string suture is performed in the free wall of the right ventricle, and a cylindrical cutter is introduced until the interventricular septum is reached (figure 5.2). During this maneuver the proximal end of the cylindrical cutter is obstructed by the operator using a finger. Peri-cutter bleeding is avoided by maintaining an appropriate tension in the purse-string suture during the introduction of the cutter. After interventricular septal contact, an aspirator is connected to the cylindrical cutter, as seen in figure 5.2. Following, a cylindrical myocardial mass is excised by rotating the cutter and maintaining a soft aspiration to avoid embolic accidents.

When ventricles are communicated, the cylindrical cutter is removed and the right ventricular wall is sutured. The volume overload causes changes in the function and

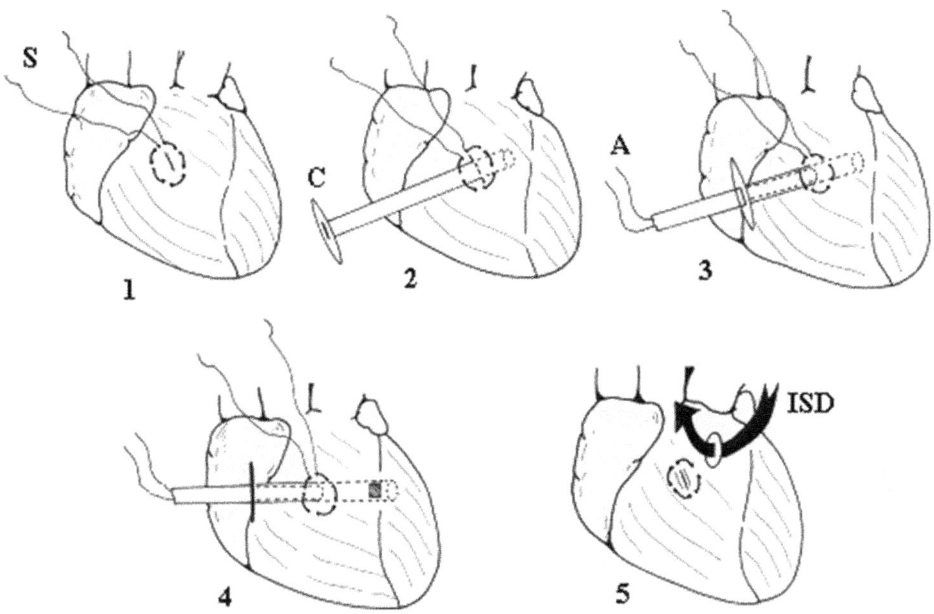

Figure 5.2. Flow-chart description of the model of an interventricular septal defect. (1) a purse-string is made in the right ventricular free wall, (2) a cylindrical cutter is inserted through an incision, (3) the cylindrical tube reaches the interventricular septum and an aspirator is connected to the tube, (4) the aspirator suctions while a piece of septal myocardium is removed, (5) the cylindrical cutter is removed and the right ventricle is sutured. Blood from the left ventricle is now passing to the right chamber (ISD).

geometry of myocytes, leading to alterations in ventricular geometry and function associated with intense neurohormonal activation. In specialized literature, similar animal models and a technique to communicate through the inter-atrial septum have been reported (Shiota *et al* 1999).

5.3.3 Cardiac arrhythmias

Animal models of cardiac arrhythmias are needed before the use antiarrhythmic drugs and catheter ablative[1] techniques in humans. Although *in vivo* and *in vitro* models have been used for over a century, they have become particularly frequent in the last few decades (Loomis and Krop 1955, Wang *et al* 1992). Moreover, validated models of cardiac arrhythmias allow one to understand the intrinsic mechanisms by which ventricular and supraventricular electrical disturbances are originated.

Animal models of induced cardiac arrhythmias have been developed in dogs, rabbits, pigs, rats, cats, goats, mice and monkeys. Arrhythmias were induced by acetylcholine administration, vagal stimulation, methacholine chloride application, aconitine administration, atrial enlargement, experimental pericarditis, atrial ischemia and rapid atrial pacing. In all cases, the purpose is to resemble the characteristics observed in clinical practice, in order to determine possible arrhythmogenic foci and to develop diagnostic and therapeutic alternatives (Schoels *et al* 1991, Stengl 2010).

Pathological conditions reproduced in animals are: atrial flutter, atrial fibrillation, Wolf–Parkinson–White syndrome, ventricular fibrillation, atrio-ventricular block, ventricular arrhythmias, long QT syndrome, among others (Hasenfuss 1998, Milan and MacRae 2005).

5.4 Models of vascular disease

Vascular disease involves arteries, veins or lymphatic vessels. There are associative diseases that involve both arteries and veins. Arterial obstructions are produced by atherosclerotic processes and less frequently by embolic episodes or congenital diseases. It is evident that the obstruction of an artery is followed by ischemia of the perfused tissues, and may determine their infarction. However, there are systemic diseases determined by the dysfunction of an ischemic organ that complicate the analysis. Furthermore, the combinations of arterial and venous abnormalities, such as arteriovenous fistulas, are also a source of heart dysfunction.

5.4.1 Renal hypertension

Many authors have developed modified animal models from the initial research on renovascular systemic hypertension reported by Goldblatt in the early 1930s mainly in rats (Goldblatt *et al* 1934). Other animal models have been used, in which the renal ischemia was produced in order to increase angiotensin production and blood pressure in systemic circulation. In 1940, Nobel Prize winners in physiology B

[1] Ablation: elimination of the focus involved in genesis of the arrhythmia.

Houssay and co-workers demonstrated the existence of angiotensin using a modified version of the Goldblatt model (Taquini 1940). They called this new hypertension-mediator 'hypertensyn' (in Spanish 'hipertensina'), and after the report by Lylle, in which the existence of the same hypertension-mediator (that they called 'angiotonin') was demonstrated (Page and Helmer 1940), both research groups decided a new name: 'angiotensin' (Braun Menéndez and Page 1958).

Small animals such as rats provided a useful tool to study systemic hypertension, both in the above-described model and those derived from genetic species, such as SHR (spontaneous hypertensive rats). However, small-animal instrumentation differs from instrumentation in large species. In the following, the hypertensive model of systemic hypertension used in the laboratory of the authors will be described.

Mongrel dogs were operated on under general anesthesia, induced by intravenous thiopentone sodium and maintained with enflurane in pure oxygen using respiratory mechanical assistance. Under sterile conditions, a right lateral laparotomy was performed and the right renal artery was uncovered after gentle dissection. A mechanical occluding device manufactured in the laboratory was placed at the origin of the artery (Fischer *et al* 1993). The occluder was designed to produce a complete occlusion of the renal artery over 24 h and was constructed using a slotted ring of laminarin[2] encased in another slotted ring made of stainless steel.

The mechanical occluder has an internal diameter of 2.7 mm, ensuring close contact with the artery, thus avoiding any luminal compromise at the time of the surgical intervention. The laparotomy was closed and a second similar surgery was performed in the contralateral side. The left artery was visualized and an electromagnetic flow probe was placed in this artery in order to monitor blood flow during the surgical procedure. Following this, a decrease of the intraluminal diameter was obtained using 4-0 silk sutured passed around the artery. Once 70% of the original blood flow was confirmed by the flow meter, the suture was tightened. The flow probe was withdrawn, the laparotomy was sutured and the animal recovered from anesthesia under veterinarian care.

After surgery, the animal received a normal diet and arterial blood pressure was non-invasively monitored. After a week, all animals showed abnormally higher levels of systemic arterial pressure (Fischer *et al* 1993).

5.4.2 Arteriovenous fistulae

Arteriovenous fistulae have been performed in experimental animals for many years in order to develop animal models focused on analyzing chronic changes of hemodynamic parameters (Liu *et al* 1991, Qing and Garcia 1992) and drug effects (Newman 1977). These mentioned animal models were developed in small and large animals (rats and dogs, respectively). The size of the animal is a factor that determines the use of different techniques to create an arteriovenous shunt.

Animal models of arteriovenous shunt are also used to induce cardiac failure, usually in dogs. Four months after the shunt construction, a state of heart failure

[2] A polysaccharide obtained from seaweed laminaria.

may be obtained. This model is characterized by fluid retention, increased pulmonary capillary pressure, ascites, and is accompanied by severe ventricular dysfunction (Taylor *et al* 1968).

The model schematized in figure 5.3 has been used in the laboratory of the authors and is characterized by a decrease in peripheral vascular resistance associated with an increase in cardiac output. Some disadvantages of this model are its high mortality that the magnitude of the anastomosis is not always predictable and a surgeon trained in micro vascular surgery must carry out the maneuvers.

5.4.3 Arterial calcification

Vitamin D_3 (1.25 dihydroxycholecalciferol) is a well-known metabolite of vitamin D, produced by the human body, currently indicated in many cases of osteoporosis. However, high doses of vitamin D_3 used in experimental animals produce acute arterial calcification accompanied by severe alteration of both the arterial structure and the mechanical function (Fischer *et al* 1991a).

In chronically instrumented dogs destined to investigate arterial wall dynamics, 5×10^5 IU of vitamin D_3 was administered daily for 10 days while maintaining a normal diet.

Arterial calcification (calcinosis) damages the elastic laminae, shown as the dark areas in figure 5.4. Electron microscopy demonstrated collagen disorganization and disruption of elastic fibers.

The mentioned structural changes were accompanied by important mechanical alterations characterized by a paradoxical decrease of arterial stiffness due to collagen fiber damage (Fischer *et al* 1991a).

5.4.4 Endothelial dysfunction

Endothelial cells are involved in smooth-muscle dynamics and are able to produce vasoconstriction and vasodilation in response to internal and/or external stimulus. The vasoactive role of endothelial cells is mediated by chemical factors such as nitric oxide, which could be modified by physiological stimuli and vascular diseases. Nitric oxide is a vasorelaxing factor that may be involved in vascular diseases produced by hyperhomocysteinemia, a risk factor of atherosclerosis.

The above-mentioned pathological condition of the arterial wall has been studied in Wistar rats, in which experimental hyperhomocysteinemia was induced. A group of three-month old Wistar rats received homocysteine thiolatone orally for 8 weeks ($50\,\mathrm{mg\,kg^{-1}\,day^{-1}}$). This determined a plasmatic hyperhomocysteinemia that induced nitric oxide inactivation (Fischer *et al* 2003).

Experimental rats are small laboratory animals that allow one to work with homogeneous groups in which pathological conditions may be induced and surgically instrumented in order to measure systemic pressure. Usually, the femoral artery and vein are cannulated and the catheters flushed with heparinized solution. One of the induced pathological conditions is obtained through intravenous nicotine administration

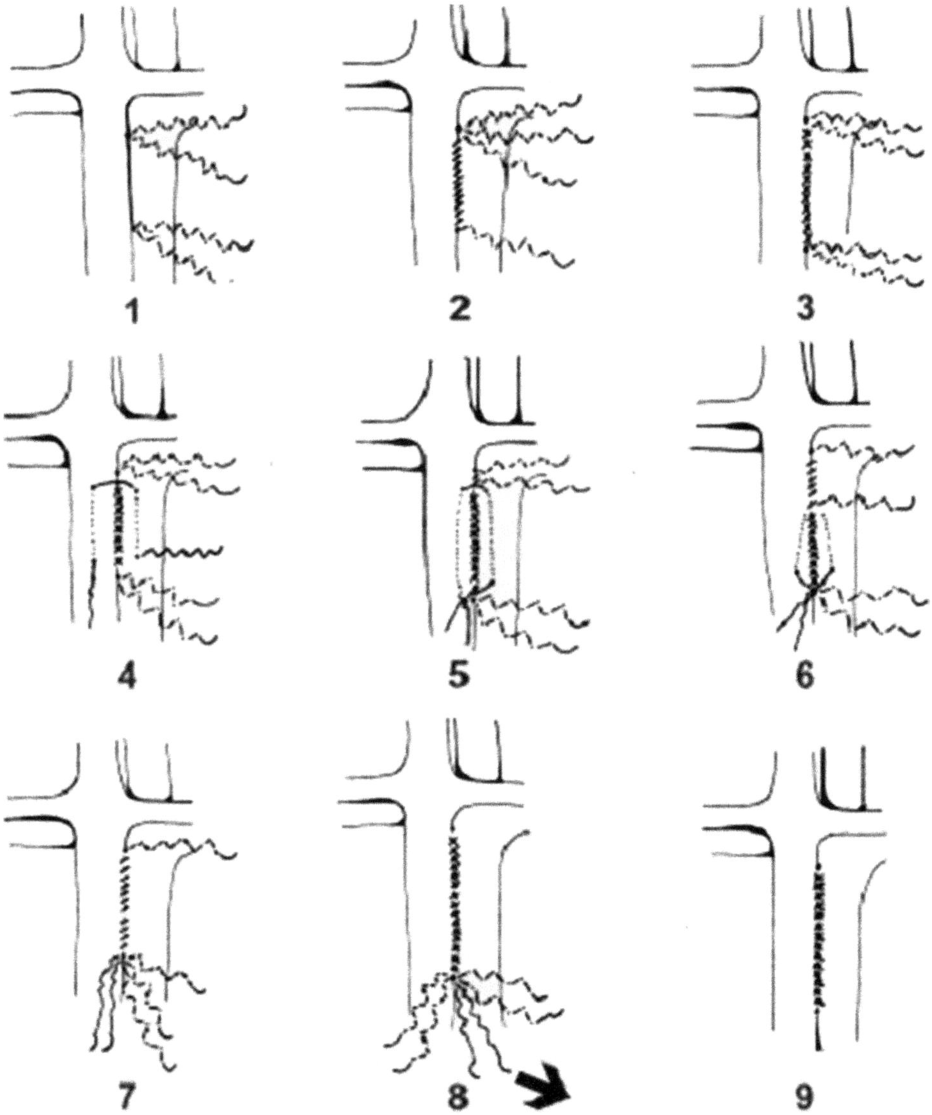

Figure 5.3. Technique to generate an aortic cava shunt. (1) A vascular infra renal segment is delimited, (2, 3) and sutured with a double dorsal polyester suture (Ti-Cron 2-0), joining the aortic and inferior vein cava walls. (4) a needle with polypropylene suture (Prolene 4-0) is inserted into the aorta in the caudal-cephalic direction and exteriorized five centimeters up for re-entering into the vein cava and exteriorized at the same level in which was first introduced, the dotted line is the intravascular polypropylene. (5, 6, 7) Subsequently, and similarly to (1, 2, 3), a ventral suture is made with polyester thread, generating an airtight space that contains the ends of the polypropylene suture, (8) the polypropylene suture is pulled in the direction of the arrow, (9) allowing the shunt to function.

(1–100 μg kg^{-1}) that results in significant increases of systemic blood pressure (Marano *et al* 1999). This animal experimentation performed in Wistar-Kyoto rats allows one to obtain hemodynamic data in a conscious animal preparation.

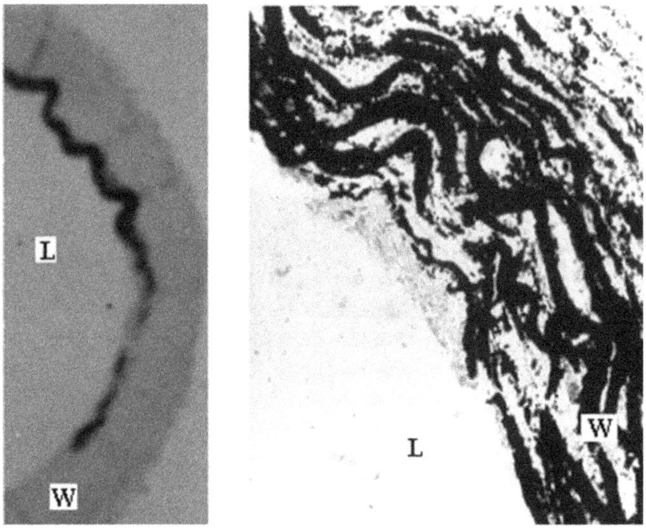

Figure 5.4. Left, the aortic wall (W) of an experimental animal showing large areas stained by the von Kossa technique near the arterial lumen (L). Right: a magnification of the same photomicrograph (×170) showing the elastic laminae stained by the von Kossa technique.

5.5 Models of cardiac failure

As mentioned above, heart failure is the last stage of almost all cardiopathies. This is due to the myocardial involvement in different diseases. Moreover, valvular diseases, coronary atherosclerotic obstructions, cardiac arrhythmias, congenital defects and other abnormalities have been corrected through surgery and endoluminal procedures. Consequently, patients survived a long time but myocardial failure determines a low cardiac output syndrome, i.e. cardiac failure produced by the only cardiac structure that could not be repaired.

Animal models of heart failure reproduce low cardiac output syndrome and the disease that originates the hemodynamic impairment. At present, circulatory assist devices are classified into two types according to the time of circulatory assistance short and long term. Consequently, both acute and chronic heart dysfunction models are needed to apply new devices.

5.5.1 Acute right ventricular failure

In our laboratory, two animal models of right ventricular failure have been used. One involved the right myocardium and the tricuspid valves (Fischer *et al* 1985) and the other was the consequence of experimental pulmonary thromboembolism that determined acute systolic blood pressure increase in the right ventricle (Fischer *et al* 1987). In the following, the former will be described.

The experimental animal, a dog in the original model, underwent surgery under general anesthesia and respiratory mechanical assistance. Anesthesia was induced with intravenous thiopentone sodium and maintained with enflurane in pure oxygen via a Bain tube. A left lateral thoracotomy allowed one to view the cardiac structures, particularly the free wall of the right ventricle.

Following the left thoracotomy, a purse-string suture was performed in the right ventricular free wall and a 1 cm ventriculotomy was performed encircled by the previous suture. Bleeding was avoided by maintaining pressure over the purse-string suture. Then, the surgeon introduced a finger to rupture the chordae tendineae, and induce tricuspid valve regurgitation. Furthermore, the right coronary artery was dissected at its origin and ligated to stop myocardial perfusion of the irrigated myocardium, i.e. the free wall of the right ventricle (Fischer *et al* 1985); see figure 5.5.

Hemodynamic failure produced by the above-described procedure was monitored in seven non-assisted animals with resulting increased right atrial pressure accompanied by decreased pulmonary arterial, aortic and left atrium pressures. Cardiac output decreased remarkably from 2.8±1.2 to 1.3±0.4 L min^{-1}. This impaired hemodynamic state was reverted using a pneumatic assist device that suctioned blood from the right atrium and injected it during the diastolic period into the pulmonary trunk (Fischer *et al* 1985).

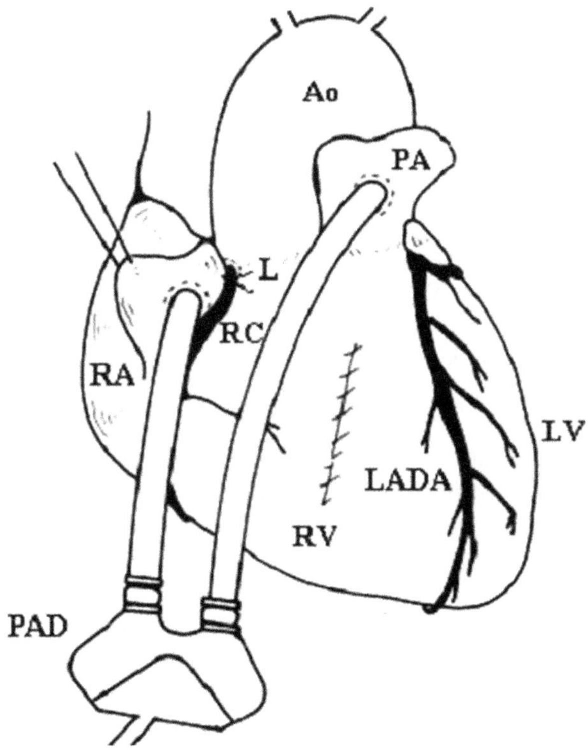

Figure 5.5. A pneumatic assist device (PAD) positioned between the right atrium (RA) and the pulmonary artery (PA). The tricuspid valve was damaged through an incision in the free wall of the right ventricle (RV) parallel to the left anterior descending coronary artery (LADA). The right coronary artery (RC) was ligated at its origin (L) while the left ventricle (LV) and aorta (Ao) remain free of any structural modifications.

5.5.2 Acute left ventricular failure

Halothane is a volatile liquid that is highly soluble in biological tissues and used to maintain anesthesia during a surgical procedure. It is currently commercially available, although its use in humans has been restricted due to its hepatic toxicity. Furthermore, halothane has a very strong negative inotropic effect, as reported in recent decades in studies where cardiac function during anesthesia was analyzed (Hamilton *et al* 1966, Sinnet *et al* 1981, Schotten *et al* 2001).

This model of heart failure was developed and reported in the laboratory of the authors following a report by Van Trigt *et al*, where anesthetics were classified according to their negative inotropic effects during their administration to experimental animals (Van Trigt *et al* 1984).

This model of cardiac depression obtained through halothane administration was used in six adult healthy Corriedale sheep. The animals weighed between 30 and 35 kg and were aged between 12 and 16 months. Anesthesia was induced with intravenous sodium thiopentone (20 mg kg^{-1}) and maintained with halothane (1%). Halothane was administered through a Bain tube during respiratory mechanical assistance using a ventilator (Neumovent 910, Tecme S. A., Cordoba, Argentina). The experiments were performed in accordance with the National Institutes of Health Guidelines for the Care and Use of Laboratory Animals.

Hemodynamic failure was produced by administering Halothane 4% in six animals. Induced heart failure was characterized by increased systemic vascular resistances and decreases of mean aortic flow, mean aortic pressure, systolic aortic pressure, diastolic aortic pressure and aortic diameter (Fischer *et al* 2011).

This reliable model of acute heart failure allows one to perform fine adjustments of the desirable myocardial depression, which is characterized by significant hemodynamic impairment, i.e. the operator can select the degree of circulatory depression according to the characteristics of the research. Moreover, the reversibility option allows one to recover and repeat the pharmacologically-induced heart failure (see figure 5.6).

The stability of this model, the option of adjusting the degree of cardiac dysfunction and the quality of signals are important factors that contribute to decrease the cost of laboratory research. Figure 5.7 shows the aortic waveforms at different degrees of cardiac impairment.

In previous works, the authors have used high doses of halothane (3% and 4%) firstly in mongrel dogs and then in sheep, resulting in severe left ventricular dysfunction, to test experimental circulatory assistance devices (Fischer *et al* 1991b, Fischer *et al* 2002, 2004, Risk *et al* 2004). Finally, no cardiac arrhythmias were observed in this model of halothane-induced heart failure.

5.5.3 Coronary microembolization

Coronary microembolism is a technique that has been used to produce irreversible chronic heart failure in dogs, pigs and sheep. The left anterior descending and circumflex arteries are used to such ends. The technique consists in injecting

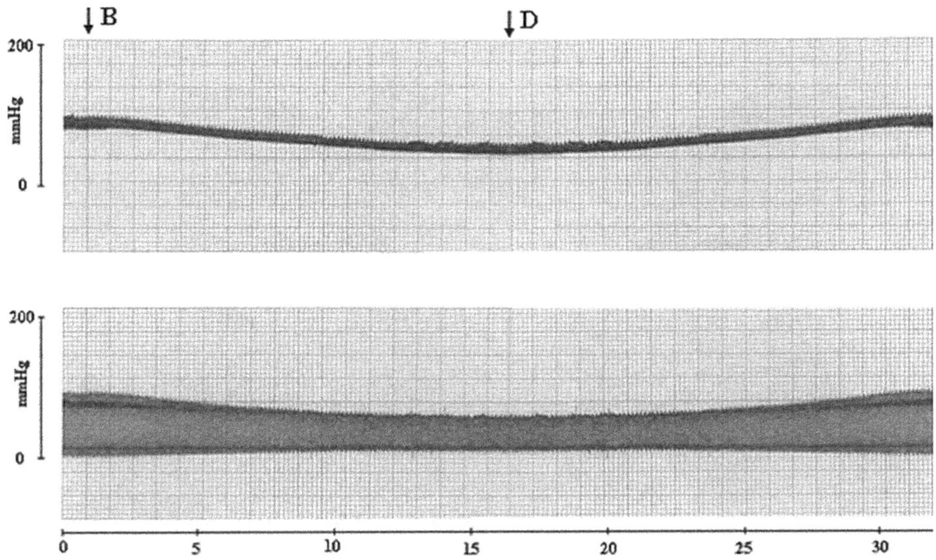

Figure 5.6. Low-speed recordings showing aortic pressure (upper panel) and left ventricular pressure (lower panel). Halothane administration (4%) beginning in B, determines a pressure reduction until the overdose is decreased (D) to 1%. Initial pressure values are recovered.

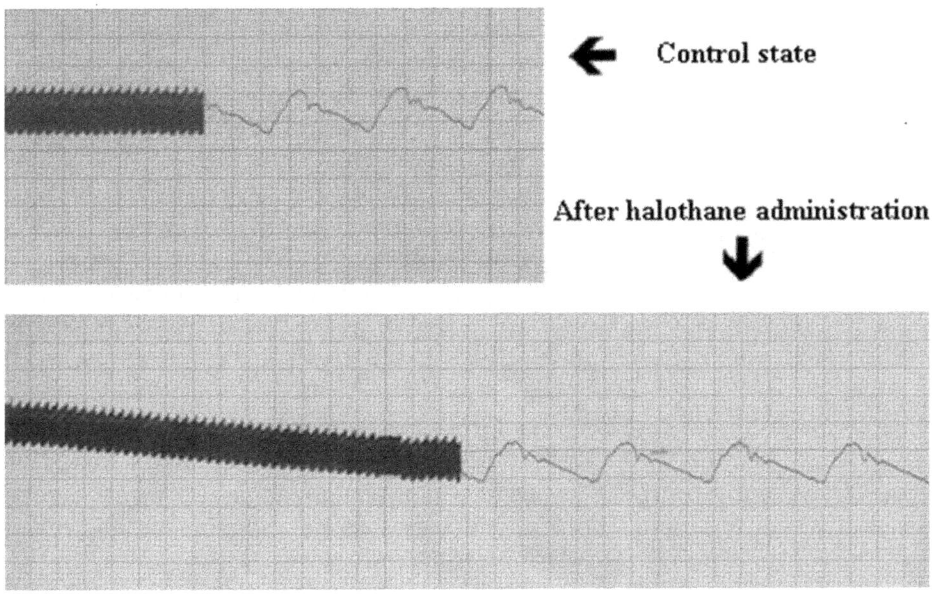

Figure 5.7. Low-speed recording and aortic steady state pressure waveform during halothane 1% administration (upper panel). An increase of halothane administration (4%) determines a transit state in which aortic pressure decreases but the waveform is maintained without cardiac arrhythmias (lower panel).

polystyrene latex microspheres (diameter between 70–100 μ) using a cardiac catheter inserted through a femoral artery (Monnet and Chachques 2005, Lavine *et al* 1991).

Around 20 000 microspheres enter the coronary artery during each injection. Four to fifteen injections are required to reach cardiac dysfunction. This is a model of myocardial ischemia, although no clear area of myocardial infarction is visible.

During coronary embolization, the left ventricular function is continuously monitored through ultrasound, although any technique able to estimate the ejection fraction or the maximum *dp*/*dt* value may be used.

This model is characterized by global myocardial damage that dilates the ventricles, has low ejection fraction, increases the end-diastolic left ventricular pressure, has prolonged isovolumetric relaxation, and causes a reduction of peak rapid filling/atrial filling velocity and integral ratios. Moreover, plasma norepinephrine levels are elevated. Heart failure remains during steady state from 3 to 6 months after the initial procedure.

This model has some limitations: it is difficult to achieve, has high mortality, cardiac arrhythmias appear and the interpretation of results is not easy (Dixon and Spinale 2009, Sabbah *et al* 1994).

5.5.4 Rapid cardiac pacing

Left ventricular pacing that results in prolonged tachycardia has been reported as a model of chronic heart failure. Rapid pacing has been used in healthy animals, and the procedure involves electro-stimulation of different areas of the canine heart: the apex, the outflow tract of the right ventricle, the free wall of the ventricles or the left atrium. After a period of 3–6 weeks, animals develop ventricular enlargement and decreased cardiac output (Yarbrough and Spinale 2003, Dixon and Spinale 2009).

Experimental chronic heart failure using rapid pacing heart stimulation has been performed in rabbits, dogs, sheep and pigs. In rabbits, electro-stimulation reaches approximately 350–400 bpm, whereas in larger animals approximately 250 bpm (Yarbrough and Spinale 2003, Hasenfuss 1998).

The myocardium can be electrically stimulated with no significant surgical trauma, and transvenous electrodes are currently used. This model has proved to reproduce the clinical signs and the neurohormonal activation normally observed in heart failure.

Animals submitted to rapid ventricular pacing have tachypnea, weight gain and ascites, biventricular dilatation, signs of pulmonary vascular congestion, and pleural effusion. These features are determined by the hemodynamic impairment, particularly a decrease in cardiac output, increases in pulmonary artery pressure, pulmonary wedge pressure, right atrial pressure and left ventricular ejection fraction. These hemodynamic changes are associated with neurohormonal activation of the renin–angiotensin system and the sympathetic system. Moreover, there is a decreased inotropic response of the myocyte, alterations in calcium homeostasis, decrease in the overall density of adrenergic β receptors in the myocardium and decreased activity of adenylate cyclase (Monnet and Chachques 2005).

5.5.5 Viral myocarditis

Dilated cardiomyopathies also originate in inflammatory processes accompanied by myocardial fibrosis. Viral infections could result in myocarditis, necrosis of myocytes and development of congestive heart failure. There is experimental data that supports the hypothesis that the influenza syndrome was responsible for a significant number of cardiomyopathies (Schnitt *et al* 1993).

The species of choice for this animal model of viral myocarditis are rats and mice. They are inoculated with Coxsackie and encephalomyocarditis viruses, resulting in an inflammatory response (Hasenfuss 1998).

The mechanisms involved in the progression of ventricular dilation and subsequent development of congestive heart failure in these models are the persistence of the viral RNA into the myocardium, the production of cytokines that influence the progression of dilated cardiomyopathy, and abnormalities in the architecture and function of the microcirculation.

Viral myocarditis has been overlooked by physicians for a long time. At present, almost 10% of patients with sudden-*onset* cardiomyopathy go through inflammatory processes, demonstrated through myocardial biopsies. Viral myocarditis has an acute start and develops into a chronic condition.

5.5.6 Myocardial toxicity

Cardiotoxicity is produced by many chemical agents such as antineoplastic agents, e.g. adriamycin and doxorubicin. Adriamycin administration to animals produced alterations in the contractile function of the myocyte (Jones *et al* 1990). The animals used to mimic heart failure produced by antineoplastic agents in humans are dogs, pigs, rabbits, goats and rats.

There is a syndrome that described the clinical findings produced by cobalt on myocardial structures. Cobalt was added to beer with fermenting purposes and produced heart failure through the generation of a cardiomyopathy. Mortality in humans produced by cobalt intoxication reaches 43%. This type of cardiomyopathy was introduced to experimental laboratories and an animal model was developed in dogs (Sandusky *et al* 1981).

5.6 Final comments

Animal models of cardiovascular dysfunction constitute a large chapter of biomedical engineering. Some of them, including those used by the authors, are summarized in this chapter.

An animal model tries to reproduce a physiological and/or a pathologic condition in an animal or an *in vitro* set-up. Scientific experimentation has been defined 'to perform changes in variables whose values are influenced by a multiplicity of factors'. These variables, e.g. hemodynamic parameters, change in both healthy and pathologic states of a human or animal model. Within healthy conditions, some variables may have normal ranges depending on the state of the subject, e.g. systolic blood pressure values higher than 150 mmHg during prolonged physical exercise is normal, but abnormal for a resting condition.

In conclusion, a variety of animal models of cardiovascular diseases can be used to study the altered biomechanical properties and, consequently, to characterize a pathological condition that can be therapeutically reversed.

References

Abarbanell A M, Herrmann J L, Weil B R, Wang Y, Tan J, Moberly S P, Fiege J W and Meldrum D R 2010 Animal models of myocardial and vascular injury *J. Surg. Res.* **162** 239–49

Barandon L, Calderon J, Reant P, Caillaud D, Lafitte S, Roques X, Couffinhal T and Dos Santos P 2010 Adjustment and characterization of an original model of chronic ischemic heart failure in pig *Cardiol. Res. Pract.* **7** 542451

Bianco R W, Wasiluk K R, Voight J M, Lahti M T, Rivard A L and Gallegos R P 2013 Large animal models in cardiac and vascular biomaterials research and assessment *Biomaterial Science* 3rd edn (Canada: Academic) ch II.3.7

Braun Menéndez E and Page I 1958 Suggested revision of nomenclatura: angiotensin *Science* **127** 242

Dixon J A and Spinale F G 2009 Large animal models of heart failure. A critical link in the translation of basic science to clinical practice *Circ. Heart Fail.* **2** 262–71

Fischer E, Levenson J, Barra J, Armentano R, Pichel R and Simon A 1993 Preventive effect of chronic converting enzyme inhibition on aortic stiffening induced by renovascular hypertension in conscious dogs *Cardiovasc. Res.* **27** 1039–44

Fischer E I, Spinelli J C, Willshaw P, Crottogini A J, de Forteza E, Clavin O, Valentinuzzi M E and Pichel R H 1988 Detection of left ventricular regional myocardial ischaemia in dogs by intraventricular conductance catheter *Cardiovasc. Res.* **22** 185–92

Fischer E I, Willshaw P, Armentano R, Besansón M I, Pichel R and Favaloro R 1985 Experimental acute right ventricular failure and right ventricular assist in the dog *J. Thorac. Cardiovasc. Surg.* **90** 580–5

Fischer E I, Willshaw P, de Forteza E, Biagetti M, Altman R, Morales M C, Pichel R and Favaloro R 1987 Animal model of pulmonary thromboembolism treated by local recirculation of streptokinase through the lung *J. Thorac. Cardiovasc. Surg.* **93** 620–7

Fischer E I C, Camus J M, Barmak W, Risk M R, Díaz A and de Forteza E 2011 Description of an animal model of acute cardiac failure: *in vivo* experiments in sheep *Latin Am. Appl. Res.* **41** 233–9

Fischer E I, Armentano R L, Levenson J, Barra J G, Morales M C, Breitbart G J, Pichel R H and Simon A 1991a Paradoxically decreased aortic wall stiffness in response to vitamin D3-induced calcinosis. A biphasic analysis of segmental elastic properties in conscious dogs *Circ. Res.* **68** 1549–59

Fischer E I C, Chachques J M, García A, Pichel R H, Morales M C and Carpentier A 1991b Temporary mechanical circulatory support for severe cardiac failure: experimental study *Int. J. Artif. Organs* **14** 466–72

Fischer E I C, Christen A I, Risk M R, Pessana F M and de Forteza E 2002 A new approach to assist postoperative heart failure in an animal model: juxta-aortic counterpulsation *Artif. Organs* **26** 819–26

Fischer P A, Dominguez G N, Cuniberti L A, Martinez V, Werba J P, Ramirez A J and Masnatta L D 2003 Hyperhomocysteinemia induces renal hemodynamic dysfunction: is nitric oxide involved? *J. Am. Soc. Nephrol.* **14** 653–60

Fischer E I C, de Forteza E, Risk M R, Nicolini G, Camus J M and Pessana F M 2004 Juxtaaortic counterpulsation: comparison with intraaortic counterpulsation in an animal model of acute heart failure *ASAIO J.* **50** 311–5

Goldblatt H, Lynch J, Hanzal R F and Summerville W W 1934 Studies on experimental hypertension, I: The production of persistent elevation of systolic blood pressure by means of renal ischemia *J. Exp. Med.* **59** 347–79

Hamilton W K, Larson C P, Bristow J D and Rapaport E 1966 Effect of cyclopropane and halothane on ventricular mechanics; a change in ventricular diastolic pressure-volume relationships *J. Pharmacol. Exp. Ther.* **154** 566–74

Hasenfuss G 1998 Animal models of human cardiovascular disease, heart failure and hypertrophy *Rev. Cardiovasc. Res.* **39** 60–76

Hodsman G P, Kohzuki M, Howes L G, Sumithran E, Tsunoda K and Johnston C I 1988 Neurohumoral responses to chronic myocardial infarction in rats *Circulation* **78** 376–81

Hongo M, Ryoke T and Ross J 1997 Animal models of heart failure. Recents developments and perspectives *Trends Cardiovasc. Med.* **7** 161–7

Jones S M, Kirby M S, Harding S E, Vescova G, Wanless R B, Dalla Libera L D and Poole-Wilson P A 1990 Adriamycin cardiomyopathy in the rabbit: alterations in contractile proteins and myocyte function *Cardiovasc. Res.* **24** 834–42

Lascano E C, Felice J I, Wray S, Kosta S, Dauby P C, Cabrera-Fischer E I and Negroni J A 2018 Experimental assessment of a myocyte-based multiscale model of cardiac contractile dysfunction *J. Theor. Biol.* **456** 6–28

Lavine S J, Prcevski P, Held C and Johnson V 1991 Experimental model of chronic global left ventricular dysfunction secondary to left coronary microembolization *J. Am. Coll. Cardiol.* **18** 1794–803

Liu Z, Hilbelink D R and Gerdes A M 1991 Regional changes in hemodynamics and cardiac myocyte size in rats with aortocaval fistulas. 2. Long-term effects *Circ Res.* **69** 59–65

Loomis T A and Krop S 1955 Auricular fibrillation induced and maintained in animals by acetylcholine or vagal stimulation *Circ. Res.* **3** 390–6

Marano G, Ramirez A, Mori I and Ferrari A U 1999 Sympathectomy inhibits the vasoactive effects of nicotine in conscious rats *Cardiovasc. Res.* **42** 201–5

Matsuoka S, Tomimatsu H, Miyauchi Y, Nakatsu T, Yuasa Y and Miyao M 1986 Effects of interventricular shunt on indices of left ventricular function *Pediatr. Res.* **20** 433–7

Milan D J and MacRae C A 2005 Animal models for arrhythmias *Cardiovasc. Res.* **67** 426–37

Moainie S L, Gorman J H 3rd and Guy T S *et al* 2002 An ovine model of postinfarction dilated cardiomyopathy *Ann. Thorac. Surg.* **74** 753–60

Monnet E and Chachques J C 2005 Animal models of heart failure: What is new? *Ann. Thorac. Surg.* **79** 1445–53

Muders F and Elsner D 2000 Animal models of chronic heart failure *Pharmacol. Res.* **41** 605–12

Mukherjee R *et al* 2003 Myocardial infarct expansion and matrix metalloproteinase inhibition *Circulation* **107** 618–25

Newman W H 1977 A depressed response of left ventricular contractile force to isoproterenol and norepinephrine in dogs with congestive heart failure *Am. Heart J.* **93** 216–21

Page J H and Helmer O M 1940 A crystalline pressor substance (angiotonin) resulting from the reaction between renin and renin-activator *J. Exp. Med.* **71** 29–42

Qing G and Garcia R 1992 Chronic captopril and losartan (DuP 753) administration in rats with high-output heart failure *Am. J. Physiol.* **263** H833–40

Rademaker M T, Charles C J, Espiner E A, Nicholls M G and Richards A M 2002 Long term Adrenomedullin administration in experimental heart failure *Hypertension* **40** 667–72

Risk M R, Ramírez A J and Fischer E I C 2004 Hemodynamic improvement and heart rate variability during aortic counterpulsation *Comput. Cardiol.* **31** 453–5

Sabbah H N, Shimoyama H, Kono T, Gupta R C, Sharov V G, Scicli G, Levine B and Goldstein S 1994 Effects of long-term monotherapy with enalapril, metoprolol, and digoxin on the progresion of left ventricular dysfunction and dilation in dogs with reduced ejection fraction *Circulation* **89** 2852–9

Sandusky G E, Henk W G and Roberts E D 1981 Histochemistry and ultrastructure of the heart in experimental cobalt cardiomyopathy in the dog *Toxicol. Appl. Pharmacol.* **61** 89–98

Schnitt S J, Stillman I E, Owings D V, Kishimoto C, Dvorak H F and Abelmann W H 1993 Myocardial fibrin deposition in experimental viral myocarditis that progresses to dilated cardiomyopathy *Circ. Res.* **72** 914–20

Schoels W, Restivo M, Caref E B, Gough W B and el-Sherif N 1991 Circus movement atrial flutter in canine sterile pericarditis model. Activation patterns during entrainment and termination of single-loop reentry *in vivo Circulation* **83** 1716–30

Schotten U, Greiser M, Braun V, Karlein C and Scheoendube F 2001 Effect of volatile anesthetics on the force frequency relation in human ventricular myocardium *Anesthesiology* **95** 1160–8

Shiota T, Jones M, Aida S, Chikada M, Tsujino H, El-Kadi T and Sahn D J 1999 Validation of the accuracy of both right and left ventricular outflow volume determinations and semi-automated calculation of shunt volumes through atrial septal defects by digital color Doppler flow mapping in a chronic animal model *J. Am. Coll. Cardiol.* **34** 587–93

Sinnet E E, Wahrenbrock E A and Kooyman G L 1981 Cardiovascular depression and thermoregulatory disruption caused by pentothal/halothane anesthesia in the harbor seal *J. Wildl. Dis.* **17** 121–30

Stengl M 2010 Experimental models of spontaneous ventricular arrhythmias and of sudden cardiac death *Physiol. Res.* **59** S25–31

Taquini A C 1940 The production of a pressor substance by the totally ischemic kidney *Am. Heart J.* **19** 513–8

Taylor R R, Covell J W and Ross J Jr. 1968 Left ventricular function in experimental aorto-caval fistula with circulatory congestion and fluid retention *J. Clin. Invest.* **47** 1333–42

Van Trigt P, Christian C C, Fagraeus L, Spray T L, Peyton R B, Pellom G L and Wechsler A S 1984 Myocardial depression by anesthetic agents (halothane, enflurane and nitrous oxide): quantification based on end-systolic pressure-dimension relations *Am. J. Cardiol.* **53** 243–7

Wang Z, Pagé P and Nattel S 1992 Mechanism of flecainide's antiarrhythmic action in experimental atrial fibrillation *Circ. Res.* **71** 271–87

Yarbrough W M and Spinale F G 2003 Large animal models of congestive heart failure: a critical step in translating basic observations into clinical applications *J. Nucl. Cardiol.* **10** 77–86

IOP Publishing

Ricardo L Armentano, Edmundo I Cabrera Fischer and Leandro J Cymberknop

Chapter 6

Hemodynamic modelization during therapeutical interventions: counterpulsation

Edmundo I Cabrera Fischer

In clinical practice, cardiovascular therapeutic interventions are done to reverse pathologic states, to reach a condition in which physiological parameters are normal or close to a healthy state allowing the patient to be as active as possible. The efficacy of invasive and non-invasive therapies should be tested before being used in humans. With this purpose, the effectiveness of a treatment is investigated using an *in vitro* set up and in animal models of cardiovascular diseases. As explained in chapter 5, cardiovascular failure can be acute or chronic and therefore the therapeutical interventions vary. It is important to consider this in prototypes developed to reverse circulatory failure in experimental animals simulating clinical diseases.

In this chapter, a circulatory assistance technique, arterial counterpulsation, will be described. This circulatory assistance technique has been widely used and is under continuous research to achieve new alternatives. Animal models used to test the effectiveness of arterial counterpulsation in cardiac failure will be summarized, also showing the state-of-art techniques of this circulatory assistance used in myocardial ischemia and heart failure.

6.1 Aortic counterpulsation

Arterial counterpulsation has been part of experimental attempts to restore hemodynamic parameters in experimental animals and in clinical practice during the last sixty years, being the most used circulatory assistance technique. It was originally conceived as a method to treat myocardial ischemia, but shortly after was considered a valid alternative to treat heart failure. The concept was very simple: physiologists of the mid-20th century were aware that left ventricular myocardial blood perfusion took place mainly during the diastolic period. Consequently, they considered that hemodynamic assistance to treat myocardial ischemia should be

doi:10.1088/2053-2563/aafb0dch6

done during this period, to increase the blood pressure gradient between the aortic and post-stenotic pressures (Kantrowitz 1990).

Arterial blood supply to left ventricular wall is essential to meet the myocardial demand of oxygen and of other elements that maintain physiological levels of contractility according to physical activity. As previously explained, the left ventricle is almost entirely perfused during the diastolic period.

As mentioned, counterpulsation is a technique that was theoretically conceived to be used to treat myocardial ischemia produced by coronary artery disease. Ischemia is produced by arterial obstruction due to atherosclerotic plaques. The aim of the technique was to increase arterial blood supply in the ischemic areas of the ventricular wall. The first experimental researches were carried out in the early 1950s, when aortocoronary by-pass and percutaneous endoluminal procedures had not been yet developed (Kantrowitz 1953, Kantrowitz and McKinnon 1959).

The efficiency of intra-aortic counterpulsation was first demonstrated in patients with cardiogenic shock due to severe myocardial ischemia, decreasing mortality, which at that time was 100%. Moreover, the improvement of patient condition was linked not only to increases of coronary diastolic blood flow, but to decreases of peripheral vascular resistance and improvement of systemic circulation (Kantrowitz *et al* 1968, Kantrowitz 2001).

Currently, arterial counterpulsation is used in acute heart failure refractory to pharmacologic therapy, or in patients at risk of developing sudden hemodynamic failure. The prophylactic use of intra-aortic counterpulsation allows one to prevent myocardial infarction in percutaneous endoluminal high-risk coronary interventions or in open heart surgeries in patients with left ventricular mechanical failure.

A well-tolerated arterial counterpulsation technique to treat acute left ventricular failure is to place a balloon catheter in the descending aorta. This two-lumen balloon catheter is inserted through a femoral artery. The correct position is confirmed using radioscopic control or a chest x-ray. The inflation and deflation of the balloon is synchronized with an electrocardiographic signal or the aortic pressure waveform that is obtained using the second lumen of the balloon catheter. After left ventricular contraction, the semilunar valves are closed and in this precise time the balloon inflation begins. Currently 40 c.c. of helium is injected in each cardiac cycle into the balloon. A console facilitates continuous monitoring of the procedure. Blood is displaced during balloon inflation, which ends before the following aortic valve opening (Kantrowitz 2001).

Since the intima layer of the arteries has an important role in the vascular dynamic control, the size of the balloon must be adequate as to not interfere with it. Damage to the aortic wall is avoided by the polyurethane architecture of the balloon, which prevents over-inflation. The size of the aortic lumen is taken into account before placing the balloon catheter, and an occlusive inflation of the balloon is avoided. All of the above-mentioned considerations should be taken into account in the development of pathologic animal models in which acute heart failure is treated using intra-aortic counterpulsation (Fischer *et al* 2005); see figure 6.1.

In clinical practice, the balloon catheter is placed in the descending aorta with its tip distal to the origin of the subclavian artery. Balloon pumping is controlled with a

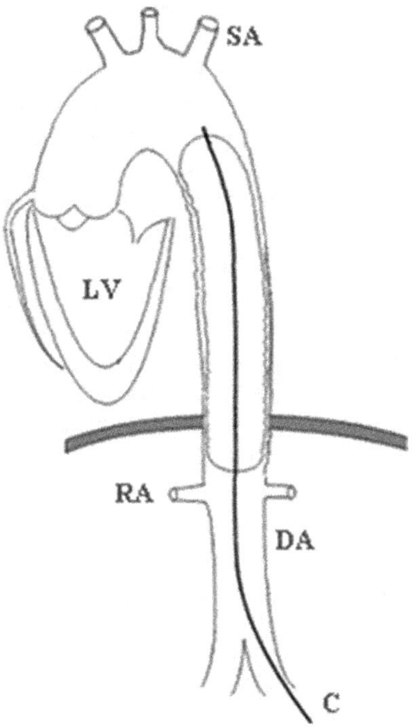

Figure 6.1. Catheter balloon introduced through the left femoral artery and placed in the descending aorta between the renal arteries and the aortic arch. LV: left ventricle, SA: subclavian artery, DA: descending Aorta, RA: renal artery, C: catheter.

console that ensures adequate balloon inflation with helium during diastole and allows one to visualize the blood pressure waveform along the cardiac cycle. During systole the balloon is collapsed, and this sudden decrease of aortic volume contributes to decrease the arterial resistance, thereby saving heart energy. Balloon inflation is synchronized using the pressure waveform or the R wave of a surface electrocardiogram, ensuring that it is completed before the diastolic period ends. The balloon undergoes a quick deflation before the next left ventricular ejection. Since at the beginning of diastolic period the aorta has the maximum blood volume, the highest blood pressure-flow changes produced by balloon inflation are obtained during the early diastole (Fischer *et al* 2005).

Intra-aortic balloon pump counterpulsation is performed for periods no longer than one month, to avoid potential complications. Aortic counterpulsation is usually maintained until a significant recovery of cardiac function is obtained or another circulatory treatment is indicated: cardiac transplant or a long-term mechanical assist device.

The balloon catheters used in adult patients are 26 cm long, and their anatomical ideal placement is between the origin of the renal arteries and the distal ostium of the left subclavian artery. As mentioned above, the console enables continuous monitoring of the procedure and also allows one to make fine adjustments to several parameters, ensuring optimum performance of the balloon catheter. One of them is the volume of helium injected into the balloon, which varies with balloon size. The injected volume indirectly determines the pressure inside the balloon. The balloon catheter is usually removed 96 h before beginning aortic counterpulsation.

The cardiac cycle can be assisted with different pumping frequencies usually expressed as the ratio of the inflation-deflation cycles with respect to the native beats of the patient. A 1:1 modality means that one inflation-deflation cycle is done in every heartbeat, 1:2 means that every other beat receives the assistance, and so on. In acute heart failure, the 1:1 modality is used, and the 1:2 assistance is only used for weaning.

6.2 Left ventricular changes during aortic counterpulsation

As the primary origin of circulatory failure is impaired myocardial contractility, the effects of circulatory assistance using intra-aortic balloon pumping are particularly relevant (see table 6.1).

In healthy subjects, heart rate, myocardial contractility, left ventricular volume and systolic blood pressure establish the myocardial oxygen demand. In coronary artery disease, myocardial oxygen supply is decreased by vascular stenosis; in cardiac failure, the end-diastolic left ventricular pressure is increased and diastolic aortic pressure is usually decreased. Diastolic intra-aortic balloon inflation produces a significant pressure augmentation that results in a significant increase of coronary blood flow and in an important decrease of left ventricular afterload. Increases of coronary blood flow determine an increase of oxygen delivered to the myocardium. Furthermore, decreases of left ventricular afterload decrease myocardial oxygen consumption (Papaioannou 2005).

Because of the above-mentioned direct effects of intra-aortic counterpulsation, there are more beneficial changes, such as the decrease of myocardial oxygen consumption due to the decrease of left ventricular afterload. Since the major determinant of myocardial oxygen consumption is left ventricular afterload, its decrease improves circulation in cardiac failure (Webb *et al* 2015).

Table 6.1. Effects of counterpulsation on left ventricular function

Direct effects	Secondary effects
↑ Diastolic aortic pressure	↓ Preload
↑ Coronary diastolic blood flow	↑ Stroke volume
↑ Coronary diastolic blood pressure	↓ Heart rate
↓ Left ventricular afterload	↓ Myocardial ischemia
↑ Right ventricular function	↓ Cardiac arrhythmias
↓ Right atrial pressure	↑ Ejection fraction
	↓ Myocardial O_2 consumption
	↓ Systolic left ventricular pressure
	↓ Left ventricular volume
	↓ Left ventricular wall stress

The volume of left ventricular ejection in each systole (i.e. stroke volume) increases as a consequence of a low aortic pressure at the end of the diastolic period (see figure 6.2).

The deflation of the intra-aortic balloon is as important as its inflation. In fact, the correct deflation of the balloon is done before the beginning of the systolic period, which decreases left ventricular afterload because of a *draining effect* of blood in the aorta. This improvement is strengthened by others that are linked to changes in the performance of the systemic arterial tree (Webb *et al* 2015).

In patients with coronary artery disease, in whom collateral circulation exists, intra-aortic counterpulsation increases blood flow to the ischemic myocardial areas. This is another consequence of the higher coronary perfusion pressure due to the circulatory assistance.

6.3 Effects of aortic counterpulsation on blood circulation

When explaining the effects of aortic counterpulsation, the 1:2 modality is used by many authors, thus the need to unify nomenclature to facilitate comparisons of findings by different authors. Kim *et al* (1996) described the effects of

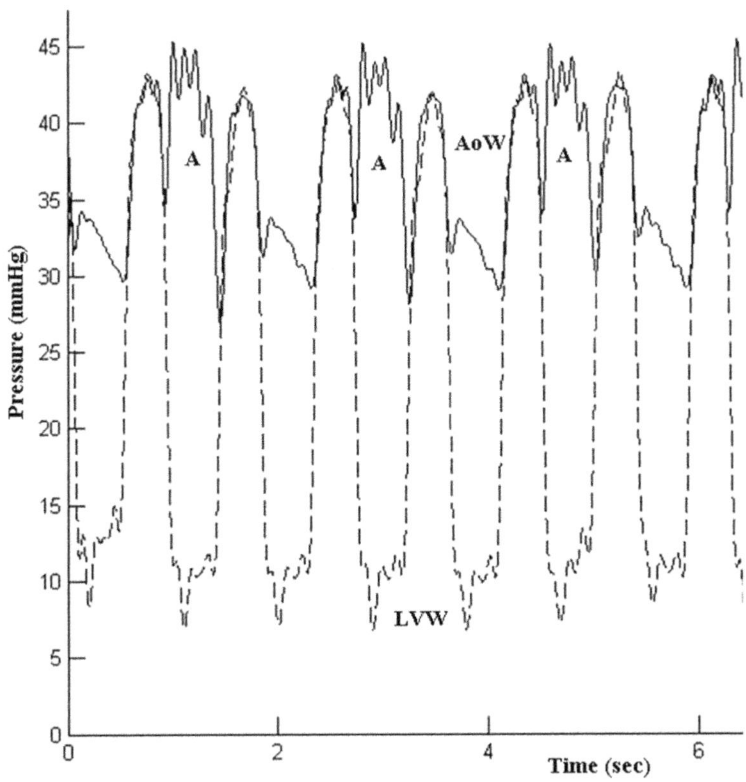

Figure 6.2. Effects of aortic counterpulsation in augmented beats (A) on aortic pressure waveform (AoW) and left ventricular pressure waveform (LVW) in an animal model of severe heart failure induced by the administration of halothane (3%). Note the decreases of end-diastolic aortic pressure in the augmented beats.

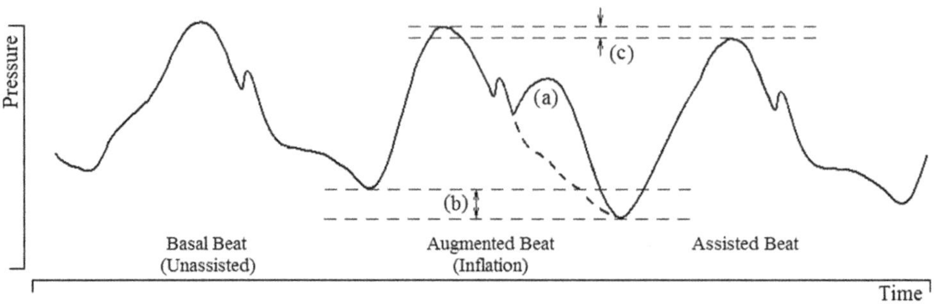

Figure 6.3. Waves of aortic pressure that show changes determined by aortic counterpulsation: (a) diastolic pressure augmentation, (b) decrease of end-diastolic aortic pressure, and (c) decrease of the peak systolic pressure of the assisted beat.

counterpulsation using the following denominations: ***basal*** beats (without intra-aortic balloon pumping: IABP), ***augmented*** beats (with IABP) and ***assisted*** beats (those that follow an augmented beat during 1:2 IABP); see figure 6.3.

Currently, aortic counterpulsation is the only technique that assists the heart in series without cardiac intervention, since the balloon catheter is placed in the descending aorta.

Heart failure determines an impairment of ventricular blood ejection into the aorta and the pulmonary artery. Left ventricular assistance is usually indicated in patients with acute heart failure. These patients show a severe impairment of hemodynamic parameters such as an increased end-diastolic left ventricular pressure, an increase in myocardial oxygen consumption, decreased cardiac output, increased systemic vascular resistance, among others. Some of these changes ensure the continuity of cardiac function even in abnormal situations, e.g. the increase of systemic vascular resistance increases the diminished arterial pressure, but decreases cardiac output due to the augmented afterload. Furthermore, increases in afterload determine increases in end-diastolic left ventricular pressures, which compromise myocardial perfusion. After the initial impairment (i.e. decreases of myocardial function), there are several factors that perpetuate the heart failure syndrome, and a vicious cycle is created.

IABP assistance aims to reestablish impaired physiological parameters, just as pharmacological treatment is used to reverse acute heart failure syndrome. IABP is generally used when pharmacological treatments fail, and its beneficial effects appear soon in successful cases (Khir *et al* 2003).

The increase of diastolic mean pressure determined by the inflation of the balloon produces an augmentation of blood flow in the thoracic and abdominal arteries, improving tissue perfusion. This effect is accompanied by the increase of diuresis, skin warming and mental activity recovery in patients with severe compromise of cardiac output.

In table 6.2, the changes in hemodynamic parameters observed during intra-aortic counterpulsation are listed. Since the clinical results of this circulatory assistance method are beyond the scope of this chapter, we summarize more than 50 years of research in this interesting field as follows: (a) intra-aortic

Table 6.2. Effects of counterpulsation on circulatory function.

Hemodynamic parameters
↑ Peripheral tissue perfusion
↓ Peripheral vascular resistances
↓ Pulmonary vascular resistances
↑ Kidney perfusion
↑ Aortic blood flow
↑ Aortic pulse pressure
↓ Aortic systolic pressure
↓ Pulmonary capillary wedge pressure
↓ Right atrial pressure
↑ Cardiac index
↓ Hematocrit
↑ Cerebral blood flow

counterpulsation improved the ominous prognosis of circulatory shock for the first time, (b) this method currently provides circulatory support, improving hemodynamic parameters and allowing a quick recuperation of severe acute heart failure, (c) development of new assist devices allows one to obtain better improvements of hemodynamic parameters than those observed with aortic counterpulsation (Papaioannou 2005).

Regardless of the new developments in the field of circulatory assistance, the simplicity and low cost of the balloon catheter pumping ensures its continuity. Moreover, new models including higher balloon volumes (e.g. 50 ml) have been reported (Webb *et al* 2015).

6.4 Indexes of aortic counterpulsation

The effectiveness of intra-aortic counterpulsation could be confirmed using hemodynamic parameters that are usually monitored in patients with severe acute heart failure. However, this is not a direct evaluation of the beneficial effects of intra-aortic counterpulsation. A method to quantify the effects of augmented diastolic pressure on subendocardial perfusion during ischemia was developed in an animal model several decades ago (Buckberg *et al* 1972). The author considered that subendocardial blood flow was directly involved with the area enclosed by the instantaneous aortic and left ventricular pressure signals during the diastolic period. Buckberg used two indexes: the tension time index (TTI) and the diastolic pressure time index (DPTI). The TTI is calculated by estimating the area under the systolic pressure signal, while the DPTI is calculated estimating the area under the diastolic aortic pressure wave and subtracting the mean left atrial pressure. The latter was assumed to be similar to the diastolic left ventricular pressure. The TTI is considered as an index of myocardial oxygen demand (Buckberg *et al* 1972).

The relationship of the above-described indexes (i.e. DPTI/TTI) was used as an index of diastolic pressure augmentation. The value of the DPTI/TTI increases with aortic diastolic pressure. During aortic counterpulsation the difference between aortic and left ventricular pressures increases.

Aortic counterpulsation produces increases of the DPTI/TTI relationship with respect to non-assisted cardiac cycles (Fischer *et al* 2005). Another method to quantify the effects of aortic counterpulsation without measuring left ventricular pressure was developed in our laboratory. Since the DPTI/TTI index needs left ventricular pressure, we explored the ability of a new index to assess counterpulsation by analyzing the diastolic and systolic areas beneath the arterial pressure curves (Fischer *et al* 1999). We called this index DABAC/SABAC (diastolic area beneath arterial curve/systolic area beneath arterial curve); see figure 6.4.

In previous research, the extent of the diastolic aortic augmentation was measured using the subendocardial viability index (DPTI/TTI) and the DABAC/SABAC index (Fischer *et al* 1999). The DABAC/SABAC index can be calculated online through specific software developed in our laboratory for experimental use.

This new index was validated by calculating the correlation between the DPTI/TTI and DABAC/SABAC indexes, to estimate the degree of association between them. In 30 counterpulsated sheep, left ventricular and aortic instantaneous pressure waves were recorded in four different states: before and after cardiac failure induction using a high dose of halothane (4%), and before and after myocardial ischemia produced by a coronary artery occluder positioned in the left anterior descending artery.

Diastolic pressure augmentation was quantified in each counterpulsated cardiac cycle using both the above-mentioned indexes. As seen in figure 6.5, the correlation coefficient showed a high degree of association between the subendocardial viability index (DPTI/TTI) and the DABAC/SABAC index. After this experimental validation of the DABAC/SABAC index it was used by other research groups in the Milwaukee Heart Institute (USA) and in Europe (Dumcius *et al* 2001, 2002). Since

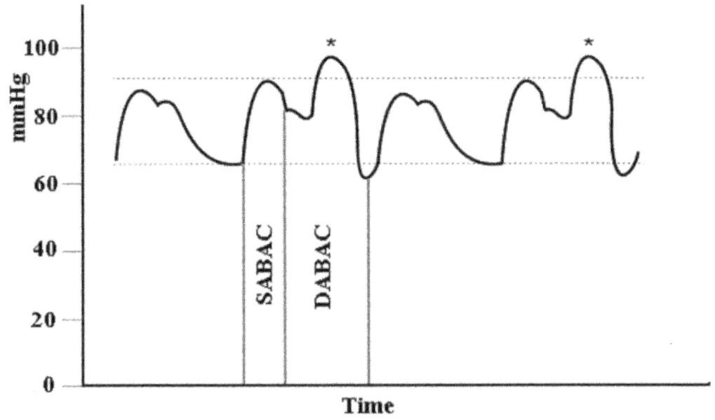

Figure 6.4. Two augmented beats (*) with decreased end-diastolic aortic blood pressure. The vertical lines limit the systolic and diastolic periods and both areas beneath the curve are calculated: SABAC: systolic area beneath the aortic curve and DABAC: diastolic area beneath the aortic curve.

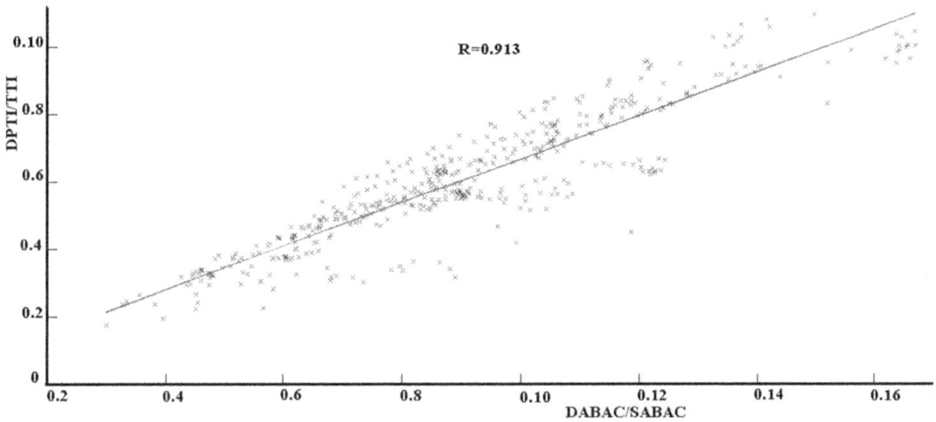

Figure 6.5. In each cardiac cycle, diastolic aortic pressure augmentation was calculated using the subendocardial viability index (DPTI/TTI) and the DABAC/SABAC index. These experimental data were obtained in counterpulsated sheep in which acute heart failure and myocardial ischemia were induced.

in clinical practice the use of left atrial or left ventricular pressure has several restrictions, the use of the DABAC/SABAC index calculated through invasive or non-invasive techniques could contribute to the simplicity of the quantification of diastolic aortic augmentation.

6.5 Arterial wall dynamics during aortic counterpulsation

There is a dynamic interaction between intraluminal pressure-flow changes and the arterial wall properties, as previously reported (Fischer *et al* 2002a). Intra-aortic counterpulsation produces hemodynamic changes in systemic vessels, and several researchers demonstrated that the vessel wall mechanical properties are modified (Stefanadis *et al* 1998, Kim *et al* 1996, Kawaguchi *et al* 1999). However, the mechanism that determines these changes in the arterial wall dynamics has not yet been clarified.

Intra-aortic counterpulsation increases arterial compliance in patients during cardiac failure, and this improvement has been attributed to a pressure-dependent mechanism. According to Kim *et al*, a reduction of the distending pressure produces a decrease of the characteristic arterial impedance and of pulse wave reflection (Kim *et al* 1996). On the other hand, Kawaguchi *et al* found a significant reduction of arterial wall elastance during intra-aortic counterpulsation with no changes in arterial pressure (Kawaguchi *et al* 1999). That is to say that the beneficial hemodynamic effects of intra-aortic counterpulsation have been confirmed in terms of arterial stiffness improvement. Moreover, a distensibility increase was demonstrated in twelve counterpulsated patients in cardiogenic shock (Stefanadis *et al* 1998), but the origin of these changes was attributed to passive or active changes in arterial wall dynamics.

These reports led to the development of an animal model in our laboratory to elucidate this controversial subject. Our results demonstrated that intra-aortic counterpulsation in experimental animals caused: (a) pressure-dependent changes in arterial wall energetic and damping properties, and (b) pressure-independent changes in arterial wall energetic and damping properties due to smooth muscle changes (Fischer *et al* 2008). The reported findings were obtained in a healthy animal model and showed a physiologic response to intraluminal stimuli.

Since aortic counterpulsation is a technique that has been developed to restore hemodynamic parameters during heart failure; we developed another model in which cardiovascular function was impaired, producing myocardial contractility depression. The analysis of hemodynamic parameters in this animal model of induced heart failure was similar to that previously described in this book. Aortic pressure, diameter and flow signals were recorded in an anesthetized animal before and after heart failure induction and during intra-aortic counterpulsation (Fischer *et al* 2009). In this research, we demonstrated a significant reduction of aortic stiffness provoked by changes in arterial smooth muscle, using variables obtained at isofrequency and isobaric conditions. That is to say that these changes were produced by the smooth muscle vascular tissue independently of arterial pressure and heart rate.

Since vascular smooth muscle tissue is the only arterial wall constituent capable of producing a quick response in mechanical terms, the above-mentioned results are not surprising. However, this smooth muscle activity is the consequence of stimuli traveling through the intima and/or adventitia layers. Thus, two different experimental studies were carried out in our laboratory: one of them to elucidate the role of the endothelial layer on arterial wall properties, and the other one to characterize the role of the adventitia, if any, on the mechanical wall properties during intra-aortic counterpulsation.

To analyze the role of the intima layer, we developed an animal model in which pressure and diameter signals were measured in the left iliac artery of seven anesthetized sheep in a basal state (i.e. non-contrapulsated cycles) and during 1:2 aortic counterpulsation in the following states: (a) in healthy animals with intact iliac arteries and without heart failure, (b) during heart failure induced by halothane 4%, in sheep with intact iliac arteries, (c) in de-endothelized iliac arteries of healthy animals without cardiac depression, and (d) in de-endothelized iliac arteries during heart failure. This animal preparation allowed us to obtain results confirming that the integrity of the endothelium is critical to modulate the response to intra-aortic counterpulsation 1:2. We concluded that 1:2 aortic counterpulsation before and after heart failure results in the dilatation of the iliac artery accompanied by a decrease of arterial stiffness (Bia *et al* 2011).

To analyze the role of the adventitia layer on the effects of aortic counterpulsation, we developed an animal model similar to that used to study the endothelium during intra-aortic balloon pumping. Pressure and diameter signals were measured in the left iliac artery of seven anesthetized sheep in a basal state (non-contrapulsated) and during 1:2 aortic counterpulsation in the following conditions: (a) in healthy animals with intact iliac arteries without heart failure, (b) in de-adventialized iliac arteries in animals without heart failure, and (c) during induced cardiac failure using halothane 4%, in animals without adventitia in the left iliac arteries (Fischer *et al* 2013).

The surgical procedure to remove the adventitia layer consisted in a gentle dissection disconnecting its weak adherences to the media layer using a pair of forceps and scissors. During the adventitia dissection, ultrasonic crystals were removed and repositioned in the same place, as previously reported (Fischer *et al* 2010).

Arterial 1:2 counterpulsation in the instrumented anesthetized animals yielded the following results: (a) In animals without heart failure, the improvement in terms of arterial wall compliance obtained with intra-aortic balloon pumping was significantly reduced by the adventitia removal, and (b) during induced cardiac failure, the impaired arterial wall distensibility, partially due to adventitia removal, was significantly improved by intra-aortic counterpulsation (Fischer *et al* 2013).

6.6 Juxta-aortic counterpulsation

Postcardiotomy left ventricular failure refractory to pharmacological treatment is a severe complication in which the only possible therapy is circulatory assistance.

Intra-aortic counterpulsation has been found to be a successful technique to assist postcardiotomy heart failure. However, descending aorta dissection, aortoiliac disease, severe femoral arteries disease, aneurysmal peripheral vessels and small peripheral arteries (i.e. children) remain as contraindications of balloon catheter femoral insertion. Consequently, other options have been studied, such as direct transaortic catheter balloon placement in the descending aorta through a puncture in the ascending aorta ensured by a purse-string suture (Santini and Mazzucco 1997, Hazelrigg *et al* 1992). This technique was used in more than 100 cases, but patients needed another operation in order to recover the balloon catheter.

In 2002 and 2004, our group reported a new method to obtain aortic counterpulsation in an animal model of cardiac failure. We used a Dacron prosthesis wrapped around the aortic arch and a balloon catheter was placed between the prosthesis and the artery in a juxta-aortic position without blood contact. The juxta-aortic position of the balloon catheter offers the advantage of avoiding the troublesome blood–biomaterial interface. This technique was thought to be useful in the early postcardiotomy period, before chest closure, in patients with severe aortoiliac disease. We demonstrated that this technique provided adequate circulatory support in an experimental animal model of cardiac failure (Fischer *et al* 2002b, 2004).

In our experimental model of juxta-aortic counterpulsation, the extra-aortic balloon catheter was inserted percutaneously through a puncture in the second intercostal space of the anesthetized animal. The second intercostal space was chosen because it has been extensively used for pneumothorax treatment (Fischer *et al* 2002b).

Juxta-aortic compression is a well-tolerated counterpulsation technique, as previously demonstrated, where chronic peri-aortic counterpulsation was obtained for long periods of time in patients subjected to dynamic aortomyoplasty (Chachques *et al* 1996). As the balloon is placed near the aortic root, the effectiveness of counterpulsation is thought to be increased because of the proximity to the aortic valve. The Dacron prosthesis is a biocompatible material and has been extensively used for grafts.

Experimental left ventricular assistance with this new technique was shown to be capable of restoring hemodynamic parameters in our animal model of acute cardiac failure. Moreover, the extent of diastolic pressure augmentations was similar to that obtained using intra-aortic counterpulsation (Fischer *et al* 2004).

6.7 Pulmonary counterpulsation

There are more counterpulsation modalities than those described in this chapter, such as biological counterpulsation that did not succeed beyond its experimental stage, as neither did this type of pulmonary artery counterpulsation. Pulmonary counterpulsation using a balloon catheter, after many attempts, is a technique that has not been widespread despite several published works (Miller *et al* 1980, Jett *et al* 1987, Fischer *et al* 1985). Perhaps the lack of a widely used counterpulsation technique in the pulmonary circuit is explained by the fact that it is a very compliant territory. Consequently, right ventricular failure is currently treated using mechanical devices that pump blood from the right atrium to the pulmonary artery, such as Excor and Thoratec assist devices.

The mechanical behavior of the pulmonary artery has been previously characterized by our group in healthy *in vivo* experimental preparations and in animal models of pulmonary hypertension (Armentano *et al* 2005).

6.7.1 Reverse blood flow during aortic counterpulsation

Intra-aortic balloon pumping displaces blood cyclically, which increases aortic diastolic pressure. This active action is accompanied by other changes that are summarized in figure 6.6.

In physiological conditions, arteries respond to increases in blood flow with a reduction of their wall stiffness and increases of their vessel diameter. Consequently, impedance decreases when blood flow increases, thus decreasing the energy consumed by the left ventricle. The nitric oxide release from endothelial cells has an active role in this dynamic and quick control of the arterial wall function. The stimulus on the endothelial cells is a combination of shear stress and strain originated by changes in the pumping function of the left ventricle (Ross Ethier and Simmons 2007).

Even though the endothelium is a single lining that limits the intraluminal space and the arterial wall, it is capable of arranging its cytoskeleton in response to changes in shear stress. This physiological condition is very different from that originated by the balloon catheter inflation. As previously reported, balloon catheter inflation determined several hemodynamic changes; blood displacement during the diastole being the main event. Increased diastolic blood flow in the aortic branches and in the abdominal aorta maintains the physiological direction, whereas flows are reversed during the diastolic period between the distal end of the balloon catheter and the aortic root (see figure 6.7).

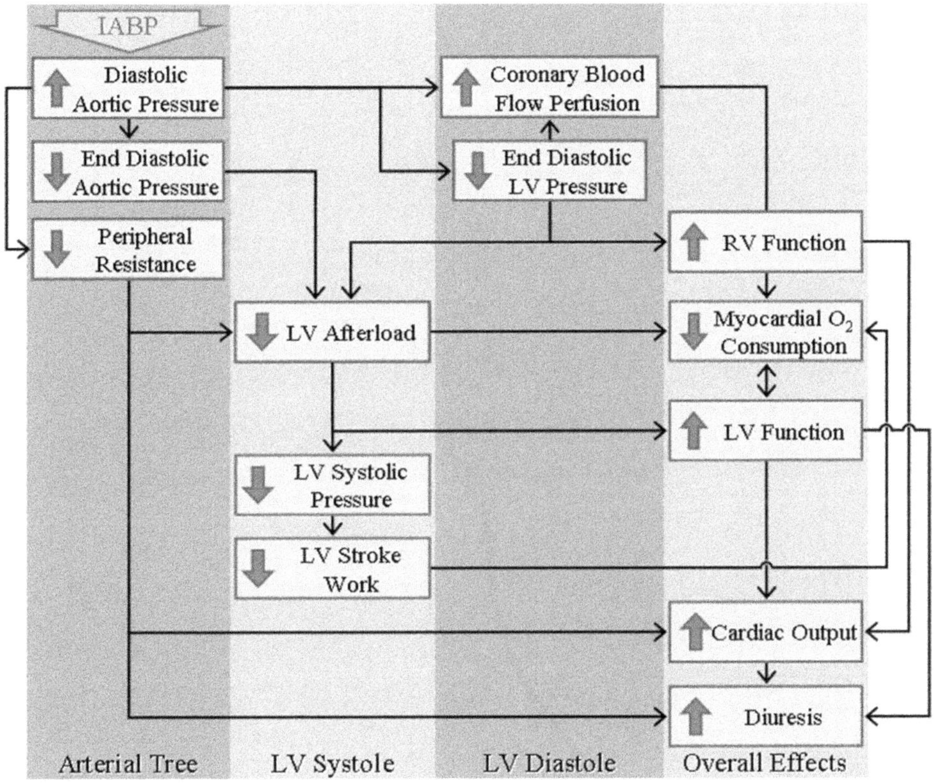

Figure 6.6. Block diagram showing the relationship between changes involved in the overall improvement due to intra-aortic counterpulsation. (a) Decreases of cardiac work through the reduction of the pressure against which the left ventricle is ejecting. (b) Increases in diastolic coronary blood flow. (c) Decreases in myocardial oxygen demand that result in a significant improvement of the pumping function. (d) An improvement of the mean aortic pressure level. Moreover, there is a blood flow augmentation in thoracic and abdominal arteries.

In an animal model of counterpulsation, experiments with a balloon catheter and pressure, flow and diameter sensors showed that increases in aortic reversal blood flow, which are associated with reversal and oscillatory shear stress, cause a smooth muscle contraction pattern accompanied by biomechanical changes (Bia *et al* 2008). These increases in reversal and oscillatory shear stress increase aortic wall viscosity and decrease isobaric arterial wall stiffness, together with a reduction of mean arterial diameter (Bia *et al* 2009). Moreover, aortic wall viscosity in the basal state (i.e. without intra-aortic counterpulsation) was $1.08 \pm 0.15 \times 10^5$ dyn s cm^{-2} versus $1.67 \pm 0.26 \times 10^5$ dyn s cm^{-2} during aortic counterpulsation ($p < 0.05$). On the other hand, the incremental elastic modulus (E_{inc}) shows the following changes ($p < 0.05$): the 2.60 ± 0.15 10^6 dyn cm^{-2} in basal state, decrease to $1.93 \pm 0.19 \times 10^6$ dyn cm^{-2} during aortic counterpulsation (Bia *et al* 2009).

These changes in the dynamic properties of the aortic wall take place in the thoracic aorta, in the space between the tip of the balloon catheter and the aortic root. The wall of this elastic artery has some differences with the descending human

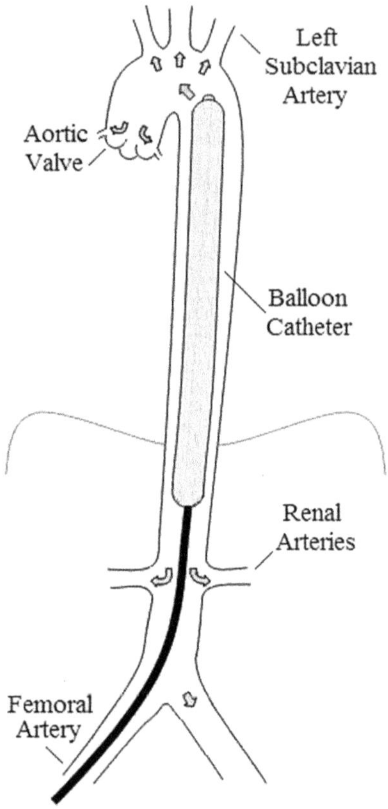

Figure 6.7. Blood flow (arrows) during balloon inflation due to the increase of the blood supplied in the aortic branches during the diastolic period, including coronary arteries. Reversed blood flow is observed in the aortic arch.

aorta at abdominal level. One of them is the difference in the collagen/elastin relationship: 0.49±0.04 in the ascending aorta versus 1.58±0.15 in the abdominal aorta (Fischer and Llaurado 1966). Furthermore, vasa vasorum are usually absent in the human abdominal aorta not observed in other adult mammals, while in the thoracic aorta vasa vasorum provide nutrition to the peripheral aortic layers (Wolinsky and Glagov 1969).

6.8 Enhanced external counterpulsation

Experiments and clinical use showed that the variation of physiological parameters contributed to explain the beneficial effects of arterial counterpulsation. ***External counterpulsation*** was first used in 1960 as a non-invasive procedure to treat myocardial ischemia, refractory to drugs. This technique was carried out by externally applying pressure during diastole using water-filled cylinders placed in the lower limbs of a patient, triggered by electrocardiography signals. The maximum applied external pressure was 250 mmHg (during approximately 250 ms), whereas the maximum negative applied pressure was −100 mmHg (Amsterdam *et al* 1977).

The hemodynamic improvement obtained with external counterpulsation was very poor and the method was abandoned. However, the intrinsic concept of the non-invasive counterpulsation remained. Three decades later, a modified version of this circulatory assistance method was reported as a technique to treat refractory myocardial ischemia. The ***enhanced external counterpulsation*** (EECP), which proved to be an adequate method to treat refractory myocardial ischemia, was introduced in clinical practice (Arora *et al* 1999).

Currently, EECP is achieved by inflating three sets of separate cuffs with atmospheric air, placed on the calves, and in the lower and upper thighs of the patient. The sequential compression begins in the cuffs placed around the calves and continues in the proximal direction. Once the three sets of cuffs are inflated at the end-diastole, they are deflated simultaneously. This sequence is synchronized with the heart cycle using a surface electrocardiogram. The pressures reached inside the cuffs are in the range of 200 and 300 mmHg (Bonetti *et al* 2003).

Currently, EEPC sessions are one hour long, once a week for 35 weeks. EECP is indicated for patients with symptomatic coronary artery disease that is refractory to medical treatment, and who are considered unsuitable candidates for myocardial revascularization. It has also been used to treat heart failure (Soran *et al* 1999).

The reported beneficial effects of EECP include: decrease of chest pain (angina pectoris), increase of exercise tolerance, increase of coronary perfusion, lower need of nitrates and an overall improved quality of life (Arora *et al* 1999, Michaels *et al* 2002). In table 6.3, the clinical effects of EECP are summarized.

The relief of angina pectoris using EECP is thought to be the result of an increase of arteriolar reactivity and arterial compliance (Levenson *et al* 2007). Furthermore, an improvement of coronary blood flow (Lawson *et al* 1992, 1996), combined with left ventricular systolic unloading, have been reported as other causes of the beneficial effects (Michaels *et al* 2002). On the other hand, adverse effects of EECP reported in the available literature include paresthesia, edema, skin abrasion, bruising, blistering, leg pain, back pain, among others (Arora *et al* 1999).

This non-invasive treatment of myocardial ischemia refractory to medical and surgical treatment is contraindicated in cases of decompensated heart failure, aortic insufficiency, severe peripheral artery disease, cardiac arrhythmias, severe hypertension, bleeding diathesis and pregnancy, myocardial infarction within the last six months, aortocoronary by-pass surgery, left main coronary trunk obstruction higher than 50%, percutaneous coronary intervention within six months, cardiac catheterization within two weeks, acute myocarditis, history of pulmonary embolisms, and history of aortic aneurisms (Arora *et al* 1999).

6.8.1 Effects of enhanced external counterpulsation on arterial wall function

EECP is similar to intra-aortic counterpulsation in terms of diastolic aortic pressure. However, EECP determines reversal blood flow all the way from the lower limbs; whose circulatory characteristics are different from the descending aorta. In fact, intra-aortic counterpulsation only reverses blood flow in the ascending aorta and the

Table 6.3. Beneficial effects of enhanced external counterpulsation.

(a)	Relief of angina pectoris (Zheng *et al* 1983, Arora *et al* 1999, Pettersson *et al* 2006, Erdling *et al* 2008).
(b)	Improvement of exercise tolerance (Arora *et al* 1999, Lawson *et al* 1996).
(c)	Reduction of myocardial perfusion defects (Lawson *et al* 1992).
(d)	Increase of coronary blood flow velocity (Michaels *et al* 2002).
(e)	Increase of intracoronary diastolic blood pressure (Michaels *et al* 2002).
(f)	Increase of plasma nitric oxide levels (Akhtar *et al* 2006).
(g)	Decrease of plasma endothelin-1 levels (Akhtar *et al* 2006).
(h)	Increase of atrial natriuretic peptide in blood (Taguchi *et al* 2004).
(i)	Arterial stiffness reduction (Nichols *et al* 2006).
(j)	Improvement of endothelial function (Bonetti *et al* 2003).
(k)	Enhanced quality of life (Feldman and Conti 2006).
(l)	Increased cardiac output (Soran *et al* 2002).
(m)	Decreased peripheral vascular resistance (Soran *et al* 2002).
(n)	Decreased myocardial oxygen consumption (Soran *et al* 2002).

aortic arch, while in the iliac arteries and downstream the diastolic blood flow increases preserving the physiological distal direction.

Since enhanced external counterpulsation is a method applied for longer periods of time than intra-aortic counterpulsation and the clinical indications are different, the individual obtained results cannot be compared.

Patients eligible for EECP treatment usually exhibit increased aortic stiffness due to aging and/or systemic hypertension. The augmented aortic stiffness is responsible for increases of oscillatory and reversal diastolic flows in peripheral arteries. Evidently, the conditions of unidirectional blood flow in peripheral arteries to which the endothelium function is usually exposed to disappear during EECP.

It is easy to quantify arterial wall stiffness in ambulatory patients that receive enhanced external counterpulsation, whereas a patient undergoing intra-aortic counterpulsation is not the ideal candidate for arterial function evaluation in clinical practice. In 2006, Nichols *et al* reported the improvement of the properties of the arterial wall after two months of enhanced external counterpulsation in patients with angina pectoris refractory to pharmacological treatment (Nichols *et al* 2006). A year later, Levenson *et al* published an interesting work where 30 patients were non-invasively counterpulsated. The authors demonstrated that after a 35 h routine of enhanced external counterpulsation, the β stiffness index significantly decreased with respect to values obtained before treatment ($P < 0.01$). According to data analysis, the obtained results were independent from systemic pressure levels and they attributed the elastic improvement to smooth muscle function changes (Levenson *et al* 2007).

More recently, Casey and Braith demonstrated that enhanced external counter-pulsation decreases arterial stiffness in the short- and long-term (Casey *et al* 2011, Braith *et al* 2012). The authors used pulse wave velocity calculations to evaluate arterial stiffness and observed that the stiffness of the aorta and the lower- and upper-limb arteries improved.

The beneficial effects of enhanced external counterpulsation have been attributed to the improvement of endothelial function, which is impaired by reversal of blood flow. This improvement could be the consequence of the increase in diastolic blood flow tending to recover the physiologic pattern (Hui *et al* 2010). The augmentation of the forward diastolic blood flow prevents the occurrence of reversal of blood flow and has important consequences on endothelial function. Nevertheless, an interesting work by Hashmi *et al* demonstrated that the improvement of endothelial function obtained after 35 h of enhanced external counterpulsation disappears one month after the seventh week of treatment (Hashemi *et al* 2008).

6.9 Final comments

Circulatory assistance involves any method capable of improving hemodynamic variables in patients suffering from a severe impairment of cardiac function that becomes refractory to medical treatment. During the last 30 years, a high level of safety and effectiveness of mechanical ventricular support of heart failure has been demonstrated by using different devices in high-risk patients (Kantrowitz *et al* 1995). Aortic counterpulsation attained using a balloon catheter is a technique in which the heart is in a series arrangement (Smith *et al* 1991) and has shown good performance in recent decades. Furthermore, other methods that use the same physiological mechanism have been developed, such as enhanced external counterpulsation and chronic balloon counterpulsation (Jeevanandam *et al* 2002).

Arterial function has barely been analyzed in counterpulsated patients with cardiac failure refractory to medical treatment. However, there are very interesting approaches that show paradoxical results, in which the increased stiffness of the arterial wall determines the best improvement in diastolic augmentation during aortic counterpulsation (Papaioannou *et al* 2004).

Arterial counterpulsation is by far a wide area of biomedical development. Future reports are necessary in order to clarify the correct use of: (a) enhanced external counterpulsation, (b) peri-aortic counterpulsation, and (c) abdominal counterpulsation.

References

Akhtar M, Wu G, Du Z, Zheng Z and Michaels A D 2006 Effect of external counterpulsation on plasma nitric oxide and endothelin-1 levels *Am. J. Cardiol.* **98** 28–30

Amsterdam E A, Lee G, Tonkon M J, DeMaria A N and Mason D T 1977 Noninvasive circulatory assistance by external counterpulsation *Advances in Heart and Disease* vol I ed T M de Dean (NY, USA: Grune & Statton) pp 209–19

Armentano R L, Bia D, Barmak W and Fischer E I C 2005 Systemic and pulmonary circulation: mechanical arterial dysfunction *Cardiovascular Failure: Pathophysiological Bases and Management* ed E I C Fischer, A Juffé Stein and J M Balaguer (Buenos Aires, Argentina: del Valle Ediciones) pp 159–70

Arora R R, Chou T M, Jain D, Fleishman B, Crawford L, KcKierman T and Nesto R W 1999 The multicenter study of enhanced external counterpulsation (MUST-EECP): effect of EECP on exercise-induced myocardial ischaemia and anginal episodes *J. Am. Coll. Cardiol.* **33** 1833–40

Bia D, Cabrera-Fischer E I, Zócalo Y and Armentano R L 2011 The endothelium modulates the arterial wall mechanical response to intra-aortic balloon counterpulsation: *in vivo* studies *Artif. Organ.* **35** 883–92

Bia D, Zócalo Y, Armentano R, Camus J, de Forteza E and Cabrera-Fischer E 2008 Increased reversal and oscillatory shear stress cause smooth muscle contraction-dependent changes in sheep aortic dynamics: role in aortic balloon pump circulatory support *Acta Physiol.* **192** 487–503

Bia D, Zócalo Y, Armentano R, de Forteza E and Cabrera-Fischer E 2009 Reversal blood flow component as determinant of the arterial functional capability: theoretical implications in physiological and therapeutic conditions *Artif. Organs* **33** 266–72

Bonetti P O, Colmes D R, Lerman A and Barsness G W 2003 Enhanced external counterpulsation for ischemic heart disease *J. Am. Coll. Cardiol.* **41** 1918–25

Braith R W, Casey D P and Beck D T 2012 Enhanced external counterpulsation for ischemic heart disease: a look behind the curtain *Exerc. Sport Sci. Rev.* **40** 145–52

Buckberg G D, Fixler D E, Archie J P and Hoffman J I 1972 Experimental subendocardial ischemia in dogs with normal coronary arteries *Circ. Res.* **30** 67–81

Casey D P, Darren T B, Nichols W W, Conti C R, Choi C Y, Khudus M A and Braith R W 2011 Effects of enhanced external counterpulsation on arterial stiffness and myocardial oxygen demand in patients with chronic angina pectoris *Am. J. Cardiol.* **107** 1466–72

Chachques J C, Radermercker M, Tolan M J, Fischer E I C, Grandjean P and Carpentier A 1996 Aortomyoplasty counterpulsation: experimental results and early clinical experience *Ann. Thorac. Surg.* **61** 420–5

Dumcius A, Bavarskis E, Chekanov V, Bytautas A and Girdauskas E 2001 Effects of thoracic aortomyoplasty using a new cardiomyostimulator for cardiac bioassist LD-PACE II, *Presented in the First Congress of the Cardiac Bioassist Association*, (*Lubeck, Germany* May 24–26)

Dumcius A, Bavarskis E, Chekanov V and Vysockas V 2002 Testing of the latissimus dorse muscle stimulation regimens in the experimental model of thoracic aortomyoplasty *Medicina* **38** 226–9

Erdling A, Bondesson S, Pettersson T and Edvinsson L 2008 Enhanced external counterpulsation in treatment of refractory angina pectoris: two year outcome and baseline factors associated with treatment failure *BMC Cardiovasc. Disord.* **8** 39–46

Feldman A M and Conti C R 2006 Prospective evaluation of EECP in congestive heart failure: the PEECH trial *J. Am. Coll. Cardiol.* **15** 37–44

Fischer E I C, Santana D B, Zócalo Y, Camus J, de Forteza E and Armentano R 2010 Effects of removing the adventitia on the mechanical properties of ovine femoral arteries *in vivo* and *in vitro Circ. J.* **74** 1014–22

Fischer E I C, Bia D, Camus J M, Zócalo Y, de Forteza E and Armentano R L 2008 Effects of intra-aortic counterpulsation on aortic wall energetics and damping: *in vivo* experiments *ASAIO J.* **54** 44–9

Fischer E I C, Willshaw P, Armentano R L, Besansón Delbo M I, Pichel R H and Favaloro R G 1985 Experimental acute right ventricular failure and right ventricular assist in the dog *J. Thorac. Cardiovasc. Surg.* **90** 580–5

Fischer E I C, Bia D, Zócalo Y, Wray S and Armentano R 2013 The adventitia layer modulates the arterial wall elastic response to intra-aortic counterpulsation: *in vivo* studies *Artif. Organs* **37** 1041–8

Fischer E I C, Barmak W and de Forteza E 2005 Aortic counterpulsation *Cardiovascular Failure: Pathophysiological Bases and Management* ed E I C Fischer, A Juffé Stein and J M Balaguer (Buenos Aires, Argentina: del Valle Ediciones) pp 159–70

Fischer E I C, Bia D, Zócalo Y and Armentano R L 2009 Smooth muscle-dependent changes in aortic wall dynamics during intra-aortic counterpulsation in an animal model of acute heart failure *Int. J. Artif. Organs* **32** 354–61

Fischer E I C, Christen A I, de Forteza E and Risk M R 1999 Dynamic abdominal and thoracic aortomyoplasty in heart failure: assessment of counterpulsation *Ann. Thorac. Surg.* **67** 1022–9

Fischer E I C, Armentano R L, Pessana F M, Graf S, Romero L, Christen A I, Simon A and Levenson J 2002a Endothelium-dependent arterial wall tone elasticity modulated by blood viscosity *Am. J. Physiol. Heart. Circ. Physiol.* **282** H389–94

Fischer E I C, Christen A I, Risk M R, Pessana F M and de Forteza E 2002b A new approach to assist postoperative heart failure in an animal model: juxta-aortic counterpulsation *Artif. Organs* **26** 819–26

Fischer E I C, de Forteza E, Risk M R, Nicolini G A, Camus J M and Pessana F M 2004 Juxtaaortic counterpulsation: comparison with intraaortic counterpulsation in an animal model of acute heart failure *ASAIO J.* **50** 311–5

Fischer G M and Llaurado J G 1966 Collagen and elastin content in canine arteries selected from functionally different vascular bed *Circ. Res.* **XIX** 394–9

Hashemi M, Hoseinbalam M and Khazaei M 2008 Long-term effect of enhanced external counterpulsation on endothelial function in the patients with intractable angina *Heart Lung Circ.* **17** 383–7

Hazelrigg S R, Auer J E and Seifert P E 1992 Experience in 100 transthoracic balloon pumps *Ann. Thorac. Surg.* **54** 528–32

Hui J C K, Lawson W E and Barsness G 2010 EECP in the treatment of endothelial dysfunction: preventing progression of cardiovascular disease *J. Geriatr. Cardiol.* **7** 79–87

Jeevanandam V, Jayakar D and Anderson A S 2002 Circulatory assistance with a permanent implantable IABP: initial human experience *Circulation* **106** 183–8

Jett K G, Picote A L and Clark R E 1987 Circulatory support for right ventricular dysfunction *J. Thorac. Cardiovasc. Surg.* **94** 95–103

Kantrowitz A, Bridgewater B and Au J 1995 Intra-aortic balloon pumping for assisted circulation: new techniques and new prospects *Assisted Circulation of Felix Unger* (Berlin, Heidelberg: Springer) pp 12–35 (printed in Germany)

Kantrowitz A 1953 Experimental augmentation of coronary flow by retardation of the arterial pressure pulse *Surgery* **34** 678–87

Kantrowitz A and McKinnon W M P 1959 The experimental use of the diaphragm as an auxiliary myocardium *Surg. Forum* **9** 266–8

Kantrowitz A, Tjonneland S, Free P S, Phillips S J, Butner A N and Sherman J L 1968 Initial clinical experience with intra-aortic balloon pumping in cardiogenic shock *J. Am. Med. Assoc.* **203** 135–40

Kantrowitz A 2001 Introduction of left ventricular assitance *Cardiovascular Failure: Pathophysiological Bases and Management* ed E I C Fischer, A I Christen and J C Trainini (Buenos Aires, Argentina: FURGF) pp 255–74

Kantrowitz A 1990 Origins of intraaortic balloon pumping *Ann. Thorac. Surg.* **50** 672–4

Kawaguchi O, Pae W E, Daily B B and Pierce W S 1999 Ventriculoarterial coupling with intra-aortic balloon pump in acute ischemic heart failure *J. Thorac. Cardiovasc. Surg.* **117** 164–71

Khir A W, Price S, Henein M Y, Parker K H and Pepper J R 2003 Intra-aortic balloon pumping: effects on left ventricular diastolic function *Eur. J. Cardiothorac. Surg.* **24** 277–82

Kim S Y, Euler D E, Jacobs W R, Montoya A, Sullivan H J, Lonchyna V A and Pifarré R 1996 Arterial impedance in patients during intraaortic balloon counterpulsation *Ann. Thorac. Surg.* **61** 888–94

Lawson W, JCK H, Soroff H S, Zheng Z S, Kayden D S, Sasvary D, Atkins H and Cohn P F 1992 Efficacy of enhanced external counterpulsation in the treatment of angina pectoris *Am. J. Cardiol.* **70** 859–62

Lawson W E, JCK H, Zheng Z S, Burger L, Jiang L, Lillis O, Soroff H S and Cohn P F 1996 Can angiographic findings predict which coronary patients will benefit from enhanced external counterpulsation? *J. Am. Coll. Cardiol.* **77** 1107–9

Levenson J, Simon A, Megnien J L, Chironi G, Gariepy J, Pernollet M G, Craiem D and Lliou M C 2007 Effects of enhanced external counterpulsation on carotid circulation in patients with coronary artery disease *Cardiology* **108** 104–10

Michaels A D, Accad M, Ports T A and Grossman W 2002 Left ventricular systolic unloading and augmentation of intracoronary pressure and Doppler flow during enhanced external counterpulsation *Circulation* **106** 1237–42

Miller D C, Moreno Cabral R J, Stinson E B, Shinn J A and Shumway N 1980 Pulmonary artery balloon counterpulsation for acute right ventricular failure *J. Thorac. Cardiovasc. Surg.* **80** 760–3

Nichols W W, Estrada J C, Braith R W, Owens K and Conti C R 2006 Enhanced external counterpulsation treatment improves arterial wall properties and wave reflection characteristics in patients with refractory angina *J. Am. Coll. Cardiol.* **48** 1208–14

Papaioannou T G, Mathioulakis D S, Stamatelopoulos K S, Gialafos E J, Lekakis J P, Nanas J, Stamatelopoulos S F and Tsangaris S G 2004 New aspects on the role of blood pressure and arterial stiffness in mechanical assistance by intra-aortic balloon pump: *in vitro* data and their application in clinical practice *Artif. Organs* **28** 717–27

Papaioannou T G 2005 Bases of intra-aortic counterpulsation *Cardiovascular Failure: Pathophysiological Bases and Management* ed E I C Fischer, A Juffé Stein and J M Balaguer (Buenos Aires, Argentina: del Valle Ediciones) pp 147–58

Pettersson T, Bondesson S, Cojocaru D, Ohlsson O, Wackenfors A and Edvinson L 2006 One year follow-up of patients with refractory angina pectoris treated with enhanced external counterpulsation *BMC Cardiovasc. Disord.* **6** 29–35

Ross Ethier C and Simmons C A 2007 *Introductory Biomechanics: From Cells to Organisms* (Cambridge: Cambridge University Press)

Santini F and Mazzucco A 1997 Transthoracic intraaortic counterpulsation: a simple method for balloon catheter positioning *Ann. Thorac. Surg.* **64** 859–60

Smith B, Barnea O, Moore T W and Jaron D 1991 Optimal control system for the intraaortic balloon pump *Med. Biol. Eng. Comput.* **29** 180–4

Soran O, Crawford L E, Schneider V M and Feldman A M 1999 Enhanced external counterpulsation in the management of patients with cardiovascular disease *Clin. Cardiol.* **22** 173–8

Soran O, Fleishman B, Demrco T, Grossman W, Schneider V M, Manzo K, Lame P A and Feldman A M 2002 Enhanced external counterpulsation in patients with heart failure: a multicenter feasibility study *Congest. Heart Fail.* **8** 204–8

Stefanadis C, Dernellis J, Tsiamis E, Stratos C, Kallikazaros I and Toutouzas P 1998 Aortic function in patients during intra-aortic balloon pumping determined by the pressure-diameter relation *J. Thorac. Cardiovasc. Surg.* **116** 1052–9

Taguchi I, Ogawa K, Kanaya T, Matsuda R, Kuga H and Nakatsugawa M 2004 Effects of enhanced external counterpulsation on hemodynamics and its mechanism *Circ. J.* **68** 1030–4

Webb C A, Weyker P D and Flynn B C 2015 Management of intra-aortic balloon pumps *Semin. Cardiothorac. Vasc. Anesth.* **19** 106–21

Wolinsky H and Glagov S 1969 Comparison of abdominal and thoracic aortic medial structure in mammals *Circ. Res.* **XXV** 677–86

Zheng Z S, Li T M, Kambic H, Chen G H, Yu L Q, Cai S R, Zhan C Y, Chen Y C, Wo S X and Chen G W 1983 Sequential external counterpulsation (SECP) in China *Trans. Am. Soc. Artif. Intern. Organs* **29** 599–603

IOP Publishing

Ricardo L Armentano, Edmundo I Cabrera Fischer and Leandro J Cymberknop

Chapter 7

Arterial wall modelization in the time and frequency domain

Ricardo L Armentano and Leandro J Cymberknop

7.1 Linear elastic theory

Solid bodies are not completely rigid, but they deform when facing forces that do not displace them, i.e. a part of a body moves with respect to another part of the same body. A body that recovers its original shape when the external forces stop is a *perfectly elastic* body. On the other hand, if it retains any permanent deformation after the forces are removed, it is a *plastic* solid.

The theory of elasticity explains the relationship between applied forces and the consequent deformations. The applied force per unit area is called *stress*, and the change in dimensions due to the stress is known as *strain*. A solid can withstand stresses, whereas liquids cannot: when faced with stress they flow, viscously or non-viscously. A force applied to a solid deforms it, and a force applied to a liquid makes it flow (Fung 1981, 1984). Often, certain materials are found that have properties similar to solids and to viscous fluids. The deformation in these materials not only depends on the stress, but also the frequency at which it is applied. These substances are called *viscoelastic materials*.

On the other hand, when there is movement, if there is a change in speed there is acceleration, and the force needed to produce that acceleration is the product of acceleration and mass. This is known as the *principle of mass*. When a viscoelastic material is subjected to tension, it can be decomposed into three basic elements: inertia, viscosity and elasticity (Peterson *et al* 1960).

7.1.1 Elasticity

Elasticity is the property of a body being able to return to its original shape after being deformed. A perfectly elastic body can be deformed in all kinds of ways, but it will regain its original dimensions as soon as the external forces cease, whereas its volume may or may not be altered by the deformations (Milnor 1982).

doi:10.1088/2053-2563/aafb0dch7

A perfectly elastic solid obeys Hooke's law, so it is also called *Hookean solid*. This law states that stress is linearly proportional to strain:

$$\sigma = E \cdot \varepsilon \Rightarrow E = \frac{\sigma}{\varepsilon}, \tag{7.1}$$

where E, the proportionality constant, is the *elastic modulus* or *Young's modulus*.

7.1.2 Viscoelasticity

Viscoelastic bodies, as described above, experience two phenomena: *stress relaxation* and *creep*, and as a consequence of them, they show hysteresis when subjected to cyclic stress and strain (see chapter 3). Stress relaxation is characterized by the decay of stress in a body with a constant deformation, and creep is the slow and prolonged deformation of a body with a constant stress. In turn, creep and stress relaxation are related to vasomotor tone. Another phenomenon that is also related to vasomotor tone and viscoelastic behavior is hysteresis. Hysteresis is seen when a body is subjected to a cyclical load: if the stress–strain relationship when loading is somewhat different to unloading, hysteresis is present (figure 7.1). Virtually all materials exhibit these phenomena, but creep and stress relaxation are not as important factors in non-biological materials, except for elastomers and some synthetic materials. Creep, stress relaxation and hysteresis are evident in biological materials, especially in tissues that contain muscle (Dobrin 1978, Fung 1981).

The study of the mechanical properties of blood vessels calls for the true understanding of the limitations of the experiments through linear elastic theory. Firstly, blood vessels and most biological materials do not have a mechanical ideal behavior, i.e. they do not obey Hooke's law, their stress–strain relationship is nonlinear.

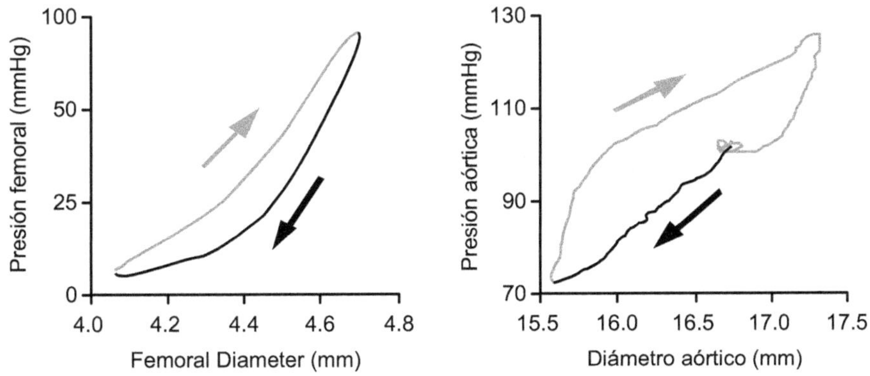

Figure 7.1. Left panel: pressure–diameter relationship showing the hysteresis enclosed area in an *in situ* isolated femoral artery of a dog. When blood flows into the artery, pressure and diameter increase (gray line). Blood then drains towards the distal territories and both variables decrease, although larger diameters can be observed for equal pressure values (black line). Right panel: stress–strain relationship for the descending thoracic aorta of a dog. As in the left panel, the systolic period (gray line) and the diastolic period (black line) have different paths.

7.2 Implementation of models in arterial mechanics

The construction of a model is a *modus operandi* in science. Once a model is described, parameters can be estimated in order to define it. The estimation of parameters allows one to characterize the behavior of a system, and the behavior of a system can be predicted through its parameters (Peterson *et al* 1960, Cobelli *et al* 1984).

Force, length and thickness are variables used to characterize the elasticity of blood vessels. When frequency is included among the observed variables, viscoelasticity can also be analyzed. Classical studies to determine the mechanical properties of blood vessels have been usually conducted in *in vitro* preparations, on segments, rings or helicoidal sections of arteries or veins. Changes in forces and lengths can be directly measured in these set-ups, but certain precautions must be considered to preserve the normal state of the vessel. Therefore, tissue samples must be kept in solutions that mimic their physiological environment in terms of ionic content, pH, O_2 and CO_2 partial pressures and temperatures (Milnor 1982).

The study of blood vessels has included elastic linear theory, and its two hypotheses: infinitely small deformations and continuous, uniform and homogeneous material structure. Dobrin has recently shown that the elastic laminae of vessels have a uniform distribution in the circumferential and longitudinal directions, and, even if there is an evident histological heterogeneity, the mechanical behavior of the arterial wall can be considered homogeneous (Dobrin 1999).

In 1954, Burton stated that parietal stress can be arbitrarily separated into three components, defined as: (a) elastic stress, that opposes the strain away from the basal circumference of the vessel, (b) active stress, which depends on the vasomotor tone and is a result of the contractile activity of the smooth muscle cells, and (c) interfacial tension (Burton 1954). It is now evident that there exists a passive elastic behavior, where the passive elements (i.e. elastin and collagen) are stressed when opposing to stretching, and an active elastic behavior, where the active elements have an ability to generate stress per se (i.e. smooth muscle cells). The study of the arterial wall can also be divided into static studies (where stress and strain changes are slow, or done step by step) and dynamic studies (where the frequency at which experiments are conducted is taken into account) (Bergel 1961a, 1961b). In order to determine the passive and active elastic behaviors, static studies are carried out; when viscosity, inertia and frequency are considered, the dynamic behavior is observed (table 7.1).

To be able to understand the elastic behavior of the arterial wall, it is necessary to know the composition of its elastic materials and how these materials interact. A detailed histologic structure description can be found in chapter 1. The predominant elastic materials of the artery walls are collagen and elastin, which are arranged as fibers, even though elastin tends to form adjacent laminae. Smooth muscle is another important component of the wall of the vessels, even though it is not considered an elastic material per se (McDonald 1974).

The simplest model to describe the mechanical properties of the arterial wall is an elastic component in series with a contractile element (SEC, *series elastic component*

Table 7.1 Mechanical properties of the arterial wall.

Static Behavior ($\omega = 0$) $E_{(\omega)} = E_{real}$	Passive Elastic Behavior	Elastin Elastic Modulus	
		Collagen Elastic Modulus	
		Relaxed Smooth Muscle Elastic Modulus (negligible)	
	Active Elastic Behavior	Activated Smooth Muscle Elastic Modulus	
Dynamic Behavior ($\omega \neq 0$) $E_{(\omega)} = E_{real} + E_{imag}$	Viscous Behavior	Viscous Modulus	Resting Smooth Muscle Viscous Modulus
			Active Smooth Muscle Viscous Modulus
	Inertial Behavior	Inertial Modulus	

ω: frequency. $E_{(\omega)}$: Complex Elastic Modulus.

and CE, *contractile element*, respectively). A second elastic element is connected in parallel to represent the connective tissue in the vascular wall (PEC, *parallel elastic component*). Two configurations are possible when combining these three elements (see figure 7.2). Model I is generally called the Voigt model, and model II, Hill model or modified Maxwell model (Dobrin 1978), even though its correct denomination is Kelvin model.

The Kelvin model best describes the mechanical properties of the arterial wall, also known as the modified Maxwell model (Dobrin and Canfield 1973, 1977). The PEC represents elastin and collagen fibers and is associated with the passive behavior of the artery. The SEC represents smooth muscle and can be defined as the algebraic sum of the extension of the compliant structures that are in series with the force-generating element (e.g. the tendon is in series with skeletal muscle, crossbridges are in series with muscle fibers). The CE is the group of myofibrils that contract. The protein titin has been linked to viscous properties in skeletal muscle and cardiomyocytes (Minajeva *et al* 2001, Kulke *et al* 2001). A new titin-like protein, smitin, has been recently described. It may have a central role in the arrangement of myosin filaments in the contractile apparatus of smooth, visceral and vascular muscle (Kim and Keller 2002). Even if the active elastic behavior is described through the study of the CE, it is not possible to separate it from the SEC. Therefore, it is described as a CE–SEC group (Barra *et al* 1993).

7.2.1 The stress–strain relationship in the arterial wall

The most general approach to characterize the elasticity of the arterial wall is through linear elastic theory, which assumes homogeneity, incompressibility and isotropy of the arterial wall (Bergel 1961a, Gow and Taylor 1968, McDonald 1974,

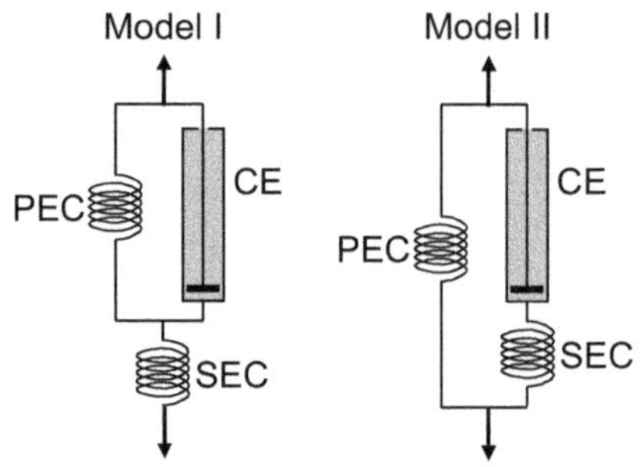

Figure 7.2. Three-element models of the arterial wall, made up of a contractile element (CE), a series elastic component (SEC) and a parallel elastic component (PEC). Model I is also known as the Voigt model, model II as the Kelvin model (also modified Maxwell model and Hill model).

Cox 1978a, 1978b, 1979, Pagani *et al* 1979, Yano *et al* 1989, Armentano *et al* 1991, 1995a). As described above, a Hookean material obeys Hooke's law:

$$\sigma = E \cdot \varepsilon, \tag{7.2}$$

where E is the elastic modulus, constant and unique, σ is the stress and ε is strain. Since the stress–strain relationship of the arterial wall is nonlinear, it is impossible to describe it with only one elastic modulus, thus the concept of *incremental modulus* is introduced:

$$\frac{d\sigma}{d\varepsilon} = E_{inc}. \tag{7.3}$$

Assuming a cylindrical geometry for the aorta, and choosing the main directions ($\breve{r}$, radial; $\breve{\theta}$, tangential and $\breve{z}$, longitudinal) and the associated stresses (σ_{rr}, $\sigma_{\theta\theta}$ and σ_{zz}) and strains (ε_{rr}, $\varepsilon_{\theta\theta}$ and ε_{zz}), the stress–strain relationship in a cylindrical coordinate system can be described as:

$$\begin{aligned}
\sigma_{rr} &= \frac{E \cdot (1-\nu)}{(1+\nu)\cdot(1-2\nu)} \cdot \varepsilon_{rr} + \frac{E \cdot \nu}{(1+\nu)\cdot(1-2\nu)} \cdot \varepsilon_{\theta\theta} \\
&\quad + \frac{E \cdot \nu}{(1+\nu)\cdot(1-2\nu)} \cdot \varepsilon_{zz} \\
\sigma_{\theta\theta} &= \frac{E \cdot \nu}{(1+\nu)\cdot(1-2\nu)} \cdot \varepsilon_{rr} + \frac{E \cdot (1-\nu)}{(1+\nu)\cdot(1-2\nu)} \cdot \varepsilon_{\theta\theta} \\
&\quad + \frac{E \cdot \nu}{(1+\nu)\cdot(1-2\nu)} \cdot \varepsilon_{zz} \\
\sigma_{zz} &= \frac{E \cdot \nu}{(1+\nu)\cdot(1-2\nu)} \cdot \varepsilon_{rr} + \frac{E \cdot \nu}{(1+\nu)\cdot(1-2\nu)} \cdot \varepsilon_{\theta\theta} \\
&\quad + \frac{E \cdot (1-\nu)}{(1+\nu)\cdot(1-2\nu)} \cdot \varepsilon_{zz},
\end{aligned} \tag{7.4}$$

where

$$C_{11} = \frac{E \cdot (1 - \nu)}{(1 + \nu) \cdot (1 - 2\nu)} \text{ y } C_{12} = \frac{E \cdot \nu}{(1 + \nu) \cdot (1 - 2\nu)} \tag{7.5}$$

and

$$\begin{aligned} \sigma_{rr} &= C_{11} \cdot \varepsilon_{rr} + C_{12} \cdot \varepsilon_{\theta\theta} + C_{12} \cdot \varepsilon_{zz} \\ \sigma_{\theta\theta} &= C_{12} \cdot \varepsilon_{rr} + C_{11} \cdot \varepsilon_{\theta\theta} + C_{12} \cdot \varepsilon_{zz} \\ \sigma_{zz} &= C_{12} \cdot \varepsilon_{rr} + C_{12} \cdot \varepsilon_{\theta\theta} + C_{11} \cdot \varepsilon_{zz} \end{aligned} \tag{7.6}$$

where υ is Poisson's ratio. Subtracting the first two equations of equation (7.6):

$$\sigma_{\theta\theta} - \sigma_{rr} = (C_{11} - C_{12}) \cdot (\varepsilon_{\theta\theta} - \varepsilon_{rr}) \tag{7.7}$$

where

$$C_{11} - C_{12} = \frac{E \cdot (1 - \nu)}{(1 + \nu) \cdot (1 - 2\nu)} - \frac{E \cdot \nu}{(1 + \nu) \cdot (1 - 2\nu)} = \frac{E}{(1 + \nu)}. \tag{7.8}$$

Substituting in equation (7.7), equation (7.8) becomes:

$$\sigma_{\theta\theta} - \sigma_{rr} = \frac{E}{1 + \mu}(\varepsilon_{\theta\theta} - \varepsilon_{rr}) \tag{7.9}$$

and the elastic modulus can be calculated as:

$$E = (1 + \nu)\frac{\sigma_{\theta\theta} - \sigma_{rr}}{\varepsilon_{\theta\theta} - \varepsilon_{rr}}. \tag{7.10}$$

If the aortic wall is considered incompressible, a Poisson's ratio of 0.5 must be adopted, but if incremental changes are considered, the elastic module in equation (7.10) can be expressed as:

$$E_{inc} = 1.5\frac{\Delta(\sigma_{\theta\theta} - \sigma_{rr})}{\Delta(\varepsilon_{\theta\theta} - \varepsilon_{rr})}. \tag{7.11}$$

Incompressibility requires a null sum of strains:

$$\varepsilon_{rr} + \varepsilon_{\theta\theta} + \varepsilon_{zz} = 0 \tag{7.12}$$

therefore the sum of incremental strains is also null

$$\Delta\varepsilon_{rr} + \Delta\varepsilon_{\theta\theta} + \Delta\varepsilon_{zz} = 0. \tag{7.13}$$

Moreover, if ε_{zz} is constant:

$$\varepsilon_{zz} = \text{constant} \Rightarrow \Delta\varepsilon_{zz} = 0 \Rightarrow \Delta\varepsilon_{rr} = -\Delta\varepsilon_{\theta\theta} \tag{7.14}$$

therefore:

$$E_{inc} = 1.5\frac{\Delta(\sigma_{\theta\theta} - \sigma_{rr})}{2 \cdot \Delta\varepsilon_{\theta\theta}} = 0.75\frac{\Delta(\sigma_{\theta\theta} - \sigma_{rr})}{\Delta\varepsilon_{\theta\theta}}. \tag{7.15}$$

The difference ($\sigma_{\theta\theta} - \sigma_{rr}$) is the combined stress (σ) of the tangential and radial stresses:

$$\sigma_{\theta\theta} - \sigma_{rr} = \sigma \tag{7.16}$$

and $\Delta\varepsilon_{\theta\theta}$ can be represented as:

$$\Delta\varepsilon_{\theta\theta} = \frac{\Delta R}{R} = \Delta\varepsilon, \tag{7.17}$$

where R is the average parietal radius between the external and internal radii (r_e and r_i, respectively):

$$R = \frac{r_e + r_i}{2} \tag{7.18}$$

and therefore, in general terms, the incremental modulus becomes:

$$E_{inc} = 0.75\frac{\Delta\sigma}{\Delta R} \cdot R \tag{7.19}$$

and when incremental changes tend to zero, they can be represented as derivatives:

$$E_{inc} = 0.75 \underset{\Delta\varepsilon \to 0}{Lim} \frac{\Delta\sigma}{\Delta\varepsilon} \Rightarrow E_{inc} = 0.75\frac{d\sigma}{d\varepsilon}. \tag{7.20}$$

7.2.1.1 Stress

The combination of the radial and tangential stresses can be calculated from the internal and external pressures of a cylinder (P_i and P_e, respectively) (Pagani *et al* 1979). The radial ($\breve{r}$) and tangential ($\breve{\theta}$) components are considered:

$$\begin{aligned} \sigma_{\theta\theta} &= \left(\frac{P_i \cdot r_i^2 - P_e \cdot r_e^2}{r_e^2 - r_i^2}\right) + \left(\frac{P_i - P_e}{r_e^2 - r_i^2} \cdot \frac{r_e^2 \cdot r_i^2}{R^2}\right) \\ \sigma_{rr} &= \left(\frac{P_i \cdot r_i^2 - P_e \cdot r_e^2}{r_e^2 - r_i^2}\right) - \left(\frac{P_i - P_e}{r_e^2 - r_i^2} \cdot \frac{r_e^2 \cdot r_i^2}{R^2}\right). \end{aligned} \tag{7.21}$$

If the external pressure is considered null, since intrathoracic pressure is close enough to intraluminal pressure, the equations in equation (7.21) are simplified:

$$\begin{aligned} \sigma_{\theta\theta} &= P_i\left(\frac{r_i^2}{r_e^2 - r_i^2}\right) + P_i\left(\frac{r_e^2 \cdot r_i^2}{r_e^2 - r_i^2} \cdot \frac{1}{R^2}\right) \\ \sigma_{rr} &= P_i\left(\frac{r_i^2}{r_e^2 - r_i^2}\right) - P_i\left(\frac{r_e^2 \cdot r_i^2}{r_e^2 - r_i^2} \cdot \frac{1}{R^2}\right), \end{aligned} \tag{7.22}$$

therefore composite stress can be expressed as:

$$\sigma = \sigma_{\theta\theta} - \sigma_{rr} = 2P\frac{(r_e \cdot r_i)^2}{r_e^2 - r_i^2} \cdot \frac{1}{R^2} \tag{7.23}$$

where P is the aortic pressure.

$$\sigma = 2P\frac{(r_i \cdot r_e)^2}{r_e^2 - r_i^2} \cdot \frac{1}{R^2}. \qquad (7.24)$$

On the other hand, in order to calculate stress, the internal radius (r_i) must be known. Assuming a constant *in vivo* arterial wall volume, r_i can be calculated from the external radius (r_e) measured experimentally, the weight (W) and the length (L) of an arterial segment (Dobrin and Rovick 1969):

$$V = \frac{W}{\delta} = \pi \cdot L(r_e^2 - r_i^2) \qquad (7.25)$$

$$r_i = \sqrt{r_e^2 - \frac{V}{\pi \cdot L}} \qquad (7.26)$$

where V is the calculated volume, assuming a density $\delta = 1.06\,\mathrm{g\,cm^{-3}}$.

7.2.1.2 Strain

The appropriate calculation for strain requires a reference value, R_0, an average parietal radius measured experimentally at an aortic pressure of 25 mmHg (Dobrin and Rovick 1969). Strain is calculated as:

$$\varepsilon = R/R_0. \qquad (7.27)$$

7.3 Elastic passive behavior

The elastic passive behavior is determined by the elastic behavior of the passive constituents of the arterial wall. The passive elastic predominant elements of the arterial wall are collagen and elastin. Vascular smooth muscle is overlooked as an elastic material (McDonald 1974). The involvement of collagen and elastin in the mechanical properties has been extensively studied *in vitro* (Cox 1976a, 1976b, Dobrin and Rovick 1969, Dobrin 1984, Ling and Chow 1977, Price 1984, Roach and Burton 1957). The nonlinearity of the passive elastic response was explained by Cox, through a collagen fiber recruitment function, i.e. the proportion of collagen fibers that participate in the mechanical response to a given transmural pressure (Cox 1978a, 1978b, 1979). The use of animal models to study the stress–strain relationship was introduced by Pagani *et al* (1979). Our laboratory works with chronically instrumented animals, which allowed to determine values for the elastic moduli of elastin and collagen fibers of a conscious animal (Armentano *et al* 1991), which were comparable to those found *in vitro*.

7.3.1 Nonlinearity of the stress–strain relationship

Since the stress–strain relationship is nonlinear, the passive elastic response cannot be described with a single elastic modulus. The most used models include a collagen

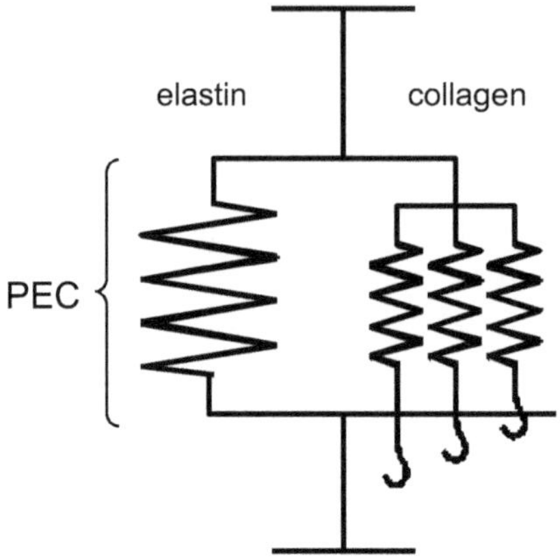

Figure 7.3. Schematic representation of the parallel elastic component (PEC). The collagen fiber recruitment as a function of strain is shown using the disconnecting hook model of Wiederhielm (1965). The collagen fiber recruitment function is represented by the number of hooked springs at different strains, simulating the elastic behavior of collagen fibers, $E_C \times f_C$ (Barra *et al* 1993).

and elastine fiber element in parallel with smooth muscle (PEC). Cox demonstrated in *in vitro* experiences that the difference in mechanical properties among different sites of the arterial tree were due to the proportion of collagen fibers acting against parietal stress. This hypothesis leads to the development of a conscious-animal model to determine the passive elastic modulus (E_{PEC}) of the arterial wall (Armentano *et al* 1991):

$$E_{PEC} = E_E + E_C \cdot f_C, \tag{7.28}$$

where E_E and E_C are the elastic moduli of elastin and collagen, respectively, and f_C is the proportion of collagen fibers that withstands the parietal stress at a given strain.

In the model represented in figure 7.3, the passive stress is:

$$\sigma_{PEC} = \sigma_E + \sigma_C, \tag{7.29}$$

where σ_{PEC} is the total passive stress, and σ_E and σ_C are the stresses taken on by elastin and collagen, respectively.

7.3.2 Elastic modulus of elastin fibers (E_E)

At low pressures, the resistance to stretching is taken on almost exclusively by elastin fibers (Roach and Burton 1957), exhibiting a linear stress–strain relationship. Beyond a certain stress value, a *break-point*, the stress–strain relationship curves upwards as more collagen fibers are recruited (Armentano *et al* 1991, Cabrera Fischer *et al* 1991). This break-point is found through successive linear regressions that consider more data in each iteration. The break-point is the stress value with the highest correlation coefficient (figure 7.4). Below the break-point stress, the elastic response of the arterial wall is linear and can be adjusted to a model where E_E is the gradient. Thus, the stress–strain relationship for elastin fibers:

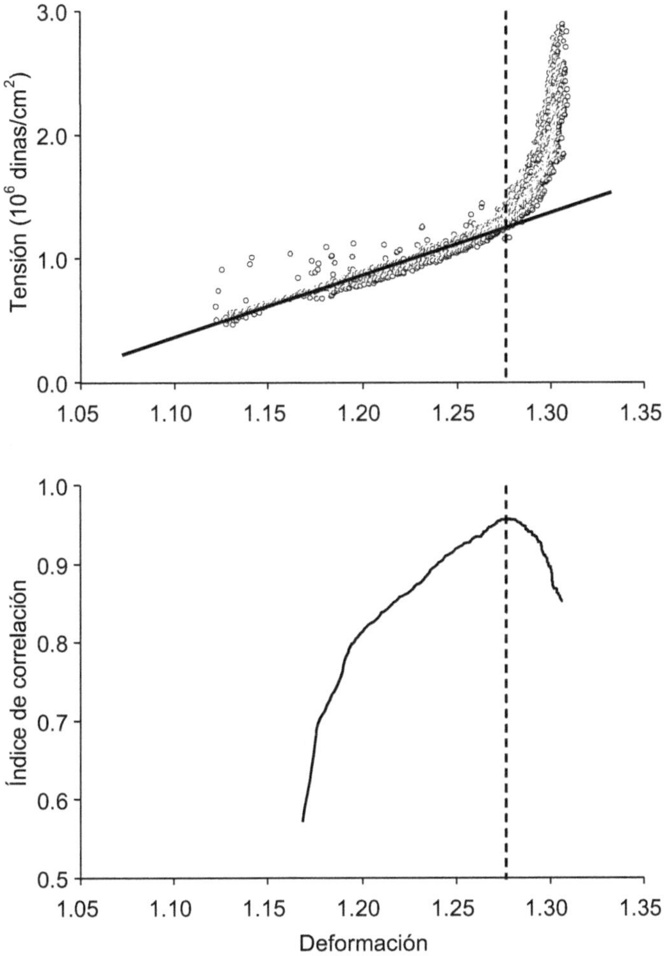

Figure 7.4. Determination of the break-point of the transition from elastin to collagen. It is found through successive linear regressions that consider more data in each iteration. The break-point (dotted line) is the stress value with the highest correlation coefficient (lower panel), and it indicates the end of the linear behavior of the stress–strain relationship (Armentano *et al* 1991).

$$\sigma_E = E_E \cdot (\varepsilon - \varepsilon_{0E}), \tag{7.30}$$

where ε_{0E} is the x-intercept, i.e. the strain at zero stress.

7.3.3 Elastic modulus of collagen fibers (E_C)

The elastic response of collagen fibers can be found by separating the stress–strain relationship of elastin from the total passive stress–strain relationship:

$$\sigma_C = \sigma_{PEC} - \sigma_E = E_C \cdot f_C \cdot \varepsilon. \tag{7.31}$$

In order to calculate E_C, the values calculated from equation (7.30) are subtracted from the measured stress–strain relationship for all strains (see figure 7.5). Collagen

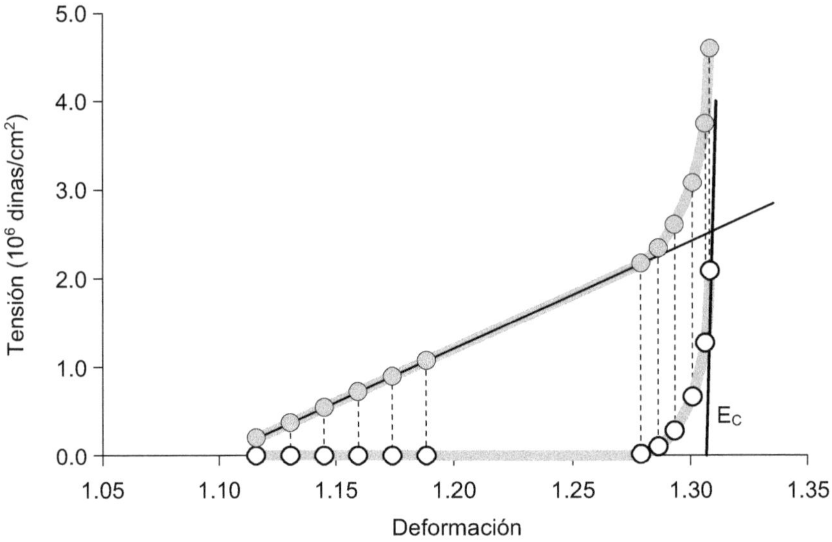

Figure 7.5. Determination of the stress–strain relationship for collagen fibers. The subtraction between the total passive stress–strain relationship (gray dots) and the straight line that represents the elastic modulus of elastin (E_E) determines the stress–strain relationship for collagen (white dots). The gradient at high stresses represents the elastic modulus of collagen fibers (E_C) (Armentano *et al* 1991).

fiber recruitment has been modeled as springs that become hooked as strains grow (figure 7.3), and the formula $E_C \times f_C$ has been adopted as the *recruitment function* (Barra *et al* 1993).

7.3.4 Recruitment function of collagen fibers (f_C)

Equation (7.31) states the stress–strain relationship of collagen fibers determined by E_C and f_C, which represents the resistance to stretching due to both the rigidity and the arrangement of collagen fibers. At high stresses all collagen fibers are considered recruited, and E_C can be calculated as the gradient of the steepest stress–strain relationship. To model the elastic response of collagen, a normal morphology function is proposed to represent the recruitment of collagen fibers as a function of strain (Armentano *et al* 1995a):

$$f_C = c_1 \cdot \tan\left(\frac{\varepsilon - c_2}{c_3}\right), \tag{7.32}$$

where c_1, c_2 and c_3 are the constant obtained from the nonlinear adjustment. Thus, replacing equation (7.32) in equation (7.31):

$$\sigma_C = E_C \cdot f_C \cdot \varepsilon = E_C \cdot c_1 \cdot \tan\left(\frac{\varepsilon - c_2}{c_3}\right) \cdot \varepsilon. \tag{7.33}$$

At low stresses, f_C is close to zero, since the collagen fibers do not withstand any stress (Burton 1954). At maximum stress, f_C is also maximal, since 100% of fibers are recruited to withstand stress, i.e. the parietal stretching.

This approach has been successfully used to describe the elastic behavior of collagen and elastin in conscious dogs (Armentano *et al* 1991). This work concludes that the elastic passive behavior is defined as:

$$\sigma_{PEC} = E_E \cdot (\varepsilon - \varepsilon_{0E}) + E_C \cdot f_C \cdot \varepsilon. \tag{7.34}$$

7.4 Active elastic behavior

The main function of elastin and function is to keep the vessel walls and the intramural pressure in equilibrium (Burton 1972). However, the elastic contribution of smooth muscle to the elastic behavior is a controversial topic. The active stress developed by smooth muscle has been overlooked as a contributor to the mechanic behavior of vessels, although it has been demonstrated that the activation of smooth muscle changes the stress–strain relationship towards high levels of stress (Aars 1971, Bader 1983, Cox 1976a, 1976b, 1978b, Dobrin and Rovick 1969, Dujardin *et al* 1980, Megerman *et al* 1986, Milnor 1982, Pagani *et al* 1978, 1979, Pieper and Paul 1969, Price 1984, Stone and Dujardin 1984, Vatner *et al* 1984). Dobrin and Rovick showed that the activation of smooth muscle increases the modulus of elasticity when observed as a function of strain, but decreases when observed as a function of stress, in isolated segments of carotid arteries of dogs (Dobrin and Rovick 1969), shedding light on previous findings that described the elastic modulus increased in some cases and decreased in others when stimulating the activation of smooth muscle. Nichols and O'Rourke suggested that the elastic modulus should be studied at steady strains (Nichols and O'Rourke 1990). The mechanics of smooth muscle has been studied in our laboratory (Barra *et al* 1993, Armentano *et al* 1995a).

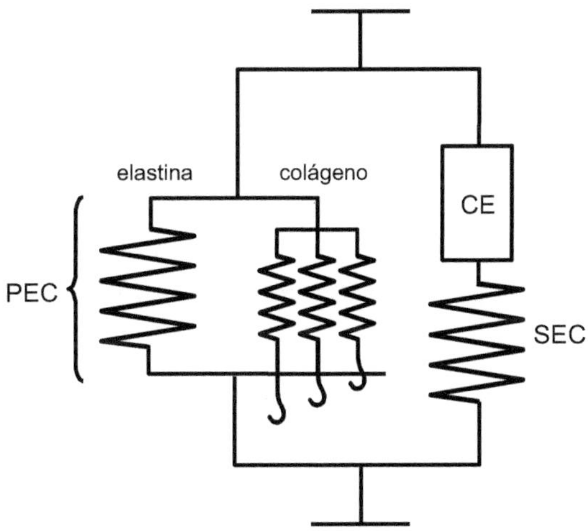

Figure 7.6. Diagram of a Kelvin model. SEC: series elastic component. PEC: parallel elastic component. CE: contractile element (Barra *et al* 1993).

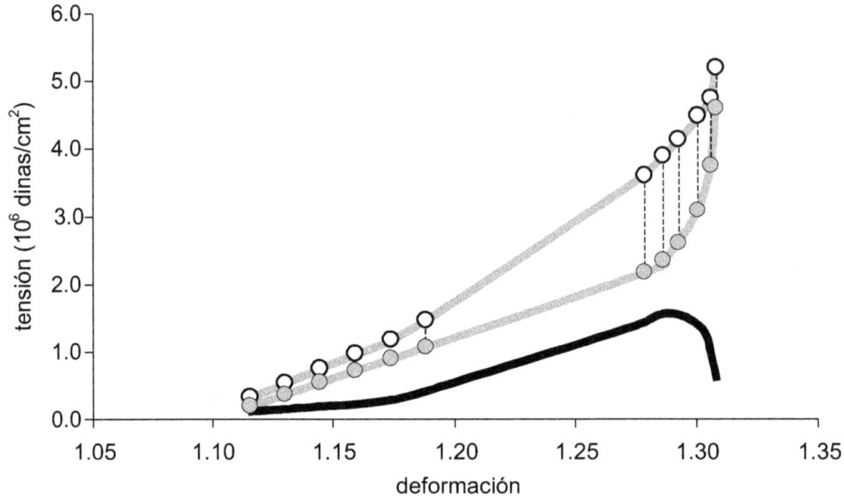

Figure 7.7. Determination of the active stress–strain relationship. The subtraction of the stress–strain relationship with activated smooth muscle (white dots) and the same values with no activation (gray dots) is the aortic muscle cell stress–strain relationship (black line) (Barra *et al* 1993).

7.4.1 Smooth muscle mechanics

The Kelvin model (figure 7.6) has been used to describe the mechanics of the smooth muscle (Barra *et al* 1993) since there is evidence that it better describes vessel walls than the Voigt model (Dobrin and Canfield 1973, 1977).

The chosen model is made up of an elastic component (SEC) in series with a force generator and viscous contractile element (CE). A parallel elastic component (PEC) is added to represent the connective tissue of the vascular wall:

$$\sigma = \sigma_{PEC} + \sigma_{SM}, \tag{7.35}$$

where σ_{SM} is the active stress in the CE–SEC set. The active stress developed by the PEC (σ_{PEC}) can be evaluated through the elastic behavior of elastin and collagen equation (7.34) without smooth muscle activation, and the total stress in the aortic wall becomes:

$$\sigma = E_E \cdot (\varepsilon - \varepsilon_{0E}) + E_C \cdot f_C \cdot \varepsilon + \sigma_{SM}. \tag{7.36}$$

The active stress in the CE–SEC set is measured by subtracting the control stress–strain relationship from the stress–strain relationship with activated smooth muscle at a constant strain (figure 7.7):

$$\sigma_{SM} = \sigma - \sigma_{PEC}. \tag{7.37}$$

7.4.2 Vascular smooth muscle activation function as a function of strain (f_{ML})

The active stress–strain relationship of the vascular smooth muscle has been characterized *in vitro* in several works (Cox 1975, 1976a, 1976b, Murphy *et al* 1980). More recently, it was obtained in conscious animals, showing that the morphology of the stress–strain curve is similar to striated skeletal and cardiac muscle, although smooth muscle is slightly more asymmetric (Barra *et al* 1993). This work demonstrated that the smooth muscle elastic modulus versus strain curve is unimodal and asymmetric, with a maximal value (E_{ML}) that represents the highest achievable elasticity at a certain activation value. To model the active stress–strain relationship of smooth muscle, the following asymmetric function, a modified Lorentzian function, was proposed (Armentano *et al* 1995a):

$$\sigma_{SM} = E_{SM} \cdot f_{SM} \cdot \varepsilon = E_{SM} \cdot \frac{m_1 \cdot \varepsilon + m_2}{m_3 + m_4 \cdot (\varepsilon - m_5)^2} \cdot \varepsilon, \tag{7.38}$$

where m_1, m_2, m_3, m_4 and m_5 are linear-adjustment constants, E_{ML} is the highest smooth muscle elastic modulus, and f_{SM} is the smooth activation function:

$$f_{SM} = \frac{m_1 \cdot \varepsilon + m_2}{m_3 + m_4 \cdot (\varepsilon - m_5)^2}. \tag{7.39}$$

7.5 Dynamic behavior

7.5.1 Determination of the purely elastic relationship

The total stress generated by the wall by opposing the deformation is commonly attributed to combined effects of elasticity, viscosity and inertia that are present in the wall. A second-degree equation (7.40) was used to describe the relationship between stress and strain, where the elastic, viscous and inertial parameters can be calculated (Peterson *et al* 1960). Bauer (Bauer *et al* 1979, 1982, Bauer 1984) developed a procedure to split the wall stress into three terms: the first depends on strain, the second one on the first time derivative of strain (velocity), and the third one on the second time derivative of strain (acceleration):

$$\sigma = E \cdot \varepsilon + \eta \cdot \frac{d\varepsilon}{dt} + M\frac{d^2\varepsilon}{dt^2} = \sigma_{\text{elastic}} + \sigma_{\text{viscous}} + \sigma_{\text{inertial}}, \tag{7.40}$$

where E, η and M are the elastic, viscous and inertial (or mass) moduli of the arterial wall, respectively. The first term is the elastic stress, the second the viscous stress and the third the inertial stress. The purely elastic stress–strain relationship by definition has no hysteresis. In order to separate the purely elastic wall properties, the viscous and inertial phenomena must be eliminated: this is done by eliminating the hysteresis from a stress–strain loop (Armentano *et al* 1995a). First, M is considered null and η values are increased from zero to a value in which the area enclosed by the loop is minimum and the direction of rotation is not altered. This value of η is recorded and M is then increased until the enclosed area disappears completely (Armentano *et al* 1995a) (figure 7.8).

The pure elastic relationship obtained through the hysteresis-elimination method can be adjusted to a logarithmic model previously used to describe large-artery properties (Armentano *et al* 1991, 1995a; Hayashi *et al* 1980, Liu *et al* 1986),

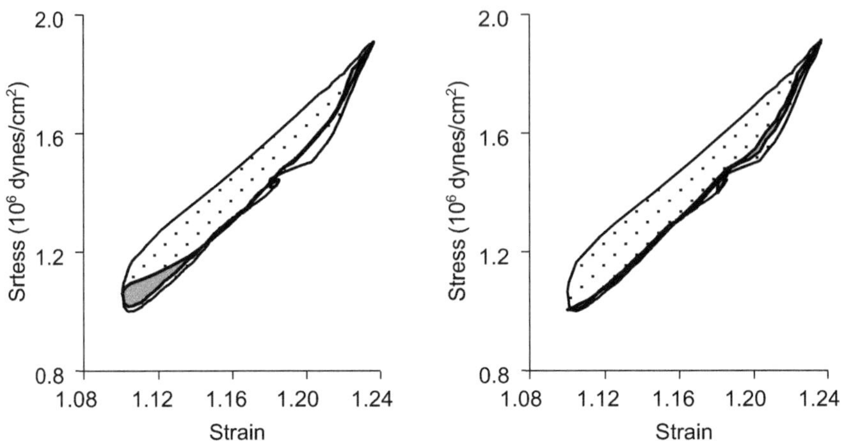

Figure 7.8. The aortic stress–strain relationship (dotted area) involves elastic, viscous and inertial properties and shows hysteresis. By eliminating the viscous stress, a new stress–strain relationship is obtained (gray area, left panel). Increments in the value of *M* decrease the enclosed area until it disappears (gray area, right panel). The loop now coincides with the diastolic stress–strain relationship.

according to the following formulas for both stress–strain and pressure–diameter relationships:

$$\begin{aligned} \varepsilon &= \alpha + \beta \cdot \ln \sigma \\ D &= \alpha + \beta \cdot \ln P, \end{aligned} \tag{7.41}$$

where α and β are two constants obtained from the fitting procedures. The elastic modulus can be calculated knowing the values of ε^* and σ^*, obtained from a logarithmic fitting of equation (7.41):

$$E_{inc} = 0.75 \frac{d\sigma^*}{d\varepsilon^*}. \tag{7.42}$$

7.5.2 Constitutive equation of the arterial wall

The model described in figure 7.6 has been used to characterize the arterial wall mechanics of conscious, chronically instrumented dogs, and its parameters were obtained by using the procedure to describe the purely elastic relationship. The constitutive equation can be formulated, taking into account the elastic response of elastin (σ_E), of collagen (σ_C) and smooth muscle (σ_{ML}), and the viscous (σ_η) and inertial (σ_M) behavior of the arterial wall (Armentano *et al* 1995a):

$$\sigma = \sigma_E + \sigma_C + \sigma_{SM} + \sigma_\eta + \sigma_M, \tag{7.43}$$

$$\sigma = E_E \cdot (\varepsilon - \varepsilon_{0E}) + E_C \cdot f_C \cdot \varepsilon + E_{SM} \cdot f_{SM} \cdot \varepsilon + \eta \cdot \frac{d\varepsilon}{dt} + M \cdot \frac{d^2\varepsilon}{dt^2}. \tag{7.44}$$

The first term characterizes the elastic behavior of elastin fibers, where ε_{0E} is the *y*-intercept. The second term is the nonlinear response of collagen fibers. Both these terms describe the passive elastic behavior of the wall (PEC). The third term exists

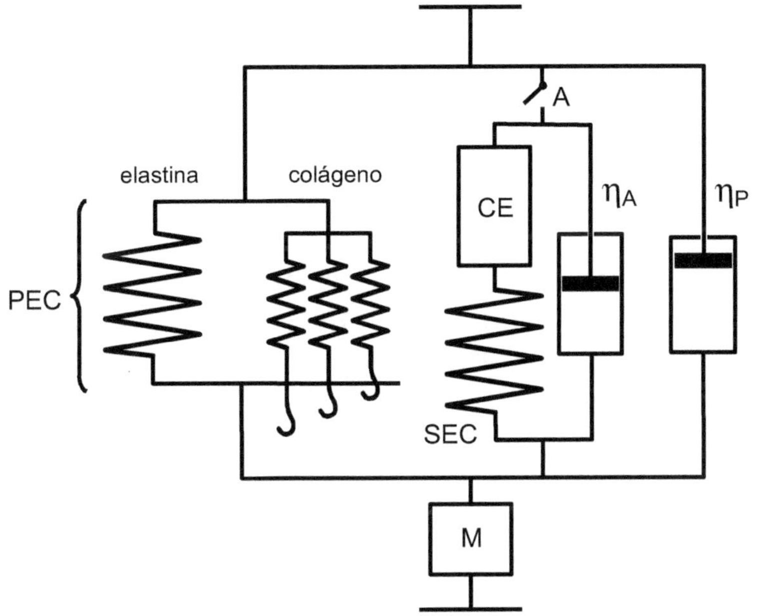

Figure 7.9. Kelvin–Voigt model linked to the constitutive equation of the arterial wall. PEC: parallel elastic component (elastin and collagen). CE: contractile element (smooth muscle). SEC: series elastic component (elastin and collagen). η_A: activated smooth muscle viscosity. η_P: passive smooth muscle viscosity. M: inertial element (wall mass). A: activation of smooth muscle switch (Armentano 1999).

only under smooth muscle activation and is similar to the collagen term, but E_{SM} is the maximum elastic modulus for smooth muscle and f_{ML} is a nonlinearity function represented by the typical morphology of smooth muscle activation. The remaining terms describe the dynamic response of the vascular wall, including hysteresis.

The model in figure 7.6 considers the contractile element as a force-generating unit with viscous properties. This element does not explicitly describe the viscous and inertial characteristics of the wall, thus certain elements that undoubtedly describe these phenomena are needed (Armentano 1999). A new model, the Kelvin–Voigt model, is introduced to better construct the constitutive equation. Figure 7.9 shows several dampers that represent the viscous elements of the arterial wall (smooth muscle), and a switch A that was added to include or exclude the contractile element from the model. The damper next to the contractile element represents the viscosity of smooth muscle during activation, whereas the second damper represents viscosity of the resting smooth muscle. A mass M was added to model the inertial properties.

Lastly, the constitutive equation can be further broadened by separating the viscous modulus into two terms: resting (η_P) and during activation (η_A):

$$\sigma = E_E \cdot (\varepsilon - \varepsilon_{0E}) + E_C \cdot f_C \cdot \varepsilon + E_{SM} \cdot f_{SM} \cdot \varepsilon + (\eta_P + \eta_A) \cdot \frac{d\varepsilon}{dt} + M \cdot \frac{d^2\varepsilon}{dt^2}. \tag{7.45}$$

Titin, a structural protein exclusive to skeletal and cardiac myofibrils, gives resting muscle its viscous properties (Minajeva *et al* 2001, Kulke *et al* 2001). A titin-like protein, smitin, has been recently described in the visceral and vascular smooth muscle of birds (Kim and Keller 2002), which may play an analogous role in the arrangement of myosin filaments in the CE. Even though the active elastic behavior should be described by studying the CE, it is not possible to segregate it from the SEC. This is why it is described as a CE–SEC set (Barra *et al* 1993).

7.5.3 Frequential analysis, cutoff frequency and dynamic range

The pulse wave that is generated in each cardiac beat abruptly changes the stress conditions in the vascular wall as it moves forward though the arterial network. However, the strain in response is delayed and produces a hysteresis phenomenon. Large arteries can be considered as a hydraulic filter whose main function is to damp or modulate the flow oscillations that exist at the beginning of the arterial network, to deliver a continuous flow to tissues. Moreover, parietal viscosity plays a main role in attenuating reflected waves by dissipating energy as heat and avoiding the arterial system to enter a resonance regime.

As previously mentioned, elasticity, viscosity and inertia of the arterial wall are mathematically linked through a second-order equation, called the constitutive equation of the arterial wall. A complex wave profile, such as arterial pressure or diameter, can be decomposed into sinusoidal waves of different amplitudes and frequencies. This decomposition process is called Fourier analysis or harmonic analysis and the Fourier transform is the tool that allows shifting from the time to the frequency domain. A time signal and its Fourier transform show two different views of the same data. Thus, the constitutive equation can be rewritten in both domains:

$$\begin{gathered}\sigma_{(t)} = E \cdot \varepsilon_{(t)} + \eta \frac{d\varepsilon_{(t)}}{dt} + M \frac{d^2\varepsilon_{(t)}}{dt^2} \\ \sigma_{(\omega)} = E \cdot \varepsilon_{(\omega)} + j\omega\eta \cdot \varepsilon_{(\omega)} + j^2\omega^2 M \cdot \varepsilon_{(\omega)}.\end{gathered} \tag{7.46}$$

The arterial system has a filtering function. The aorta is the main damper, and its function can be characterized through a transfer function. This transfer function is the quotient of the output and input signals. The study of the input/output relationship is analogous to observing the cause–effect relationship. In this case, the input signal is stress and the output signal is strain:

$$\begin{gathered}\sigma_{(\omega)} = \varepsilon_{(\omega)} \cdot (E + \eta \cdot j\omega + M \cdot j^2\omega^2) \\ \frac{\sigma_{(\omega)}}{\varepsilon_{(\omega)}} = E_{(\omega)} = E + \eta \cdot j\omega + M \cdot j^2\omega^2.\end{gathered} \tag{7.47}$$

The transfer in the frequency domain is represented by $H_{(\omega)}$. A null frequency has a transfer function $H_{(0)}$, and represents the static behavior of the system:

$$H_{(0)} = \frac{\varepsilon_{(0)}}{\sigma_{(0)}} = \frac{1}{E}. \tag{7.48}$$

The dynamic behavior of the system for non-zero frequencies the transfer function is:

$$\frac{1}{E_{(\omega)}} = \frac{\varepsilon_{(\omega)}}{\sigma_{(\omega)}} = H_{(\omega)} = \frac{1}{E + \eta \cdot j\omega + M \cdot j^2\omega^2} = \frac{1}{E} \cdot \frac{\frac{E}{M}}{\frac{E}{M} + \frac{\eta}{M} j\omega + j^2\omega^2}$$
$$H_{(\omega)} = H_{(0)} \cdot \frac{\frac{E}{M}}{\frac{E}{M} + \frac{\eta}{M} j\omega + j^2\omega^2}. \tag{7.49}$$

If inertial effects are considered negligible (Peterson *et al* 1960), equation (7.49) is reduced to a first-order linear system. In this kind of system, the transfer function decreases with increasing frequencies as a function of E/η. A usual approach in physical sciences to analyze first-order systems is to determine the frequency at which $H_{(\omega)}$ falls 3 dB with respect to $H_{(0)}$, i.e. a cutoff frequency of −3 dB (Peterson *et al* 1960, Armentano 1999). At this frequency $H_{(\omega)}/H_{(0)}$ is 0.707, or $1/\sqrt{2}$. Therefore, in a viscoelastic system with negligible mass, the transfer function between stress and strain can be expressed as (Armentano 1999):

$$\frac{1}{E_{(\omega)}} = H_{(\omega)} = \frac{\varepsilon_{(\omega)}}{\sigma_{(\omega)}} = \frac{1}{E + \eta \cdot j\omega} = \frac{1}{E} \cdot \frac{1}{1 + j\omega\frac{\eta}{E}} = H_{(0)} \cdot \frac{1}{1 + j\omega\frac{\eta}{E}}. \tag{7.50}$$

And the cutoff frequency (f_{cutoff}) of −3 dB:

$$\left|\frac{H_{(\omega)}}{H_{(0)}}\right|_{f_{cutoff}} = \frac{1}{\sqrt{2}} = 0.707; \; \left|H_{(\omega)}\right|_{f_{cutoff}} = \frac{1}{\sqrt{2}} H_{(0)}; \; \left|\omega\frac{\eta}{E}\right|_{f_{cutoff}} = 1. \tag{7.51}$$

If f_{cutoff} is known, E and η can be calculated, and vice versa (Peterson *et al* 1960), therefore:

$$\omega_{cutoff} = \frac{\eta}{E} = 1; \quad 2\pi f_{cutoff} \cdot \frac{\eta}{E} = 1; \quad f_{cutoff} = \frac{1}{2\pi} \cdot \frac{E}{\eta}. \tag{7.52}$$

Another frequently used approach in physical sciences is to evaluate the properties of the system from the constitutive equation. The differential equation must be converted into a polynomic equation to determine the roots and analyze the response of the system (Peterson *et al* 1960). The Laplace transform is a well known technique to solve differential equations, where the temporal domain is changed to the s domain, also called the *s plane* (Smith 1997). The s domain is a complex plain, where real numbers are represented in the horizontal axis and the imaginary numbers in the vertical axis of a rectangular coordinate system.

Therefore, using the Laplace transform and assuming a linear-system hypothesis, the constitutive equation can be rewritten in the s plane:

$$\begin{aligned} \sigma_{(t)} &= E \cdot \varepsilon_{(t)} + \eta \frac{d\varepsilon_{(t)}}{dt} + M \frac{d^2\varepsilon_{(t)}}{dt^2} \\ \sigma_{(\omega)} &= E \cdot \varepsilon_{(\omega)} + j\omega\eta \cdot \varepsilon_{(\omega)} + j^2\omega^2 M \cdot \varepsilon_{(\omega)} \\ \sigma_{(s)} &= E \cdot \varepsilon_{(s)} + \eta \cdot s \cdot \varepsilon_{(s)} + M \cdot s^2 \cdot \varepsilon_{(s)}, \end{aligned} \tag{7.53}$$

where s is a complex variable $s = r + j\omega$. This coordinate system can identify any point through the variables r (the real-axis distance) and ω (the natural frequency, in the imaginary axis). The transfer function in the s plane, $H_{(s)}$, is:

$$\begin{aligned} H_{(s)} &= \frac{\varepsilon_{(s)}}{\sigma_{(s)}} = \frac{1}{E + \eta \cdot s + M \cdot s^2} \\ &= \frac{1}{E} \cdot \frac{\frac{E}{M}}{\frac{E}{M} + \frac{\eta}{M}s + s^2} = H_{(0)} \cdot \frac{\frac{E}{M}}{\frac{E}{M} + \frac{\eta}{M}s + s^2}. \end{aligned} \tag{7.54}$$

Although finding the transfer function is key to Laplace analysis, a particular notation is needed, as the numerator and the denominator must be represented as polynomials:

$$\omega_n = \sqrt{\frac{E}{M}}; \quad \xi = \frac{\eta}{2\sqrt{E \cdot M}}, \tag{7.55}$$

where, ω_n is the natural resonance frequency without oscillations, ξ is the damping ratio. As:

$$2 \cdot \xi \cdot \omega_n = 2\frac{\eta}{2\sqrt{E \cdot M}} \cdot \frac{\sqrt{E}}{\sqrt{M}} = \frac{2\eta\sqrt{E}}{2\sqrt{E}\left(\sqrt{M}\right)^2} = \frac{\eta}{M} \tag{7.56}$$

the transfer function in the s plane can be rewritten as:

$$H_{(s)} = H_{(0)} \frac{\omega_n^2}{s^2 + 2 \cdot \xi \cdot \omega_n + \omega_n^2} \tag{7.57}$$

whose denominator $s^2 + 2 \cdot \xi \cdot \omega_n + \omega_n^2$ is a polynomial as $as^2 + bs + c$, whose roots s_1 and s_2 can be found through $s_{1,2} = -b \pm \sqrt{b^2 - 4ac}/2a$, and:

$$
\begin{aligned}
s_{1,2} &= -\omega_{1,2} = \frac{-2 \cdot \xi \cdot \omega_n \pm \sqrt{(2 \cdot \xi \cdot \omega_n)^2 - 4 \cdot \omega_n^2}}{2} \\
s_{1,2} &= -\omega_{1,2} = \frac{-2 \cdot \xi \cdot \omega_n \pm \sqrt{4 \cdot \omega_n^2 \cdot \xi^2 - 4 \cdot \omega_n^2}}{2} \\
s_{1,2} &= -\omega_{1,2} = \frac{-2 \cdot \xi \cdot \omega_n \pm \sqrt{4 \cdot \omega_n^2(\xi^2 - 1)}}{2} \\
s_{1,2} &= -\omega_{1,2} = \frac{-2 \cdot \xi \cdot \omega_n \pm 2 \cdot \omega_n^2\sqrt{\xi^2 - 1}}{2} \\
s_{1,2} &= -\omega_{1,2} = -\xi \cdot \omega_n \pm \omega_n\sqrt{\xi^2 - 1}\,.
\end{aligned}
\tag{7.58}
$$

Replacing equations (7.55) in equation (7.58),

$$
\begin{aligned}
s_{1,2} &= -\frac{\eta}{2\sqrt{E}\sqrt{M}} \cdot \frac{\sqrt{E}}{\sqrt{M}} \pm \sqrt{\frac{E}{M}}\sqrt{\frac{\eta^2}{4 \cdot E \cdot M} - 1} \\
s_{1,2} &= -\frac{\eta}{2(\sqrt{M})^2} \pm \sqrt{\frac{\eta^2 \cdot E}{4 \cdot E \cdot M^2} - \frac{E}{M}} \\
s_{1,2} &= -\frac{\eta}{2 \cdot M} \pm \sqrt{\left(\frac{\eta}{2 \cdot M}\right)^2 - \frac{E}{M}}\,.
\end{aligned}
\tag{7.59}
$$

The parameters E, η and M can be calculated for two cutoff frequencies (Peterson *et al* 1960):

$$
\omega_1 = -s_1; f_1 = \frac{\omega_1}{2\pi}; \; \omega_2 = -s_2; f_2 = \frac{\omega_2}{2\pi}. \tag{7.60}
$$

If the cutoff frequency of the first pole (ω_1) is small with respect to the other pole (ω_2), the cutoff frequency (−3 dB) is approximately defined by ω_1, and therefore, as $f_2 \gg f_1$, the system can be approximated to a single-constant system where $f_1 = -3$ dB (Armentano 1999). The cutoff frequency, therefore, defines the frequency range (dynamic range) that the system accepts as an input with no distortion at the output, whereas frequencies beyond the cutoff frequency will be damped or attenuated by the system. This damping function is undertaken by large vessels.

7.5.4 Damping function

The mechanical properties of arteries are a determinant factor in the hemodynamics of the system. The aorta, the pulmonary artery and large distribution vessels are easily and quickly distended in each ejection of the heart, temporarily holding 50% of the systolic discharge (Dobrin 1978). The vessels then draw back during diastole. These dimensional changes make the mechanical properties of the wall a determining factor in the morphology of the arterial pressure wave. Large arteries transmit the pressure wave and are the main source of vascular impedance, i.e. dynamic resistance to oscillatory components of blood flow (Dobrin 1978). Even though the vascular wall has a mass and is viscous, the existence of a flow across capillaries after cardiac ejection done in each cardiac cycle is almost exclusively due to the elastic properties of elastin in the vascular walls. However, the distribution phenomenon of the vascular system is not limited to the elastic characteristics of the vessel, nor to the viscous of inertial characteristics. Flow distribution is a complex phenomenon where wave reflection takes part. Wave reflection is an interesting yet complex field, since it requires a complicated physical and mathematical approach and a set of simplifying hypotheses (Fung 1984). This explanation exceeds the aim of this chapter. In a simplified manner, ejection produces a pressure wave that is transmitted along the arterial system (incident wave). This wave travels along vessels and distends their walls circumferentially, overcoming the resistance of the wall. However, waves *collide* against bifurcations, narrowings and arterioles, where resistance is maximal, and are consequently reflected towards the heart. The countless amount of reflected waves form a *reflected wave*, that interferes with the incident wave (Milnor 1982).

As mentioned above, the heart delivers energy to the vascular system during systole. A part of that energy is kinetic, and accelerates the ejected blood volume and eases its flow. A big portion of the volume remains stored during systole as potential energy, as arteries proximal to the heart increase their diameter. During the diastolic period, the stored elastic energy guarantees a continuous blood flow towards the periphery and a high pressure, that is, higher than in the ventricle.

Energy is dissipated in each cardiac cycle. The energy delivered by the heart and received by the arterial system is not entirely used to accelerate a blood volume and to keep a fraction of that volume within the arteries, but is also lost as heat. This energy loss is associated with viscous effects and is about 15%–20% of the energy delivered by the heart (Shadwick 1999). The dissipated energy helps attenuate the velocity of the pulse wave, which is propagated along the wall as a circumferential distension wave (Fung 1984). The viscoelastic properties of the arterial wall, together with blood viscosity, prevent the system from becoming resonant, which would happen if the circulatory system were perfectly elastic and blood were non-viscous (Shadwick 1999).

In summary, the functions carried out by arteries are to make up a low-resistance distribution system and dampen the systolic charge, delivering a constant flow towards the periphery. The mechanical properties of the vascular wall make the *cushioning function* of the arteries possible. Blood pressure is kept at high levels due to wall elasticity, and flow continues even when there is no ejection during the diastolic period, whereas viscosity is responsible for attenuating the reflection phenomena and avoiding resonance in the system (McDonald 1974, Milnor 1982, O'Rourke 1982, Fung 1984, Shadwick 1999).

References

Aars H 1971 Diameter and elasticity of the ascending aorta during infusion of noradrenaline *Acta Physiol. Scand.* **83** 133–8

Armentano R L, Levenson J, Barra J G, Cabrera Fischer E I, Breitbart G J, Pichel R H and Simon A C 1991 Assessment of elastin and collagen contribution to aortic elasticity in conscious dogs *Am. J. Physiol.* **260** H1870–7

Armentano R L, Barra J G, Levenson J, Simon A and Pichel R H 1995a Arterial wall mechanics in conscious dogs: assessment of viscous, inertial, and elastic moduli to characterize the aortic wall behavior *Circ. Res.* **76** 468–78

Armentano R L 1999 Détermination *in vivo* des caractéristiques hémodynamiques artérielles, application a l'hypertension *PhD Thesis* Université Paris 7 – Denis Diderot

Bader H 1983 Importance of the gerontology of elastic arteries in the development of essential hypertension *Clin. Physiol. Biochem.* **1** 36–56

Barra J G, Armentano R L, Levenson J, Cabrera Fischer E I, Pichel R H and Simon A 1993 Assessment of smooth muscle contribution to descending thoracic elastic mechanics in conscious dogs *Circ. Res.* **73** 1040–50

Bauer R D, Büsse R, Schabert A, Summa Y and Wetterer E 1979 Separate determination of the pulsatile elastic and viscous forces developed in the arterial wall *in vivo Pflügers Arch.* **380** 221–6

Bauer R D, Büsse R and Schabert A 1982 Mechanical properties of arteries *Biorheology* **19** 409–24

Bauer R D 1984 Rheological approaches of arteries *Biorheology* **(Suppl I)** 159–67

Bergel D H 1961a The static elastic properties of the arterial wall *J. Physiol.* **156** 445–57

Bergel D H 1961b The dynamic elastic properties of the arterial wall *J. Physiol.* **156** 458–69

Burton A C 1954 Relation of structure to function of the tissues of the wall of blood vessels *Physiol. Rev.* **34** 619–42

Burton A C 1972 *Physiology and Biophysics of the Circulation* (Chicago, IL: Year Book Medical Publishers) pp 63–75

Cabrera Fischer E I, Armentano R L, Levenson J, Barra J G, Morales M C, Breitbart G J, Pichel R H and Simon A C 1991 Paradoxically decreased aortic wall stiffness in response to vitamin D_3-induced calcinosis: a biphasic analysis of segmental elastic properties in conscious dogs *Circ. Res.* **68** 1549–59

Cobelli C, Carson E R, Finkelstein L and Leaning M S 1984 Validation of simple and complex models in physiology and medicine *Am. J. Physiol.* **246** R259–66

Cox R H 1975 Arterial wall mechanics and composition and the effects of smooth muscle activation *Am. J. Physiol.* **229** 807–12

Cox R H 1976a Mechanics of canine iliac artery smooth muscle *in vitro Am. J. Physiol.* **230** 462–70

Cox R H 1976b Effects of norepinephrine on mechanics of arteries *in vitro Am. J. Physiol.* **231** 420–25

Cox R H 1978a Passive mechanics and connective tissue composition of canine arteries *Am. J. Physiol.* **234** H533–41

Cox R H 1978b Regional variation of series elasticity in canine arterial smooth muscles *Am. J. Physiol.* **234** H542–51

Cox R H 1979 Comparison of arterial wall mechanics in normotensive and spontaneously hypertensive rats *Am. J. Physiol.* **237** H159–67

Dobrin P B and Rovick A A 1969 Influence of vascular smooth muscle on contractil mechanisms and elasticity of arteries *Am. J. Physiol.* **217** 1644–51

Dobrin P B and Canfield T R 1973 Series elastic and contractile elements in vascular smooth muscle *Circ. Res.* **33** 454–64

Dobrin P B and Canfield T R 1977 Identification of arterial smooth muscle series elastic components in intact carotid artery *Am. J. Physiol.* **232** H122–30
Dobrin P B 1978 Mechanical properties of arteries *Physiol. Rev.* **58** 397–460
Dobrin P B 1984 Mechanical behaviour of vascular smooth muscle in cylindrical segments of arteries *in vitro Ann. Biomed. Eng.* **12** 497–510
Dobrin P B 1999 Distribution of lamellar deformations. Implications for properties of arterial media *Hypertension* **33** 806–10
Dujardin J P, Paul L T and Pieper H P 1980 Effect of acute volume loading on aortic smooth muscle activity in intacts dogs *Am. J. Physiol.* **238** H379–83
Fung Y C 1981 *Biomechanics. Mechanical Properties of Living Tissues* (New York: Springer)
Fung Y C 1984 *Biodynamics. Circulation* (New York: Springer)
Gow B S and Taylor M G 1968 Measurements of viscoelastic properties of arteries in the living dog *Circ. Res.* **23** 111–22
Hayashi K, Handa H, Nagasawa A, Okumura A and Morikate K 1980 Stiffness and elastic behavior of human intracraneal and extracraneal arteries *J. Biomech.* **13** 175–84
Kim K and Keller T C S III 2002 Smitin, a novel smooth muscle titin-like protein, interacts with myosin filaments *in vivo* and *in vitro J. Cell Biol.* **156** 101–12
Kulke M, Fujita-Becker S, Rostkova E, Neagoe C, Labeit D, Manstein D J, Gautel M and Linke W A 2001 Interaction between PEKV-titin filaments. Origin of a viscous force component in cardiac myofibrils *Circ. Res.* **89** 874–81
Ling S C and Chow C H 1977 The mechanics of corrugated collagen fibrils in arteries *J. Biomech.* **10** 71–7
Liu Z, Brin K and Yin F C P 1986 Estimation of total arterial compliance: an improved method and evaluation of current methods *Am. J. Physiol.* **251** H588–600
McDonald D A 1974 *Blood Flow in Arteries* 2nd edn (London: Edward Arnold)
Megerman J, Hasson J E, Warnock D F, L'Italien G J and Abbott W M 1986 Noninvasive measurements of nonlinear arterial elasticity *Am. J. Physiol.* **250** H181–8
Milnor W K 1982 *Hemodynamics* (Baltimore, MD: Williams & Wilkins)
Minajeva A, Kulke M, Fernandez J M and Linke W A 2001 Unfolding of titin domains explains the viscoelastic behavior of skeletal myofibrils *Biophys. J.* **80** 1442–51
Murphy R A 1980 Mechanics of vascular smooth muscle *Handbook of Physiology* section 2: The Cardiovascular System ed D F Bohr, A P Somlyo and H V Sparks Jr vol II (Bethesda, MD: American Physiological Society) pp 325–51
Nichols W W and O'Rourke M F 1990 *McDonald's Blood Flow in Arteries* (London: Edward Arnold)
O'Rourke M F 1982 *Arterial Function in Health and Disease* (New York: Churchill Livingstone) pp 153–69
Pagani M, Baig H, Sherman A, Manders W T, Quinn P, Patrick T, Franklin D and Vatner S F 1978 Measurement of multiple simultaneous small dimensions and study of arterial pressure-dimension relations in conscious animals *Am. J. Physiol.* **235** H610–7
Pagani M, Mirsky I, Biag H, Manders W T, Kerkhof P and Vatner S F 1979 Effects of age on aortic pressure-diameter and elastic stiffness-stress relationships in unanesthetized sheep *Circ. Res.* **44** 420–9
Peterson L H, Jensen R E and Parnell J 1960 Mechanical properties of arteries *in vivo Circ. Res.* **8** 622–39

Pieper H P and Paul L T 1969 Responses of aortic smooth muscle studied in intact dogs *Am. J. Physiol.* **217** 154–60
Price J M 1984 Length-dependent activation and sensitivity in arterial ring segments *Ann. Biomed. Eng.* **12** 481–96
Roach M R and Burton A C 1957 The reason for the shape of the distensibility curve of arteries *Can. J. Biochem.* **35** 681–90
Shadwick R E 1999 Mechanical design in arteries *J. Exp. Biol.* **202** 3305–13
Smith S W 1997 *The Scientist and Engineer's Guide to Digital Signal Processing* (San Diego, CA: California Technical Publishing)
Stone D N and Dujardin J P 1984 Changes in smooth muscle tone influence characteristic impedance of the aorta *Am. J. Physiol.* **246** H1–7
Vatner S F, Pasipoularides A and Mirsky I 1984 Measurement of arterial pressure-dimension relationships in conscious animals *Ann. Biomed. Eng.* **12** 521–34
Wiederhielm C A 1965 Distensibility characteristics of small blood vessels *Fed. Proc.* **24** 1075–84
Yano M, Kumada T, Matsuzaki M, Kohno M, Hiro T, Kohtoku S, Miura T, Katayama K, Ozaki M and Kusukawa R 1989 Effect of diltiazem on aortic pressure-diameter relationship in dogs *Am. J. Physiol.* **256** H1580–7

IOP Publishing

Biomechanical Modeling of the Cardiovascular System

Ricardo L Armentano, Edmundo I Cabrera Fischer and Leandro J Cymberknop

Chapter 8

Pulse propagation in arteries

Ricardo L Armentano and Leandro J Cymberknop

8.1 Introduction

Intermittent expulsion of blood by the left ventricle results in pressure and flow waveforms in the circulation. The understanding and characterization of this pulse behavior is generating a clinical interest due to the important implications for risk prediction and the mechanisms of action of therapeutic agents. Indeed, the sudden expulsion of blood from the ventricle to the aorta in every systolic ejection produces a pressure wave that propagates along the arteries to the periphery, called a pulse wave or arterial pulse. Thus, the arterial pulse can be defined as 'the transmission of a pressure change in the arterial wall and in the blood when it flows through a system of elastic vessels'. The velocity of propagation of the arterial pulse wave is greater than blood flow velocity in the arteries. Such propagation velocity is greater in small arteries than in vessels close to the heart. In general, the stiffer the artery, the faster the arterial pulse, and the more elastic the artery, the slower the arterial pulse.

The study of wave propagation of pressure and flow and its breakdown into incident and reflected waves are highly important in physiological assessment and clinical practice (Hughes *et al* 2008). At the exit of the left ventricle, incident waves are generated cycle by cycle and reflected waves originate from distant points where structural maladaptation occurred: dimensions, branching or changes in stiffness. Reflected pressure waves generated at maladaptation points are added to the incident wave, while flow waves cancel out. The pressure waveform can change considerably depending on the reflections, generating an increase in their maximum (systolic) values. These increased pressure values are the cause of severe traumatism of the arterial conducting system (Hughes *et al* 2008).

In theory, undulatory motion appears with an equilibrium state in a system. The wave is a disturbance that pulls the system apart from its equilibrium state. Waves that need a deformable or elastic material medium to propagate are called mechanical waves. Unlike oscillations, a wave consists of a motion in numerous different points of a system. These motions are coupled in such a way that an

doi:10.1088/2053-2563/aafb0dch8

original disturbance is transmitted to the neighboring portions of matter and from these to the following, thus propagating through the medium. Depending on the relationship between the motions of particles of the material's medium and the direction of wave propagation, waves can be classified into:

- Transverse waves, if particle oscillations in the medium are perpendicular to the direction of propagation of the wave.
- Longitudinal waves, if particle oscillations in the medium are produced in the same direction as wave propagation.

Not all points in the medium are reached at the same time by the disturbance because the wave propagates at a certain velocity (wave velocity) in such a way that the particles that are furthest from the disturbance site of origin will start moving with a certain delay. The medium does not move as a whole as the wave propagates. The particles in the medium perform limited motions around their equilibrium positions. Thus, there is no transport of matter in undulatory motion. In order to be able to set these media, through which waves propagate, in motion, energy should be added to the system performing mechanical work on it. Waves transport this energy from one region of the medium to the other. Therefore, energy is the only thing that is transmitted in a wave (Hughes *et al* 2008).

A wave can also consist of the propagation of

- A single pulse (wave pulse) characterized by having a beginning and an end and therefore, a limited extension. The particles of the medium move only during the time interval used by the pulse to move through it. The pulse waveform can widen as the wave propagates (wave dispersion) though, in many practical cases, this deformation is negligible and the pulse waveform is kept unaltered.
- A succession of identical or nonidentical pulses (waves train). If disruptions are periodic, there will be a train of periodic waves, whose most simple and important case is that of harmonic waves, in which each particle of the medium exhibits simple harmonic motion. Ideally, a periodic wave does not have either a beginning or an end, and therefore it has an unlimited extension. Unlike the pulse, it does not disperse as it propagates.

The general equation that describes the undulatory motion propagating with a defined velocity v and without distortion along an axis $+X$ or $-X$ is

$$\frac{d^2\xi}{dt^2} = \mathrm{v}^2 \frac{d^2\xi}{dx^2}, \qquad (8.1)$$

which is a basic wave equation. The solution to this equation can be expressed as

$$\begin{aligned} \xi(x,\, t) &= f(x - \mathrm{v}t) \\ \xi(x,\, t) &= f(x + \mathrm{v}t) \end{aligned} \qquad (8.2)$$

or a combination of both. It is easy to demonstrate that a harmonic wave of the following type

$$\xi(x, t) = \xi_0 \mathrm{sen} k(x - \mathrm{v}t) \tag{8.3}$$

satisfies the wave equation.

Brief historical review: Although the development of the conceptual analysis and measurement of the parameters involved in pulse wave propagation has evolved dizzily in the last 30 years, it must be noted that such propagating features have been proposed and used for a more rational comprehension of propagating phenomena for a long time. For example, the oldest document dealing with this issue is attributed to the Ebers Papyrus, 1550 BC, which proposes a certain relationship between pulsatility and heartbeats. The ancient Chinese, Egyptian and Indian cultures established relationships between blood pulsations observed at different points and heartbeats. For example, hundreds of years ago, Chinese medicine practitioners used the palpation of pulsations in the radial artery as a means to diagnose their patients' physiological state (Li 1987). More recently, in 1628, Harvey described the pulsatile nature of blood as a consequence of an intermittent input flow, which occurs during one third of the heart cycle, now known as systole, in combination with an essentially stable flow through the periphery (Li 1987).

In 1773, Hales registered the magnitude of blood pressure around which oscillations develop but it was not until 1863 when Chaveau and Marey registered blood pressure that we learned about pulse form. Although the concept of the reflected wave was analyzed by Harvey early on, the description of the reflected wave influence on the modification of pulse form in patients with increased arterial pressure is attributed to Frederick Mahomed (1872–74). Apparently, the concept of the artery as a reservoir is attributed to Hales. The reservoir function resulted in one of the most popular theories in the study of blood circulation known as the fire pump or Windkessel model. One of the adherents and a fervent advocate of such theory was Frank, who used such concepts in later works (Li 1987, Parker 2009, Nichols and O'Rourke 2005).

The application of Windkessel theory leads to modeling of the artery as a simple elastic tube where pressure pulsations in any site of the arterial tree must occur simultaneously. In other words, this implies that the pressure pulse propagates with infinite velocity. In practice, this hypothesis has been rejected because of the simple measurement of the velocity. The finite velocity of propagation was considered in 1775 by Euler, who developed a formula for its calculation. This formula is currently known as the Moens–Korteweg formula, whose creators were in charge of its modification a century later (Parker 2009, Nichols and O'Rourke 2005).

It must be stated that since the second half of the twentieth century, and with the advent of new techniques for measurement, modern concepts of pulse transmission have been developed such as those dealt with by Mc Donald in 1960 and 1974, and Taylor in 1960 (Nichols and O'Rourke 2005, 2008), as well as Womersley's revealing works on oscillating flow theory (Womersley 1957).

Among the most complete revisions on such physico-mathematical developments are those of Noordergraaf (1969, 1978), Finkelstein and Ross Collins (1982), and O'Rourke (O'Rourke 1982, 1990).

Modeling has been a necessary and essential step towards the understanding of the properties of the cardiocirculatory system (Wetterer and Kenner 1968, Welkowitz 1977), the reason by which the biomedical sciences are converging to the path that brought so much success to the engineering sciences and physics. In order to avoid harmful consequences, a series of general strict norms must be fulfilled for the application of these models in medicine as established by Cobelli's works (Cobelli *et al* 1984, Carson and Cobelli 2001) and the Modeling in Biomedical Research notes (NIH Conference 1989).

With the advent of technological advances in instrumentation for the measurement of pressure, flow, dimensions and velocity profiles, for application in humans, the concept of pulse wave propagation and its resulting effects is being constantly updated.

8.1.1 Characteristics of pulse propagation

Both pressure pulse and flow suffer morphological modifications in their propagation along the arterial tree caused by the following factors:

- nonuniform vascular geometry,
- nonuniform vascular elasticity,
- damping, and
- reflected waves.

These factors also modify the flow and pressure pulse wave velocities because they are a function of arterial stiffness, dimensions and blood density (Milnor 1982, Li 1987, Nichols and O'Rourke 2005). Indeed, vascular branching provides the circulatory system with a very particular type of geometry in which when the flow and pressure waves find discontinuities, due to an obturation, a branching or nonuniform elasticities, reflections are generated that modify the waveforms during propagation (O'Rourke 1976, 1982, 1990, O'Rourke and Kelly 1993).

On the other hand, the vascular wall becomes stiffer in the periphery, producing an increase in wave dispersion that, consequently, affects reflections (Burton 1972).

A parameter to consider—due to its enormous influence in the pulse wave—is viscosity, present both in the wall and the fluid. The resulting effect is an attenuation, which will be directly proportional to the frequency of the signal. The incisura dicrota possesses the greatest frequential richness of the pulse wave and, thus, it will be progressively dampened as it progresses. Thus, when the flow reaches the femoral artery, the high frequency characteristics of the wave disappear: in these sites, a waveform smoothing can be observed. When the pulse reaches the arterioles, it is so dampened that its waveform looks like a pure sinusoid (Li 1987).

Of all the factors previously mentioned, the most important is the reflected wave, which is the primary cause of wave distortion in the arterial system. For instance, it has been suggested that the reflections are of the same type as those taking place in a tube closed at one end, the arterioles being the sites with the greatest reflection, and that in such a case, the reflected flow and pressure waves are

180° out of phase (Taylor 1959, O'Rourke 1982, O'Rourke and Kelly 1993). The ejection of blood by the heart produces flow and pressure waves and these pulsations are transmitted to the entire arterial tree. The velocity at which these waves travel and the changes in their forms and amplitudes are determined by blood viscosity, vessels' elasticity, difference in lengths, distensibilities along the entire system, and branching distribution. These properties interact and it is only possible to identify the individual effects theoretically. The blood flow ejected by the left ventricle with every heartbeat produces an incident arterial pressure pulse. Due to the nature of the system, secondary waves, called reflected waves, are added to this original pulse. These waves have a retrograde flow generated in the imperfections of the terminations (Westerhof *et al* 1972). Such waveforms show different patterns at different sites of the arterial system and in the same artery under different circumstances. These secondary waves are of lesser amplitude than primary waves and they are perfectly differentiable from the high frequency noise caused by the closure of the aortic valve. In some cases, the amplitude of these reflected waves can be of high magnitude as is the case of the peripheral arteries close to the reflection sites (O'Rourke and Kelly 1993). One of the most original and novel approaches proposed that the reflected wave works as negative feedback in the arterial system (Quick *et al* 2002).

The reflected wave is generated at the sites where arterial branching abounds as well as in the sudden changes in dimensions, such as in the arterial terminations and in the multiple sites where low resistance conduits end in high resistance arterioles. Therefore, there is no specific site of reflection; rather, a reflected wave would be the result of multiple reflections originated at different sites of the periphery of the body, which, in addition, has an effective length as in every distributed phenomenon (Li 1987, Campbell *et al* 1989). The reflected wave is the main cause of the aging-related increase in systolic blood pressure, and it is responsible for the substantial differences in systolic pressure between the central and peripheral arteries in young people. The transmitted and reflected waves cause a delay of the pulse between the peripheral and central arteries, and pulse amplification (an increase in pulse pressure) between both sites (O'Rourke 1982, O'Rourke and Kelly 1993).

Under normal circumstances, in experimental animals and young human subjects, the reflected wave returns to the ascending aorta from the body periphery when ventricular ejection ends. The foot of the secondary wave then appears in the ascending aorta to correspond in high frequencies to the incisura produced by the closure of the aortic valve. Such a moment of occurrence is desirable because the increase of the ascending aorta pressure caused by the wave reflection happens in the diastole and not in the systole. Such increase in diastolic pressure and its resulting increase in the perfusion pressure of the coronary arteries on the left ventricle, without augmenting its afterload, is a highly advantageous situation. Finally, it could be suggested that the reflected wave optimizes the ventricle-arterial interaction in normal individuals (O'Rourke 1982, O'Rourke *et al* 1987, O'Rourke and Kelly,1993).

8.1.2 Definition of the constituent elements of the hydraulic opposition to cardiac ejection

The main function of the systemic circulation is to maintain a constant blood flow through the capillaries, in such a way as to facilitate nutrient diffusion. The major distribution arteries work as a hydraulic low-pass filter to keep that flow constant (Burton 1972, O'Rourke 1982, O'Rourke and Kelly 1993).

As cardiac rejection is received and dampened mainly in the aorta, where more than 60% of the arterial compliance lies, a new frame of reference was established for its analysis, which is called ventricular–aortic coupling (Elzinga and Westerhof 1991). This consists of two important concepts: the role of the heart as a pump that is connected to a hydraulic load and the perfusion of the heart as an organ (Nichols and O'Rourke 1990, Milnor 1975, O'Rourke *et al* 1987).

Considering the ventricle function primarily as a hydraulic pump, it is necessary to quantify the pressure in the cavity next to the left ventricle during systole. This pressure opposes the ejection of blood from the ventricle and determines myocardial oxygen requirements. During systole, the pressure in the left ventricle is almost equivalent to aortic pressure. The differences between both pressures start in the period between the end of ventricular contraction and the opening of the aortic valve; continuing in the interval after the closing of the aortic valve and during ventricular relaxation, when the aortic pressure curve shows a predominantly slow fall (O'Rourke *et al* 1987).

In medical practice, the opposition to the ejection is characterized as the mean pressure generated by the aorta during systole. Considering the heart as both a pump and an organ, the aortic pressure wave must be analyzed through two characteristic values, namely: the mean pressure during systole, which is vital for the activity of the left ventricle as a pump, and the mean pressure during diastole, which is important for coronary perfusion (O'Rourke 1982, O'Rourke and Kelly 1993).

To conceptually analyze the circulatory system, three very important components are used: the left ventricle, the arterial system and the arteriole-capillary bed. The hydraulic opposition to the flow ejected by the heart occurs in the last two, that is, in the arterial system which represents the blood macrocirculation and in the arteriole-capillary bed, which contains the blood microcirculation. In the macrocirculation, the opposition to flow is governed by the mechanical properties of the arterial wall and the geometric characteristics of this territory in terms of vessel branching. In the arteriole-capillary territory, the opposition to flow is governed by the rheological properties of blood and the dimensions of these small vessels (O'Rourke and Taylor 1967, O'Rourke and Kelly 1993, Bensalah 1985).

In order to globalize the hydraulic load shown by the systemic circulation, the macro and microcirculatory effects are usually grouped into three basic predominant parameters: peripheral resistances, compliance and reflected wave (Murgo and Westerhof 1987). The elastic characteristics of the arterial wall are included in the arterial compliance group (mainly aorta), the peripheral resistances include the resistance to a stationary system (mainly arterioles) and the reflected wave includes the ramifications and growing stiffness of the arterial tree. With the help of analogous hydraulic-electric models, each of these parameters can be estimated separately and information on hydraulic load through each of their conceptual components can be obtained (Nichols *et al* 1980, 1987).

8.1.2.1 Peripheral resistance

Energy dissipation is generally associated with viscous phenomena and, therefore, to the dissipation of heat by friction. In the case of the arterial system, peripheral resistance (R_P) occurs in the arteriole-capillary bed and two physical magnitudes have a significant influence on it: blood viscosity and vessel dimensions.

$$R_P = \frac{\text{Mean pressure}}{\text{Mean Flow}} = \frac{8 \cdot \mu \cdot L}{\pi \cdot R^4}, \tag{8.4}$$

where μ is blood viscosity, L is the length of the arterial segment analyzed and R is the artery radius.

8.1.2.2 Arterial compliance

Arterial compliance is defined as the variation of vessel volume per unit of arterial pressure variation. It characterizes the dampening performance of pulsatility, thus fulfilling the main function of the great vessels that consists in acting as a hydraulic low-pass filter, producing an attenuation in the pulsatility imposed by the heart so that a continuous flow can reach the tissues. Among the most accurate methods for the noninvasive determination of arterial compliance is tonometry, used to obtain instantaneous pressure, and the automatic analysis of B-mode ultrasound images, used to obtained the waveform of the instantaneous arterial diameter. Its analytical expression is as follows:

$$C = \frac{D_M}{2 \cdot \rho \cdot VOP^2}, \tag{8.5}$$

where D_M is the mean arterial diameter, ρ is the blood density and PWV is the propagation velocity of the pressure wave.

8.1.2.3 Reflected wave

The pulse wave propagated through the arterial tree is broken down into two waves with opposite directions of propagation (incident wave and reflected wave, figure 8.1).

The characteristic resistance (Z_C) represents the value of resistance that would be needed as a load in the system so that reflections, or the system impedance in high frequencies, are not produced. Under these circumstances, the characteristic resistance in the arterial system exclusively represents the intrinsic properties, rather than the ramifications typical of the geometry or the peripheral resistance. It is calculated as follows:

$$Z_C = \frac{\rho \cdot VOP}{\frac{\pi}{4} D_M^2}, \tag{8.6}$$

where ρ is the blood density (assumed to be constant), PWV is the pulse wave velocity determined by the simultaneous recording of two pressure signals separated

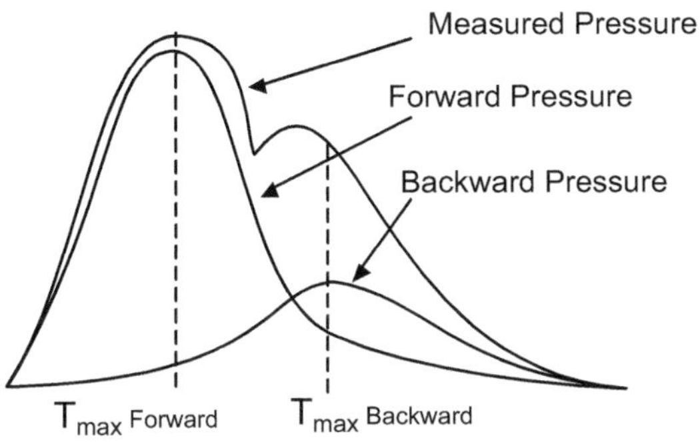

Figure 8.1. Pressure wave breakdown into an incident and a reflected wave.

by a known distance (Armentano *et al* 1994) and D_M is the mean diameter of the artery measured using a vascular ultrasound machine. Although the value of Z_C is not clinically relevant, it allowed the determination of the reflection coefficient in these studies.

8.1.3 Arterial impedance

Cardiac ejection is an essentially dynamic event and its analysis will require a deeper knowledge on the type of pulse, mainly in relation to its morphology. To analyze a pulsatile regime and to properly characterize it, mathematicians have shown that it is possible to characterize any complex wave (regardless of its shape) as a sum of more simple periodic functions, such as the sine and cosine functions, which is known as the Fourier's theorem (Patterson and Brown 1987). In other words, any form of complex wave is the result of the sum of sinusoidal functions of different amplitude and frequency but which are an exact multiple of the fundamental frequency or global frequency of the periodic phenomenon. Such a technique is commonly used in the engineering sciences and has made it possible to understand very complex phenomena. But engineers have gone a little further. They created a parameter that contains all the necessary information about the hydraulic load in each of the sinusoids that make up the main wave. In other words, the pressure waveform entering the arterial tree is the resulting sum of a series of sinusoidal pressure sources or generators of different amplitude and frequency which, in turn, generate a flow signal for each of them; and the sum of the latter will be the measured fluid.

The parameter referred to previously is called ***impedance***, which could be defined, without much mathematical rigor but with much conceptual strength, as the arterial system's opposition to the pulsatile flow provided by the heart (Armentano *et al* 1994, O'Rourke and Taylor 1967, O'Rourke and Kelly 1993, Finkelstein and Ross Collins 1982).

Since pressure and flow are periodic signals, a figure is not enough to characterize them fully. If those waves are characterized by only one value, we might talk about a maximum (or systolic) value, a minimum (or diastolic) value, a mean value, etc. However, in no case does this value provide the whole information contained in the waveform. For a deep understanding of a complex signal, like flow or pressure, such waves are broken down into an infinite number of pure sinusoidal functions of different growing amplitude and frequencies which, algebraically added up, allow a fully reliable reconstruction of the output signal. Each of these components is called harmonic and they consist of two values, one for modules and another for phases. Harmonic zero represents the offset of the signal or mean value, as it is known in medicine. The first or fundamental harmonic represents the most valuable component of the signal because it is generally the greatest in amplitude and it contains the same frequency as the original signal. The second harmonic has twice the frequency of the original signal. The third harmonic has thrice the frequency and so on (Patterson and Brown 1987).

The mathematical tool used to calculate the decomposition of the signal into its harmonic components is called the Fourier transform and it allows one to know all such components with only one calculation. This is also known as harmonic analysis and when this procedure is used, it is said to be an analysis in the frequency domain in order to differentiate it from the one performed in time, which is referred to as time domain analysis.

The simplest way to understand this phenomenon is to think of acoustic phenomena, in which a pure or simple sound is caused by simple sinusoidal vibrations. In general, sounds produced by musical instruments are not simple since the fundamental sound in them is accompanied by a series of harmonics, whose number or intensity characterizes the instrument or source of the sound. The lowest frequency (lowest pitch) is the fundamental sound because it imposes its frequency to the resulting complex sound. The timbre of a sound depends on the number and the intensity of harmonics that accompany the fundamental sound.

Definition

Arterial impedance (Z) is defined as the quotient of pressure and flow. Considering the previous formulae, this results in:

$$Z = \frac{P}{Q} = \frac{\rho c}{A} \cdot \frac{f(t - x/c) + g(t + x/c)}{f(t - x/c) - g(t + x/c)}. \tag{8.7}$$

Arterial impedance is the opposition of the arterial system to the pulsatile flow imposed by the heart and, since it expresses the relation between two periodic waveforms (pressure and flow), it is useful to analyze it in the frequency domain. Thus, impedance will be the quotient of the pressure and flow modules of each of the harmonics, and phase will be the difference between each of the corresponding phases. For this reason, impedance will be represented with a module diagram and a phase diagram (Comolet 1984, Finkelstein and Ross Collins 1982, Nichols *et al* 1980, 1987).

The advantage of impedance is that it includes all the components that are part of the arterial blood system. This concept considers two important characteristics of blood circulation: one related to macrocirculation, to the mechanical characteristics of the arterial wall and to the geometric characteristics of that territory; and one related to the resistance to flow within the microcirculation and to the rheological properties of blood (Bensalah 1985). For this reason, impedance quantifies the hydraulic load of the circulation viewed from the ventricle.

There are special cases that are extremely important and which will be dealt with below. These are the concepts of input impedance, load impedance, longitudinal impedance and characteristic impedance, which derive from the global definition provided above.

The procedure generally used to determine input impedance consists in measuring instant pressure $p(t)$ at a certain point and flow $q(t)$ simultaneously. Then, assuming that the signals obtained are periodic, they are analyzed using the Fourier transform in order to obtain the harmonic components that make up the signal,

$$\begin{aligned} p(t) &= P_0 + \sum_{n=1}^{N} P_n \cdot \cos(n \cdot \omega \cdot t + \phi_n) \\ q(t) &= Q_0 + \sum_{m=1}^{N} Q_n \cdot \cos(n \cdot \omega \cdot t + \theta_m), \end{aligned} \tag{8.8}$$

where P_0 corresponds to the mean value of $p(t)$; Q_0, to the mean value of $q(t)$; N is the number of harmonics considered in the analysis; and ω is the heart fundamental frequency expressed in rad s^{-1}.

The quotient of the pressure harmonic and the flow harmonic gives the harmonic of the impedance at that frequency,

$$Z(j \cdot \omega \cdot n) = \frac{P_n \cdot e^{j(n \cdot \omega \cdot t + \phi_n)}}{Q_n \cdot e^{j(n \cdot \omega \cdot t + \theta_n)}} = \frac{P_n}{Q_n} e^{j(\phi_n - \theta_n)}. \tag{8.9}$$

The previous equation refers to one specific harmonic. If Z_n is the quotient of P_n and Q_n, and φ_n is the difference between ϕ_n and θ_n, impedance $Z(j \cdot \omega \cdot n)$ can be defined for each frequency in terms of its module and phase,

$$Z(j \cdot \omega \cdot n) = Z_n \cdot e^{j\varphi_n}. \tag{8.10}$$

In theory, an infinite number of harmonics can be considered when developing a Fourier series. In practice, however, it has been observed that a limited number of harmonics provide insufficient information about the pressure and flow signals studied.

Within this conceptual framework, the concept of characteristic impedance defined above is the impedance that should be observed in the absence of reflections. It is obtained in the frequency domain by calculating the average of the last three harmonics.

8.1.4 Wave reflection

The reflection coefficient (Γ) is defined as the relation between the reflected pressure and the incident pressure or between the reflected flow and the incident flow:

$$\Gamma = \frac{P_r}{P_i} = \frac{Q_r}{Q_i}. \tag{8.11}$$

Considering the reflected and incident elements of the formula above, the reflection coefficient of the load (where Z_L is the load impedance) can be expressed as the quotient of the two elements:

$$\Gamma_L = \frac{\dfrac{Z_L A}{\rho c} - 1}{\dfrac{Z_L A}{\rho c} + 1} \tag{8.12}$$

based on the previous definitions, this can also be expressed as:

$$\Gamma_L = \frac{Z_L - Z_0}{Z_L + Z_0} \tag{8.13}$$

since

$$Z_0 = \frac{\rho c}{A}. \tag{8.14}$$

It should be noted that if the system terminates in its characteristic impedance, the reflection coefficient is null and there is no reflected wave. This is known as the adapted system. The following special cases can be mentioned:

(a) Tube closed at one end

$$Z_L = \infty \Rightarrow \Gamma_L = 1 \tag{8.15}$$

(b) Open tube

$$Z_L = 0 \Rightarrow \Gamma_L = -1 \tag{8.16}$$

(c) Tube terminated with Z_0

$$Z_L = Z_0 \Rightarrow \Gamma_L = 0. \tag{8.17}$$

If the arterial system is terminated in its characteristic impedance, there will be no reflections.

8.1.5 Reflection coefficient

Vascular impedance is a complex magnitude that must be analyzed in the frequency domain and, as mentioned above, it is related to the rheological and mechanical properties of the circulatory system.

Waves travel without reflection provided the diameter and elasticity of the conduit are uniform; but if the conduit is ramified or has sections with different mechanical properties, waves are partially reflected back to their site of origin (Newman *et al* 1983). Under such conditions, a pressure wave P_m at any point is the sum of an incident wave (P_f) and a reflected wave (P_b), $P_m = P_f + P_b$. As mentioned above, the relation between the reflected wave and the incident wave is called reflection coefficient. This relation can also be analyzed in the frequency domain. In that case, the calculation consists in obtaining the quotient of the harmonics corresponding to the reflected wave and the incident wave and, therefore, there will be a module diagram and a phase diagram. If the phase angle of the reflection coefficient is null, the incident and reflected pressure waves will be exactly in phase, which is an ideal situation. The reflection coefficient value for each harmonic is expressed in terms of its module and phase. The value that the module can take for the fundamental component is between 0 and 1, while the phase angle can take any value between 0° and 360°.

As already stated, one way to express such a coefficient, without resorting to frequency analysis, is the following:

$$\Gamma = \frac{Z_L - Z_0}{Z_L + Z_0}. \tag{8.18}$$

8.1.6 Separation of incident wave and reflected wave

The role of reflected waves in the determination of the arterial pressure and flow waveforms can easily be observed by applying a simple algorithm through which the incident and reflected wave components can be obtained separately. This separation can be achieved using an analogy with a power transmission line (Westerhof *et al* 2009, Murgo and Westerhof 1987). In such a case, the relevant equations are as follows:

$$\begin{aligned} P_m &= P_f + P_b \\ Q_m &= Q_f + Q_b \\ P_f &= Z_0 \cdot Q_f \\ P_b &= -Z_0 \cdot Q_b, \end{aligned} \tag{8.19}$$

where P is pressure, Q is flow, m is the measured wave, f is the incident wave, b is the reflected wave and Z_0 is the characteristic impedance.

The measured pressure wave (P_m) is equivalent to the sum of the incident wave (P_f) and the reflected wave (P_b). The measured flow wave (Q_m) is also equivalent to the sum of the incident wave (Q_f) and the reflected wave (Q_b). The pressure and flow incident and reflected waves are related by the characteristic impedance of the arterial system. In major arteries like the aorta, Z_0 is determined by the inertial effects and compliance, the combination of which makes Z_0 a real number. The given relations predict that pressure and flow incident waves will be identical, while the reflected waves will be identical but with opposite signs because pressure phenomena are additive, that is, they add up, and flow phenomena are subtractive, that is, they are subtracted. Since pressure and flow are measured quantitatively and characteristic impedance is calculated from the impedance spectrum, the equations can be solved, thus obtaining the incident and reflected waves. Working on the previously mentioned relations, we have:

$$\begin{aligned} P_f &= Z_0 \cdot Q_f = \frac{(P_m + Z_0 \cdot Q_m)}{2} \\ P_b &= -Z_0 \cdot Q_b = \frac{(P_m - Z_0 \cdot Q_m)}{2}. \end{aligned} \tag{8.20}$$

Another method used to obtain the incident and reflected waves without using flow measurement is the following:

$$P_m = P_f + P_b \tag{8.21}$$

as previously defined. If a total occlusion with $Q = 0$ (null flow) is performed distal but immediately close to the pressure sensor, a reflection coefficient will be obtained whose absolute value will be the unit, =1, thereby obtaining:

$$P_{m_o} = P_o = 2 \cdot P_f. \tag{8.22}$$

Since the whole incident wave will be reflected, we get:

$$P_f = \frac{P_o}{2}. \tag{8.23}$$

If we now subtract P_f from the pressure measured without occlusion, the following will be obtained:

$$P_b = P_m - \frac{P_o}{2}. \tag{8.24}$$

Therefore, the incident and reflected waveforms would be obtained through an externally generated total occlusion. Using this method, it is possible to know the flow, measured indirectly.

Another method is wave velocity analysis (Hughes *et al* 2008, Hughes and Parker 2009). The basic equation in one dimension that describes the conservation of mass and momentum in an elastic tube, with negligible dissipation, can be solved using the method of characteristics. The equations are presented in terms of the section A area, the velocity of the fluid U, pressure P and density ρ:

$$\begin{aligned} \frac{\partial A}{\partial t} + \frac{\partial (U \cdot A)}{\partial x} &= 0 \\ \frac{\partial U}{\partial t} + U \cdot \frac{\partial U}{\partial x} &= -\frac{1}{\rho}\frac{\partial P}{\partial x}, \end{aligned} \tag{8.25}$$

where the longitudinal direction is x. Assuming that the section is a function of pressure only, both equations can be summarized to find the solution.

Any perturbation applied on the tube propagates in the positive (x_+) and negative (x_-) directions at a velocity given by $U \pm c$, where U is the velocity of the fluid and c is wave velocity. For a temporary perturbation, a change in pressure is associated to a change in velocity as follows:

$$-dP = \pm \rho \cdot c \cdot dU. \tag{8.26}$$

The intensities of the pressure and velocity waves are always added up, whether they are incident or reflected. This analysis can be performed throughout the cardiac cycle, basically composed of an ejection and a relaxation phase. Since intensities are added, the method can be used to separate them:

$$dP = dP_+ + dP_-$$
$$dU = dU_+ + dU_-. \tag{8.27}$$

Finally, by replacing values, we obtain:

$$dP_\pm = \frac{(dP \pm \rho \cdot c \cdot dU)}{2}$$
$$dU_\pm = \frac{(dU \pm dP/\rho \cdot c)}{2}. \tag{8.28}$$

The pulse wave value is determined by means of the graph showing pressure as a function of velocity and by calculating the slope of the curve during early systole, where there are no reflected waves. In this way, according to (Hughes and Parker 2009), the slope value obtained corresponds to the $\rho \cdot c$ value (Hughes *et al* 2008, Hughes and Parker 2009), see figure 8.2.

Pulse wave and characteristic impedance are related through the following equation:

$$c = \frac{Z_0 \cdot A}{\rho}. \tag{8.29}$$

8.1.7 Measurement of the propagation coefficient.

The propagation coefficient (γ) describes the transmission characteristics of the pressure wave harmonics traveling along an artery

$$P_x = P_0 e^{-\gamma x} = P_0 e^{-(a+i[\omega/c])x}, \tag{8.30}$$

where P_x is the pressure distal to P_0 separated at a distance x, ω is the angular frequency (s^{-1}), a is the attenuation coefficient (cm^{-1}), and c is the phase velocity ($cm\ s^{-1}$) of the propagated wave. The propagation coefficient for each harmonic in

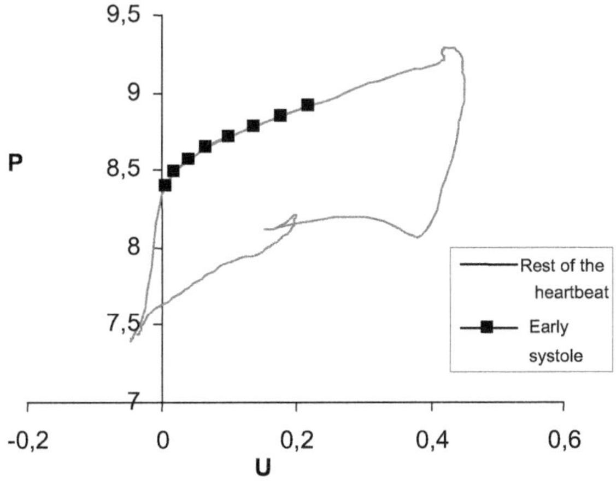

Figure 8.2. PU loop from which the $\rho \cdot c$ value is obtained.

the pressure wave is calculated using the three-pressure method (Gessner and Bergel 1966), which mathematically removes the reflection effect. Therefore (Gessner and Bergel 1966),

$$\gamma = \frac{1}{\Delta x} \cos h^{-1}\left(\frac{P_1 + P_3}{2P_2}\right), \tag{8.31}$$

where P_1, P_2, and P_3 are the complex harmonics of the three pressures measured, that is, proximal, medial and distal, respectively, Δx is the separation between sensors, and h is the thickness of the vascular wall *in vivo* (Gessner and Bergel 1966).

The real and imaginary parts of the complex propagation coefficient provide a measure of attenuation (a, in cm^{-1}), related to the viscosity that attenuates the pressure wave, and a measure of velocity c (in cm s^{-1}), an indicator of arterial stiffness (Bergel and Schultz 1971, Milnor 1982).

8.1.8 Determination of reservoir and excess pressures

Reservoir and excess pressures (P_{res} and P_{exc}, respectively) can be calculated through the 'known pressure only' method (Aguado-Sierra *et al* 2008, Westerhof *et al* 2009) since there is no input flow (Q). In this case, a three-element Windkessel model can be considered, where P_{exc} is the difference between P and P_{res} and it is related to the characteristic impedance of the model (Z_0, a resistance for the present analysis). P_{exc} is proportional to the flow (similar in form). The impedance made up of the system's peripheral resistance (R) and arterial compliance (C) is related to P_{res}. Both parameters (R and C) are usually obtained during the diastole, where Windkessel models of two or three elements behave similarly (Aguado-Sierra *et al* 2008, Westerhof *et al* 2009). The ordinary differential equation governing the relation between P_{res} and input flow Q can be expressed as follows:

$$C\frac{dP_{res}(t)}{dt} = Q(t) - \frac{P_{res}(t) - P_{\infty}}{R}, \tag{8.32}$$

where P_{∞} is the pressure at which flow through the microcirculation ceases. P_{∞} is greater than zero and closer to the diastolic pressure value than to the venous pressure value (Aguado-Sierra *et al* 2008, Westerhof *et al* 2009). Since P_{exc} is proportional to flow, parameter $Q(t)$ can be substituted with the expression $aC(P - P_{res})$, where a is a constant value. Then, the reservoir pressure can be obtained by solving the resulting differential equation:

$$d\frac{[P_{res}(t) - P_{\infty}]}{dt} + \left(a + \frac{1}{\tau}\right)(P_{res}(t) - P_{\infty}) = a[P(t) - P_{\infty}], \tag{8.33}$$

where τ is the time constant of the two-element Windkessel model (the product of R and C). The constant and P_{∞} can be obtained by adjusting the last third of the diastolic period to the exponential decay (Aguado-Sierra *et al* 2008, Westerhof *et al* 2009).

$$P_{dia}(t) - P_{\infty} = (P_0 - P_{\infty})e^{-\frac{t}{\tau}}, \tag{8.34}$$

where P_{dia} is the pressure measured during the last third of the diastole, while P_0 is the initial value of such interval. Parameter a was determined iteratively from the value that minimizes the quadratic difference between the estimated decay during P_{dia} and the expression of P_{res}. The start of the diastolic period was calculated by determining the time value where dP/dt is minimal. Such calculated time value has a better correlation with the closing of the aortic valve. Once parameter a was obtained, the resulting P_{res} was also used to obtain P_{exc}, as mentioned above (figure 8.3):

$$P_{exc}(t) = P(t) - P_{res}(t). \tag{8.35}$$

8.1.9 Physiopathological alterations in propagation characteristics

In 1878, Moens and Korteweg described what is currently known as the Moens–Korteweg equation for the pulse wave velocity of an elastic tube, such as a blood vessel. The conventional method used to determine wave velocity (PWV) includes measures of the time elapsed (T) between the start of both pulse signals (wave foot)

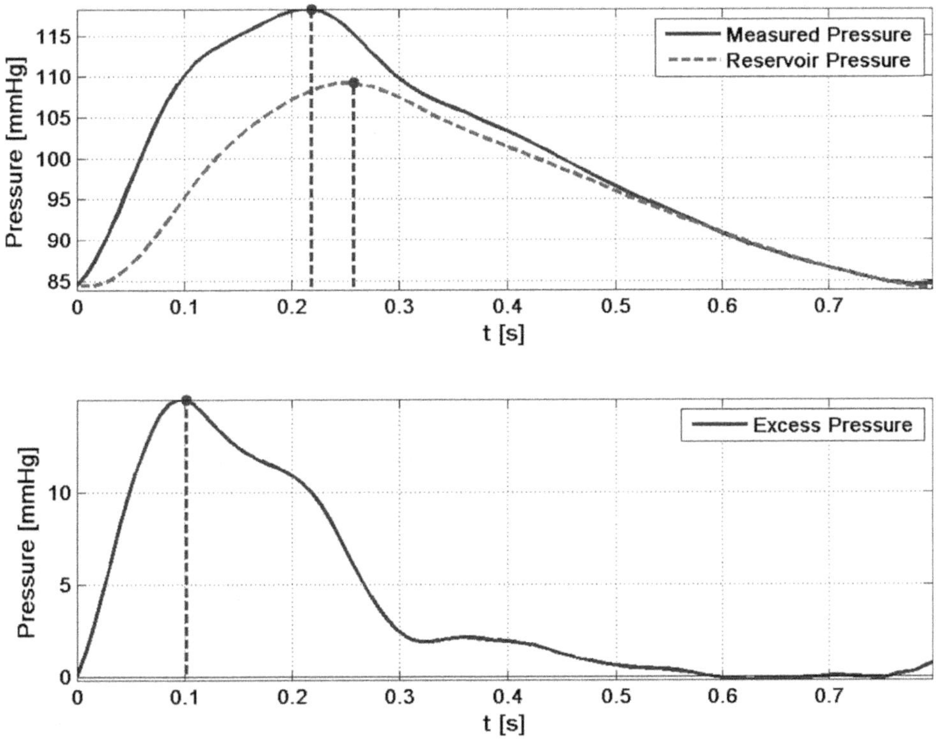

Figure 8.3. Upper panel: example of measured arterial pressure. Solid line: aortic pressure. Dotted line: reservoir pressure. Lower panel: excess pressure. Maximum pressure values and their times of occurrence were calculated for all pressures.

and the distance (L) separating the two measurement sites. Time T that quantifies the time mismatch between both waves must be carefully determined at the start of each wave where the reflection possibilities are almost null and therefore this mismatch between wave foots would only be related to the propagation of the incident wave, unaffected by reflection issues and artifacts (Chiu *et al* 1991, Bramwell and Hill 1922, Simon *et al* 1991, Pruett *et al* 1988, Nichols and O'Rourke 2005).

Aortic PWV is a direct measure of arterial stiffness in the aorta. It is a parameter that can be measured directly and in real time. Measurements are taken simultaneously at the carotid and femoral arteries and the aortic pulse wave is then represented. The stiffer the aorta, the higher its pulse velocity. An increase in aorta pulse velocity is associated with:

- Stroke in the hypertensive population.
- Atheroma plaques in the coronary arteries.

Pulse wave velocity has an independent predictive value in patients with kidney failure, coronary disease, uncomplicated hypertension and in the general population in relation to:

- Global mortality.
- Cardiovascular mortality.
- Cardiovascular morbidity.
- Coronary disease.
- Cerebrovascular disease.

It is for cardiovascular events that the predictive value of arterial stiffness and wave reflection becomes more significant. There is evidence that the carotid-femoral PWV is an intermediate end point for cardiovascular events, both fatal and nonfatal. Aortic PWV has a better predictive value than the classic risk factors included in risk scales. Central pressure and the augmentation index (Nichols and O'Rourke 2005, Hughes *et al* 2008) have an independent predictive value of all causes of mortality in patients with kidney injury, hypertension and coronary disease.

The arrival time of the reflected wave depends on a series of cofactors including artery length and pulse wave velocity (PWV), which have a prominent role. When physical development ceases, which means there will be no changes in anatomical lengths, a progressive increase in PWV is observed with aging in humans (Simon and Levenson 1991, Simon *et al* 1991, O'Rourke 1990, O'Rourke and Kelly 1993). This is correlated with an increase in arterial stiffness and is attributable to the effects of an increase in parietal stress, which might cause the rupture of the arterial wall elastic layer (O'Rourke and Kelly 1993). Changes in aortic PWV caused by aging can occur independently of changes in blood pressure caused by a modification in the stiffness of the vascular wall itself due to modifications in the parietal constituents. Actually, both pressure and parietal effects affect PWV simultaneously. The effects of a PWV increase on the reflected wave and, therefore, on the aortic pressure wave, can be observed using drugs that increase or decrease mean arterial pressure. When the mean pressure decreases, the reflected wave is seen later, and when it increases, there is an early appearance of the reflected wave, which is located in the systolic portion of the pressure wave. These pressure waves with late systoles affect left ventricular pressure as well as aortic pressure, which leads to a distortion of the optimal transfer as proposed by the ventricular–aortic coupling (O'Rourke *et al* 1987, Nichols *et al* 1987).

The effects of the reflected wave on the afterload can be quantified by calculating the increase of the pressure wave in the time domain. In the frequency domain, this is done by calculating the relation between pressure and flow, known as vascular impedance. The hemodynamic effects of the increase in pressure can be separated into an increase in peripheral resistance (observed in the vascular impedance diagram as an increase in the impedance module for the harmonic zero), an increase in the characteristic impedance (observed as an increase in the impedance module for high harmonics) and an early reflected wave (which moved the impedance curve towards the right) (Nichols *et al* 1980).

Under adequate normal circumstances, the reflected wave maintains the aortic pressure during the start of the diastole without losing pressure during the systole. Therefore, there is an increase in diastolic pressure that does not modify systolic blood pressure. If wave reflection occurs early, there is an increase in systolic pressure and a decrease in pressure during the diastole (Kelly *et al* 1989a, 1989b).

The effects of an early reflected wave can be understood by comparing the pressure waves in young subjects (type C) and elderly subjects (type A) with the same mean arterial pressure (Kelly *et al* 1989a, 1989b) as shown in the figure 8.4.

This figure shows an increase in the systolic pressure peak, an increase in the mean systolic pressure and an increase in the end systole pressure (type A), all accompanied by a decrease in mean pressure. The changes in systolic pressure increase the myocardium's oxygen demand, and a change in diastolic pressure tends to decrease the amount of blood perfused to the myocardium. An increase in systolic pressure increases left ventricular afterload, decreases ventricular ejection and can generate left ventricular hypertrophy as a secondary consequence (O'Rourke 1982, O'Rourke *et al* 1987).

It is important to stress that in both cases mean arterial pressure is the same and, for this reason, peripheral resistance could be similar in both subjects, which indicates that such characteristics are primarily an effect of the major arteries.

An early reflected wave is clearly an undesirable phenomenon in adult subjects, especially if they are hypertensive. Therefore, pharmacological manipulation is expected to achieve a delay or reduction of it.

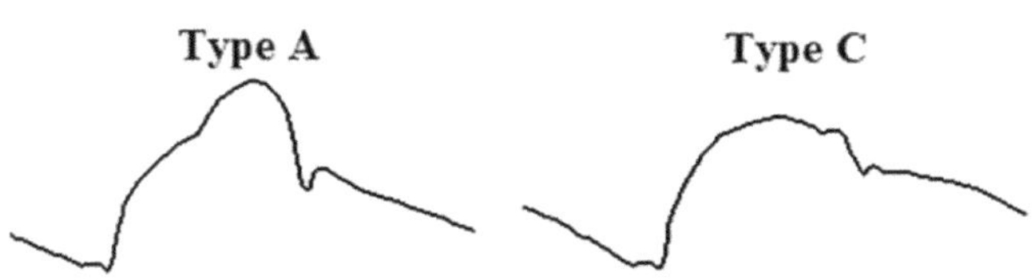

Figure 8.4. Pressure signals obtained from (a) elderly subjects, (b) young subjects.

It has been found that peripheral resistance, the reflection coefficient and wave pulse velocity are increased and that arterial compliance is decreased in hypertensive patients in relation to the normal group (Ting *et al* 1991, Nichols *et al* 1987, Liu *et al* 1986, 1989). These results are in line with alterations in compliance and reflection as indicated by the studies conducted by Simon (Simon and Levenson 1991, Simon *et al* 1991). These structural modifications might be due to a mismatch in the blood vessel wall or diameter in regional variations in the activation of the vascular smooth muscle, as suggested by Ting *et al* (1990, 1991). The increase in the mismatch index in hypertensive groups is of paramount importance because it suggests a higher mismatch of a possible optimal coupling between the heart and the artery (Elzinga and Westerhof 1991, O'Rourke *et al* 1987) caused by a greater reflected wave. Since this wave travels at a higher speed, it increases mean systolic pressure, causing a higher afterload and decreasing mean diastolic pressure, which reduces coronary perfusion pressure to the ventricle.

Many studies have recorded changes in arterial pressure in relation to aging. It has been documented that systolic pressure increases with age (Bia *et al* 2011) although variations in pressure related to age may not be uniform and might show differences depending on the characteristics of the population (Nichols and O'Rourke 2005). In contrast, minimal changes have been registered in relation to diastolic pressure, observing a reduction over 60 years of age (Nichols and O'Rourke 2005). An analysis of the reservoir/excess pressure components has shown that both increase with age (Bia *et al* 2011), but with different profiles (figure 8.5). The increase observed in the reservoir and excess pressure are consistent with previous publications based on recent studies (Davies *et al* 2010).

Reservoir pressure is related to systemic properties. As a result, changes related to reservoir pressure are caused by the combination of variations of the same kind. In opposition, excess pressure is more closely related to local behavior since the systemic response (a reservoir component) is not part of the evaluation. Therefore, different and complementary information may be obtained by analyzing both pressures (Bia *et al* 2011).

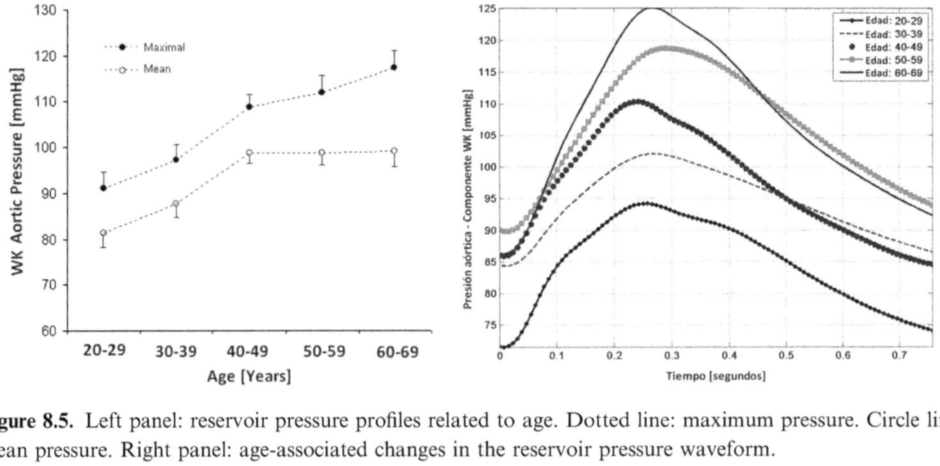

Figure 8.5. Left panel: reservoir pressure profiles related to age. Dotted line: maximum pressure. Circle line: mean pressure. Right panel: age-associated changes in the reservoir pressure waveform.

In relation to this, it would be more appropriate to process one specific pressure waveform (levels and morphology), by previously identifying its reservoir and excess components. It should be noted that an arterial pressure wave (and/or a change suffered by it) is the result of combinations of different components (Bia *et al* 2011). In this context, knowledge of the pressure profiles expected according to age as well as their individualized components would be very valuable to differentiate normal changes (related to aging) from those caused by vascular pathologies.

References

Aguado-Sierra J, Alastruey J, Wang J J, Hadjiloizou N, Davies J and Parker K H 2008 Separation of the reservoir and wave pressure and velocity from measurements at an arbitrary location in arteries *Proc. Inst. Mech. Eng.* H **222** 403–16

Armentano R L, Baglivo H, Cabrera Fischer E I and Sanchez R (ed) 1994 *Hipertensión Arterial Limítrofe ('Borderline'). Es un estado prehipertensivo? Implicancias experimentales, clínicas y pronósticas* (Buenos Aires: Centro Editor de la Fundación Favaloro)

Bensalah A 1985 Détermination atraumatique de l'ímpedance d'entrée arterielle. Application clinique *Thése de Docteur es Sciences* (Paris, Francia: Université Paris VII)

Bergel D H and Schultz D L 1971 Arterial elasticity and fluid dynamics *Prog. Biophys. Moll. Biol.* **22** 1–36

Bia D, Cymberknop L, Zocalo Y, Farro I, Torrado J, Farro F, Pessana F and Armentano R L 2011 Age-related changes in reservoir and excess components of central aortic pressure in asymptomatic adults *Conf. Proc. IEEE Eng. Med. Biol. Soc.* **2011** 6454–7

Bramwell J C and Hill A V 1922 The velocity of the pulse wave in man *Proc. R. Soc. Lond.* **93** 298–306

Burton A C 1972 *Physiology and Biophysics of the Circulation* (Chicago, IL: Year Book Medical Publishers)

Campbell K B, Lee L C, Frasch H F and Noordergraaf A 1989 Pulse reflection sites and effective length of the arterial system *Am. J. Physiol.* **256** H1684–9

Carson E and Cobelli C 2001 *Modelling Methodology for Physiology and Medicine* (Academic) pp 218–21

Chiu Y C, Arand P W, Shroff S G, Feldman T and Carroll J P 1991 Determination of pulse wave velocities with computerized algorithms *Am. Heart J.* **121** 1460–70

Cobelli C, Carson E R, Finkelstein L and Leaning M S 1984 Validation of simple and complex models in physiology and medicine *Am. J. Physiol.* **246** R259–66

Comolet R 1984 *Biomécanique Circulatoire* (París: Masson)

Davies J, Baksi J, Francis D, Hadjiloizou N, Whinnett Z and Manisty C *et al* 2010 The arterial reservoir pressure increases with aging and is the major determinant of the aortic augmentation index *Am. J. Physiol. Heart Circ. Physiol.* **298** H580–6.

Elzinga G and Westerhof N 1991 Matching between ventricle and arterial load *Circ. Res.* **68** 1495–500

Finkelstein S M and Ross Collins V 1982 Vascular hemodynamics impedance measurement *Prog. Cardiovasc. Dis.* **24** 401–18

Gessner U and Bergel D H 1966 Methods of determining the distensibility of blood vessels *IEEE Trans. Biomed. Eng.* **13** 2–10

Hughes A D, Parker K H and Davies J E 2008 Waves in arteries: A review of wave intensity analysis in the systemic and coronary circulations *Artery Res.* **2** 51–9

Hughes A D and Parker K H 2009 Forward and backward waves in the arterial system: impedance or wave intensity analysis? *Med. Biol. Eng. Comput.* **47** 207–10

Kelly R, Hayward C, Avolio A and O'Rourke M 1989a Noninvasive determination of age-related changes in the human arterial pulse *Circulation* **80** 1652–9

Kelly R, Hayward C, Ganis J, Daley J, Avolio A and O´Rourke M 1989b Non-invasive registration of arterial pressure pulse waveform using high-fidelity applanation tonometry *J. Vasc. Med. Biol.* **3** 142–9

Li J K-L 1987 *Arterial System Dynamics* (New York: New York University Press) pp 6–21

Liu Z, Brin K and Yin F C 1986 Estimation of total arterial compliance: an improved method and evaluation of current methods *Am. J. Physiol.* **251** 588–600

Liu Z, Ting C T, Zhu S and Yin F C 1989 Aortic compliance in human hypertension *Hypertension* **14** 129–36

Milnor W K 1982 *Hemodynamics* (Baltimore, MD: Williams and Wilkins) 56–96

Milnor W R 1975 Arterial Impedance as ventricular afterload *Circ. Res.* **36** 565–70

Murgo J and Westerhof N 1987 Arterial reflections and pressure waveforms in humans *Ventricular Vascular Coupling Clinical, Physiological and Engineering Aspects* (New York: Springer)

Newman D L, Greenward S E and Bryant Moodie T 1983 Reflection from elastic discontinuities *Med. Biol. Eng. Comput.* **21** 687–701

Nichols W W and O'Rourke M F 2008 The life and times of Donald A. McDonald *Artery Res.* **2** 1e8

Nichols W W, O'Rourke M F, Avolio A P, Yaginuma T, Murgo J, Pepine C J and Conti C R 1987 Age-related changs in left ventricular/arterial coupling *Ventricular Vascular Coupling Clinical, Physiological and Engineering Aspects* (New York: Springer)

Nichols W W and O'Rourke M 2005 Properties of the arterial wall: theory. Properties of the arterial wall: practice *McDonald's Blood Flow in Arteries: Theoretical, Experimental and Clinical Principles* 4th edn (London: Edward Arnold) ch 3, pp 49–65, ch 4, pp 67–93

Nichols W W and O'Rourke M F 1990 Aging, high blood pressure and disease in humans *McDonald's Blood Flow in Arteries: Theoretical, Experimental and Clinical Principles* 3rd edn (Lea and Febiger) pp 398–420

Nichols W W, Pepine C J, Geiser E A and Conti C R 1980 Vascular load defined by the aortic input impedance spectrum *Fed. Proc.* **39** 196–201

NIH Conference 1989 *Modeling In Biomedical Research: An Assessment of Current and Potential Approaches* (Washington, DC: U.S. Department of Health and Human Services)

Noordergraaf A 1969 *Hemodynamics. Biological Engineering* (New York: McGraw-Hill)

Noordergraaf A 1978 *Circulatory System Dynamics* (New York: Academic)

O'Rourke M F, Avolio A P and Nichols W W 1987 *Ventricular Vascular Coupling Clinical, Physiological and Engineering Aspects* (New York: Springer)

O'Rourke M F and Kelly R P 1993 Wave reflection in the systemic circulation and its implications in ventricular function *J. Hypertens.* **11** 327–37

O'Rourke M F and Taylor M G 1967 Input impedance of the systemic circulation *Circ. Res.* **20** 365–79

O'Rourke M F 1990 Arterial stiffness, systolic blood pressure, and logical treatment of arterial hypertension *Hypertension* **15** 339–47

O'Rourke M F 1982 *Arterial Function in Health and Disease* (New York: Churchill Livingstone) 153–69

Parker K H 2009 A brief history of arterial wave mechanics *Med. Biol. Eng. Comput.* **47** 111–8

Patterson P E and Brown L 1987 Biomechanical waveform analysis in the frecuency domain *Eng. Med. Biol. Mag.* **6** 12–6

Pruett J D, Bourland J D and Geddes L A 1988 Measurement of pulse wave velocity using a beat sampling tecnique *Ann. Biomed. Eng.* **16** 341–7

Quick C M, Berger D S and Noordergraaf A 2002 Arterial pulse wave reflection as feedback *IEEE Trans. Biomed. Eng.* **49** 440–5

Simon A and Levenson J 1991 Use of arterial compliance for evaluation of hypertension *Am. J. Hypertens.* **4** 97–105

Simon A, O'Rourke M F and Levenson J 1991 Arterial distensive and its effects on wave reflection and cardiac loading in cardiovascular disease *Coronary Artery Dis.* **2** 1111–20

Taylor M G 1959 Wave travel in arteries *Thesis* (London: University of London)

Ting C T, Chang M S, Wang S P, Chiang B N and Yin F 1990 Regional pulse wave velocities in hypertensive and normotensive humans *Cardiovasc. Res.* **24** 865–72

Ting C T, Chou C Y, Chang M S, Wang S P, Chiang B N and Yin F 1991 Arterial hemodinamics in human hypertension - Effects of adrenergic blockade *Circulation* **84** 1049–57

Welkowitz W 1977 *Engineering Hemodynamics: Application to Cardiac Assist Devices* (Lexington, MA: Lexington Books)

Westerhof N, Lankhaar J W and Westerhof B E 2009 The arterial Windkessel *Med. Biol. Eng. Comput.* **47** 131–41

Westerhof N, Sipkema P, Van Den Bos G C and Elzinga G 1972 Forward and backward waves in the arterial system *Cardiol. Res.* **6** 648–56

Wetterer E and Kenner T 1968 *Grundlagen der Dynamik des Arterienpulses* (Berlin: Springer)

Wormersley J R 1957 Oscillatory flow in arteries: the constrained elastic tube as a model of arterial flow and pulse transmission *Phys. Med. Biol.* **2** 178

Chapter 9

Damping in the vascular wall

Ricardo L Armentano and Leandro J Cymberknop

It is widely accepted that arteries damp the pulsatility of the pressure and flow incident (anterograde) waves generated in each ventricular ejection, as blood circulates from the large arteries to the peripheric circulation. Essentially, this was shown when the pulsatility or amplitude of flow and pressure waves in the input (large central arteries) and the output (microcirculation) of the arterial system were registered. Consequently, the whole arterial system has been modeled as a system working as a lowpass hydraulic system, that is, it reduces the high levels of pulsatility generated by the heart. That important function determines that blood reaches the microcirculatory system with low levels of pulsatility.

However, although this function of the arterial system is widely accepted, the mechanisms through which the arteries perform these functions have not been fully unraveled. In this context, our group has been working from a theoretical and experimental perspective, with the aim of deepening knowledge of the mechanisms used by each arterial segment (like a cell) to contribute to the global damping of pressure and flow waves (Armentano *et al* 2003, 2007).

The objective of this chapter is to provide the reader with the theoretical and experimental foundations on which our work is based. To that purpose, we will deal with the fundamental theoretical physiological foundations. Without a doubt, a detailed account of the theory underlying our analysis (e.g. the theory of filters) is beyond the scope of this chapter so the following content is the basics to understand our work. The reader who is interested in delving into these topics can widen their knowledge by reading the references at the end of the chapter. In the second part, we will finish the chapter showing a series of results that were validated in scientific papers published in international refereed journals, thus allowing us to move forward in the topic (Armentano *et al* 2003, 2006, 2007, Bia *et al* 2005a, 2005b, 2005c, 2006, 2007, Pessana *et al* 2004, Zócalo, 2006, 2007). It is worth noting that everything that the reader will find here has the strengths and weaknesses of any approach attempting to describe or characterize something as complex as reality

doi:10.1088/2053-2563/aafb0dch9

through physical–mathematical models, even more, considering that our objective was to generate a solid conceptual framework, but as simple as to be able to be used in the clinical practice.

The identification of the fundamental dynamic properties of the arterial wall (e.g. viscoelasticity, natural vibration frequencies, damping fractions) constitutes the foundation to characterize the real conditions of such structure, and to estimate the response that it may provide under a specific hemodynamic condition (e.g. hyper-pulsatility). In addition, characterizing such properties would enable the assessment of the need to implement any structural intervention measure, to avoid structural and/or functional failures (e.g. aneurysm). In this context, the aim for the approach presented here is to theoretically and experimentally estimate the dynamic properties of the 'arterial wall' structure, through non-invasive methodologies (realistic dynamic tests), with emphasis on its abilities to dampen or filter the pulsatility and to protect itself against them. In addition, we think that knowing these properties will be essential to predict the ability of the arterial wall to face different hemodynamic conditions in healthy subjects and/or with a vascular pathology, or in vascular grafts from soft tissue. In other words, just as the integration of analytical and experimental methods leads to the development of studies to predict the seismic vulnerability of buildings, we believe that a similar approach could be used to measure the vulnerability of the arterial wall in detail.

The application of tests typical of structural dynamics, such as free vibration tests and forced vibration tests induced by harmonic or environmental excitement, leads to the identification of the dynamic properties of different structures and to the measurement of their vulnerability in high frequency oscillations. However, these tests, widely used for materials and structures' strength studies, require experimental techniques that make their application to the non-invasive study of human arteries difficult. Consequently, our team has worked to access this information through studies in which the vibrations to which the 'arterial wall' structure is subjected to measure its response are the actual signals (pressure and/or flow waves) with which the system is confronted in its physiological hemodynamic condition. Undoubtedly, this approach poses different limitations, such as the lack of control over the excitation signal, but it provides insuperable advantages, such as the fact that it can be applied non-invasively in human clinics.

9.1 Physiological bases of wall damping and filtering

In this section, our aim is to establish the conceptual basis supporting our group's work and to establish the theoretical framework required to understand the methodological approach and the results that will be dealt with below.

9.1.1 The arterial wall as an oscillating system; energy and elastic and viscous work.

In each ejection, the left or right ventricle generates pressure and flow incident waves (they travel towards the arterial system or load) propagating from the heart through the large, medium and small arteries to the microcirculation or periphery. On propagating through the conducting arteries, at each site where the incident waves find a discontinuity in the mechanical and geometrical properties of the arterial tree (e.g. bifurcations, stenosis, arterial terminations, arterioles) reflected or retrograde waves are generated (they travel towards the generator or ventricle), which travel from the reflection site to the heart. It is worth noting that the 'reflection' phenomenon occurs when a wave, on encountering a new medium through which it cannot pass totally or partially, changes the propagation direction. The continuous existence of incident and reflected waves determines that, at any arterial site, the pressure and flow waves are formed by the overlapping of incident waves and reflected waves (figure 9.1).

This characteristic of the arterial system determines that each surface area of the endoluminal face of the arterial wall is subjected to forces (e.g. perpendicular to the wall) generated by incident and reflected waves (e.g. pressure waves) that will impose a certain level of pressure ('pressure blow or impact'), which will result in a distension of the artery. In other words, the endoluminal surface of the arterial wall will be cyclically facing pressure waves (disturbances of the mean or stable pressure level propagating through space) which, with each impact against the wall, will apply a force on its surface that will modify the motion or resting state of the arterial wall, producing an acceleration, by modifying its velocity. In other words, each pressure wave will give energy to the arterial wall.

Although the term energy has many meanings and definitions, it is clear that they are all related to the idea of an ability to do, transform or put into motion, or to the ability to perform a task. In the arterial case, the energy 'delivered' by the pressure (or flow) wave to the arterial wall, once force is applied on it, will allow the artery to move, distending all its wall constitutive elements (e.g. elastin fibers, collagen, muscle cells). Given the fact that some of these elements contribute to the mainly elastic behavior of the arterial wall and others, to the viscous behavior, it can be schematically said that the energy applied on the arterial wall will allow it to perform the required work (force × movement) to distend its elastic components (elastic work) and its viscous components (viscous work). It must be considered that the basic unit of work in the international system of units (IS) is 'newton × meter', called 'joule', and it is the same unit that measures energy. Consequently, the energy provided (e.g. by the pressure wave) is the ability to perform work (in the arterial wall) or that the work generates a variation of energy (in the arterial wall). That is why, in our work, we could indistinctly refer to the calculation of the elastic work or elastic energy, or to the calculation of the viscous work or viscous energy.

9.1.2 Damping or filtering function: arterial self-protection

9.1.2.1 Damping: role on the ventricular afterload and the microcirculatory flow
In this context of arteries subjected to pulsatile conditions of pressure and flow, it is widely accepted that one of the main functions of the arterial system, in addition to carrying blood towards the periphery (conducting or conduit function), is to damp pulsatility (damping function). A damper could be defined as a *'device that absorbs energy, used normally to reduce undesired oscillations of a periodic movement or to absorb energy coming from blows or impacts'*. Consequently, accepting that the

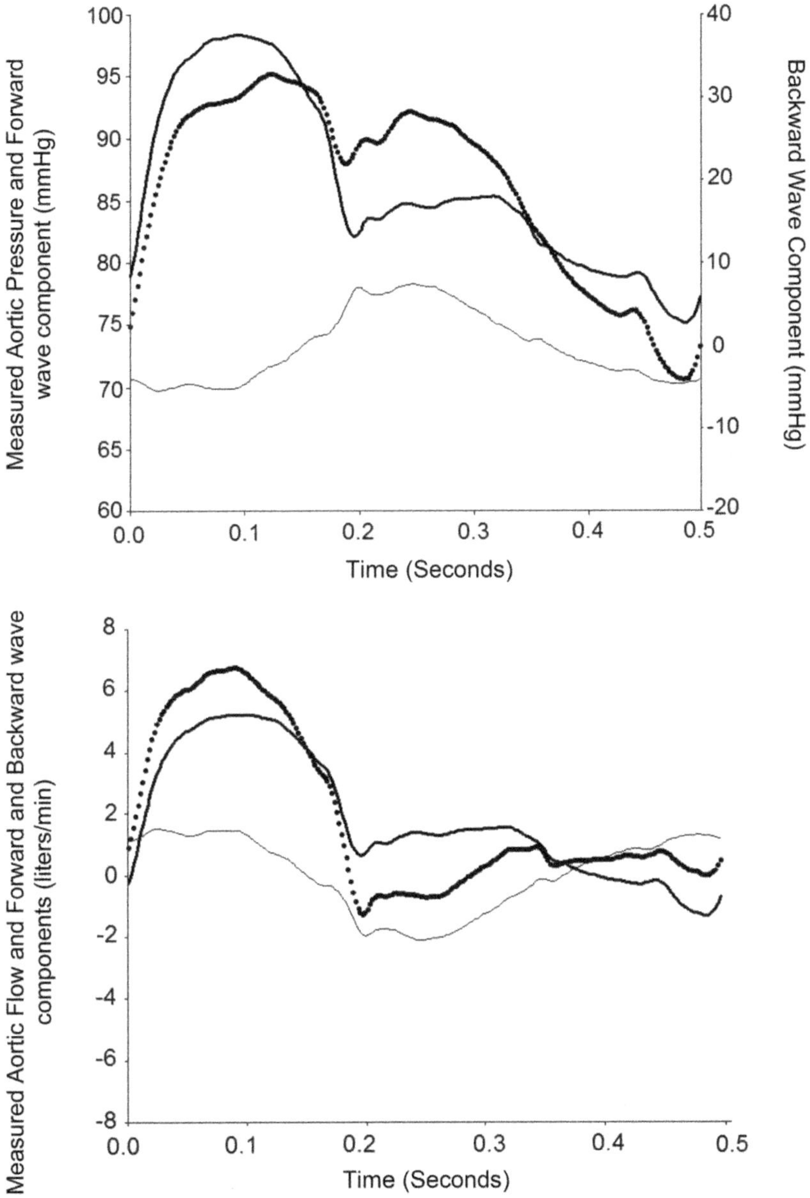

Figure 9.1. Aortic pressure and flow waves measured in a sheep. In each graph, the wave measured with a pressure or flow sensor, and its incident (in addition to the stationary component) and reflected component are illustrated.

arteries work as dampers means accepting that the arterial wall's aim is to reduce the oscillations imposed by the pressure and/or flow waves that 'impact' against their walls. In order to act as efficient dampers, arterial walls present a viscoelastic behavior that, as we have seen in the relevant chapters, lets them store and dissipate energy in each pulse.

Traditionally, the physiological importance of the damping ability of the arterial wall has been acknowledged due to the effects on the ventricular afterload (central effects) and/or due to its effects on the microcirculatory system (peripheral effects). On the one hand, an artery with a high ability to damp will reduce the levels of ventricular dynamic afterload in each cardiac ejection and it will make blood flow reaching the interchanging vessels (capillaries) either continuous or systo-diastolic, instead of only systolic. Thus, it has been acknowledged that a suitable damping function is important to keep the ventricular work and myocardial oxygen consumption levels low, and to maintain high levels of tissue oxygenation (Nichols and O'Rourke 1998).

9.1.2.2 Damping: role in wall self-protection

In addition to the heart and microcirculation functions mentioned, a suitable damping ability is essential for the arterial wall to have a suitable 'self-protecting ability'. Unfortunately, this physiological role played by the arterial wall has barely been considered to date. Previous studies have shown that, like other inorganic and/or organic material subjected to continuous oscillation and vibration, the pressure and flow waves sooner or later generate fatigue on the materials constituting the arterial wall. It must be noted that the stress of the arterial wall, like in other materials, refers to a phenomenon by which the rupture of the materials under cyclic dynamic loads is produced more easily than with static loads. An example of this is what happens with some metals (e.g. wire), whose structure can be easily broken if they are subjected to repeated bending while it is more difficult to break them by subjecting them to static forces. Evidently, it must be understood that, under normal conditions, the arterial wall is far from its breaking point, or a shear–stress relationship which would cause it to rupture since it has a high security factor. However, like other materials, the exposure of the arterial wall to a chain of or continuous oscillations around a central position (determined by the mean arterial pressure) for a considerable period of time could produce the erosion or damage of the wall structures and, consequently, the tissue response to that overload, even if the breaking point is not reached.

The idea that the 'arterial wall', in addition to being a structure that works on the ventricular afterload and/or on the microcirculation, is a structure that must self-protect from the pulsatile conditions existing in the circulatory system, and that the level or ability to self-protect can be modified by acute and/or chronic, permanent and/or temporary changes, is the core idea that has driven most of our studies in the last few years (Armentano *et al* 2003, 2006, 2007, Bia *et al* 2005a, 2005b, 2005c, 2006, 2007, Pessana *et al* 2004, Zócalo, 2006, 2007).

In this context, in which the arterial wall must 'protect itself' or 'avoid facing' the high frequencies of the pressure and flow waves, it is conceptually possible to model it as a 'viscoelastic damper' and/or an 'electronic filter', in charge of eliminating or attenuating high frequency oscillations which, contained in the pressure wave, could be transferred to the diameter wave, and consequently cause vibration or frequency alterations—dependent on the wall components (Armentano *et al* 2006, 2007, Bia *et al* 2005a, 2005b, 2005c, 2006, 2007, Pessana *et al* 2004, Zócalo, 2006, 2007).

9.1.2.3 Damping: classification of the main types.
A structural system subjected to a state of dynamic loads undergoes displacement. When the external excitement disappears, as a result of viscous friction forces, the structure comes to rest. The motion of the structures subjected to variable forces during a period of time depends, in particular, on the damping properties, that is, on the dissipation of energy through the material constituting the structure, between the bonds of their different elements, between them and the medium surrounding them. Consequently, damping is defined as the ability of a structure to hold up the energy transmitted by an external action through its friction forces.

9.1.2.4 Coulomb damping or pure friction
Coulomb damping or pure friction describes the physical phenomenon of friction between dry surfaces, which is independent of the motion velocity once it has started. So, Coulomb damping occurs when friction between particles of a structure holds up or absorbs the external actions. Consequently, it consists of a friction damping that possesses direction of the displacement and sign opposite to that of velocity.

This type of damping occurs due to friction in the connections or supporting points. It is constant, independent of velocity or amount of displacement, and usually it is treated as 'internal viscous damping', when the level of displacement is small, or as 'hysteretic damping' when it is high (Alarcón 1989, Cornejo 2002, Rodríguez 2001).

9.1.2.5 Internal viscous or frequency-dependent damping
Internal viscous or frequency-dependent damping is a widely used way of describing structures' damping; it refers to the loss of kinetic energy of a body that moves inside a fluid. It is described as: $Fa = x \cdot c$, Fa being the force produced by the damper, c the damper constant, and x the relative velocity between both ends of the damper. Although the model does not accurately reflect the structure's behavior, it provides a linear equation that substantially reduces the cumbersome numerical calculations required for its analysis.

In viscous damping, the damping force is proportional to the movement velocity. Consequently, in these systems the dissipated energy or attenuation or damping coefficient varies linearly with velocity or frequency. However, since in most materials damping varies very slowly in relation to frequency, using viscous damping to model the energetic dissipation in such materials would lead to an underestimation or overestimation at low and high frequencies, respectively.

Viscous damping is widely used in classical damping devices (e.g. automobiles). In general, through viscous fluid sheets that circulate through narrow holes, resisting forces that are proportional to the movement velocity and of opposite sign are generated, which tend to damp oscillation. In the course of a cycle, the work of such forces, which is positive, represents viscous damping (Alarcón 1989, Cornejo 2002, Rodríguez 2001, Varanasi 2002, 2004).

9.1.2.6 Structural hysteretic or frequency-independent damping

Structural hysteretic or frequency-independent damping is a type of common damping that occurs when an element is subjected to reversals in the load orientation and the material is already within the inelastic or nonlinear range. Not all the deformation energy accumulated in the element during the filling phase is converted to kinetic energy in the discharge cycle, which is reflected by the fact that the discharge curve has a different trajectory from that of the load curve. Consequently, this type of damping is called 'hysteretic' because it is based on the study of the hysteresis cycle of the energy dissipation of the system in question, and it consists of a behavioral response of the constituting materials. Then, it is defined as the ability to absorb the external actions due to a correct configuration of its transversal sections (e.g. dimensions, materials quantity, etc). In hysteretic damping, the damping force is proportional to the movement and of opposite sign to velocity. In a cycle, the exterior force delivers a positive work corresponding to the dissipated energy of the structure: that is the damping as a consequence of the hysteresis. The loss coefficient generally increases with the cycle's amplitude. In addition, in this type of damping, the rate of damping decreases very slowly with frequency or, as a first approach, it remains almost constant in a wide range of values. That is why the hysteretic damping can be considered as one that has a constant damping rate, or is independent from the loading frequency. On certain occasions, in order to use a 'hysteretic damping' system, a simple mechanical model formed by a spring of stiffness k is used, in parallel to a damper of constant c and a mass m subjected to an oscillating load $\mathrm{Pe}^{i\alpha t}$ (Alarcón 1989, Cornejo 2002, Rodríguez 2001, Varanasi 2002, 2004).

The last two types of damping (viscous and hysteretic) are the most commonly found, even coexisting in some materials or structures (figure 9.2). In the case of the arterial wall, for a tridimensional, multi-element structure with viscoelastic properties, any of the three types of damping could ideally contribute to pulse wave attenuation. In this sense, the Coulomb or friction damping (e.g. friction between the elastic sheets), velocity-dependent damping (e.g. mediated by the displacement of intra-wall viscous liquids such as the liquids in cell matrices and/or in cell cytoplasm), and hysteretic structures (e.g. smooth muscle cells) are present in each loading and unloading cycle of the arterial wall.

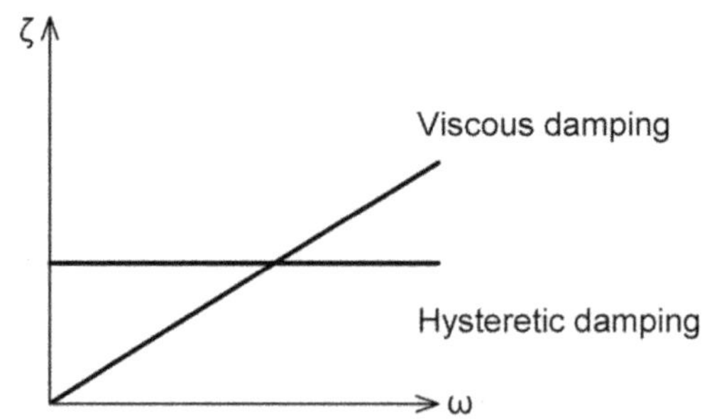

Figure 9.2. Differences between the loss coefficient (ζ), attenuation or damping coefficient for viscous and hysteretic damping, in relation to its response as a function of frequency. It can be observed that in the hysteretic damping, the loss coefficient corresponds to a constant of the material.

Considering the types of damping described above, two related coefficients, which we will use in our work, can be described:

The *loss coefficient* (ζ) is a dimensionless coefficient typical of the damping effect, and it is given by the relation between the dissipated energy during a cycle and the maximum potential energy multiplied by 2π:

$$\zeta = \text{Dissipated energy in a cycle}/2 \cdot \pi \cdot \text{Maximum potential energy}.$$

In the case of the hysteretic damping, it could also be written as follows:

ζ: Dissipated energy in a complete loading/unloading cycle/2 · π. Elastic deformation energy in relation to force and maximum deformation in the cycle (figure 9.3: $\zeta = A_L/4\pi A_T$) (Cornejo 2002).

9.1.3 The arterial wall as a mass–spring–damper system

The existence of structural components of the arterial wall with elastic behavior (e.g. elastin fibers) and with viscous behavior (e.g. cytoplasmatic liquid of the muscle cells, liquid of extracellular matrix), is key in the determination of the damping ability of the arterial wall. In this respect, these components determine that the wall behaves schematically as a spring–dashpot type damper. Although numerous springs and viscous damper arrangements can be made to model the arterial wall (some were presented in chapters 4 and 5), the Kelvin–Voigt model is a simple model which is sufficient to our aim (figure 9.4).

In this model, the helical spring is a deformable elastic element that keeps the wall in its equilibrium position, and its mission is to absorb the impact suffered by the arterial wall from the pressure wave. However, if the spring were alone, when the

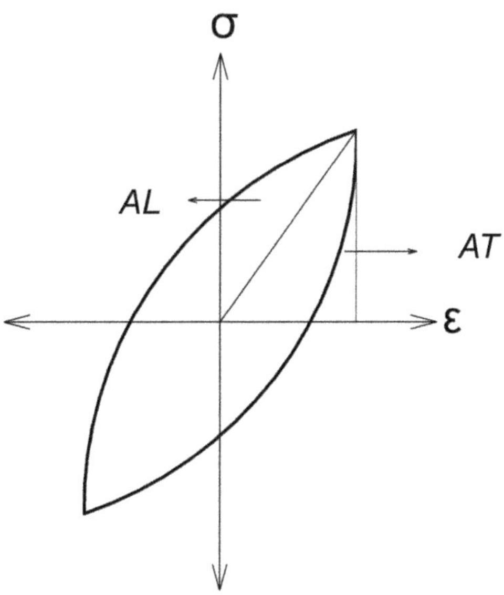

Figure 9.3. Damping rate or loss coefficient of the hysteretic model for a hysteretic stress (σ)–strain (ε) relationship.

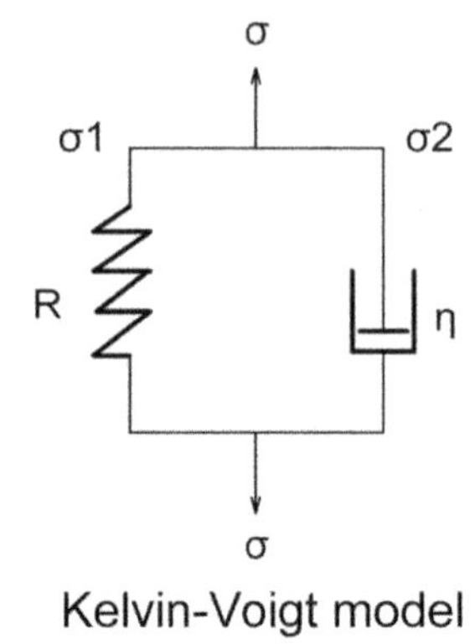

Figure 9.4. Kelvin–Voigt model representing the arterial wall as a spring–viscous dashpot type damper. R: spring or elastic element. η: viscous damper. σ: wall stress distributed in the elastic (σ_1) and viscous (σ_2) component.

arterial wall received the pressure impact, it would be transmitted to the spring, which would compress during systole absorbing such impact. Once the spring is compressed, it will 'return' the energy received (elastic energy) and will tend to return to its initial shape, leading to stretching. However, if this was not controlled, it could be highly abrupt. If this occurred, the arterial wall could 'bounce' against the pressurized blood in the artery, and then lead to a series of compression–stretching cycles in oscillating motions that could generate real harmful vibrations of the arterial wall components.

The dampers or viscous components of the arterial wall will serve to control these bounces. They absorb the energy of the springs and, as expressed by its name, they damp or attenuate the abrupt (of high frequency or velocity) reactions of the spring so that the arterial wall does not enter a permanent oscillation regime. In other words, the existence of the viscous component of the arterial wall would allow it to reach its required stability.

In sum, the main objective of the spring or elastic component of the arterial wall is to absorb energy. To that end, it 'absorbs' the impact in the arterial wall generated by the pressure wave and accumulates the energy of this impact through its deformation. Its mission will be completed by the damper, or viscous component, which 'damps', causing part of the energy delivered to the wall by the pressure wave not to be stored in the elastic component (systolic dissipation or release of energy), which is lost as heat. In addition, it allows the energy absorbed by the spring to be released as heat (diastolic dissipation or release of energy).

Another way of understanding the damper's behavior would be that while the elastic component transforms the kinetic energy into potential energy and vice versa, the viscous components transform the kinetic energy into thermal energy, in other words, they generate heat.

In addition to this approach, the spring–dashpot system mass or the arterial wall mass could be considered, which also contributes to its stabilization against oscillations caused by the pressure wave. However, as we will see, the contribution of the arterial wall mass to the level of damping reached can be considered negligible.

Wall dissipation and storage energies.

The viscous dissipation energy (W_D) in the arterial wall (per area unit) during a quarter of a cardiac cycle, is defined as:

$$W_D = \frac{\omega \cdot \eta \cdot A}{\pi},$$

where ω is $2\pi \cdot$ heart rate, and $\omega\eta$ represents the viscous losses (due to heat in the wall), and A is the mean cross-sectional pulsatile area.

The maximum value of elastic strain energy per area unit, stored in the wall during a quarter of a cycle (strain work or elastic potential energy storage, W_A) and returned without losses during diastole, is defined as:

$$W_A = \frac{2 \cdot A \cdot E}{\pi},$$

where E is the arterial elastic modulus (the inverse of arterial compliance) and A is the mean cross-sectional pulsatile area.

These two energies represent storage and dissipation per cardiac cycle. The first one is closely related to the elasticity of elastic fibers of the arterial wall (collagen and smooth muscle), while the dissipation energy is closely related to the wall viscosity modulus, indicating the smooth muscle's role and its remodeling in pathologies such as arterial hypertension (Armentano *et al* 2006).

9.1.3.1 The need for an adequate balance between the spring (elasticity) and the damper (viscosity).

For a suitable characterization, first it is necessary to measure the 'suspension stiffness' (determined by the 'rigidity' of the spring) and 'damping stiffness' (determined by the 'rigidity' of the dashpot), and their relationship. In other words, it is necessary to characterize the elasticity and viscosity of the arterial wall. 'Rigid' springs (springs with a high elastic constant) will produce rapid oscillations, due to which they will need a 'rigid' damper (e.g. springs with a high viscosity) to reduce such oscillations rapidly. Conversely, a 'soft' spring will need a 'soft' damper (e.g. dampers with a low level of viscosity) so that the spring effect does not slow down excessively. If, for example, a soft spring and a hard damper were used, the arterial wall strain would be more easily achieved (rapid pressure–diameter transfer) when the pressure wave impacts the arterial wall, but it would take longer to return the artery to its initial position, since the high viscosity would make the spring recovery much slower. Consequently, like in the suspension and damping equipment of industrial use (e.g. in the automotive industry), the spring–damper equilibrium or, in other words, the elastic response–viscous response, must be kept at least theoretically. As a consequence, to a certain point, the level of elasticity and the level of viscosity of an artery, that is, the degree of stiffness of the spring and the damper, are directly related.

On the other hand, depending on the type of oscillation, the characteristics of the spring and damper must be adjusted. In this sense, small undulations need a low level of elasticity and viscosity, and large undulations require slower and more rigid springs and dampers.

Consequently, depending on the arterial segment considered and the levels of oscillations, a compromise should be found between the lightness and stiffness of the spring and damper. In this sense, as we will see further in this chapter, by studying different arterial segments from the sheep lung and systemic circuit and the human systemic circuit, we found that despite the large variations in the levels of elastic and viscous responses between different arteries, the 'elastic response/viscous response' relationship remained constant. In addition, this response remained unaltered in hypertensive patients, in whom the remodeling process of the arterial wall had modified their elastic and viscous response levels. However, this relationship was modified due to acute changes of pressure and/or modifications of the arterial smooth muscle tone. Consequently, this relationship could be considered a 'new' biological constant, characteristic of constitutive elements of the arterial wall and of the level of the existing smooth muscle tone (Armentano *et al* 2006, 2007, Bia *et al* 2005a, 2005b, 2005c, 2006, 2007, Zócalo, 2006, 2007).

9.1.4 The arterial wall modeled as a filter

9.1.4.1 Transfer function of the arterial wall

So far, we have analyzed the wall's damping function, representing the arterial wall through a mechanical system or model of the spring–dashpot type, with a negligible mass. However, it is also possible to model this function, thinking of it as the action of an electronic filter.

Representing the arterial wall as an electronic filter means considering it as an element that discriminates a certain frequency or range of frequencies of an input signal passing through it, being able to modify both its amplitude and its phase, and producing certain changes in the output signal. For the case of the arterial wall, in our model, the pressure or stress applied on the arterial endoluminal surface was adopted as the input signal and the diameter wave or resulting arterial strain, as the output signal.

The way a filter behaves is described by its 'transfer function', since it is this function that determines the way in which the applied signal or input signal changes in amplitude and in phase when passing through the filter. Consequently, to characterize the 'vascular wall' filter, one of the first objectives established was, as we will see, to determine the wall pressure–diameter 'transfer function', in different situations and in different arteries. In other words, the transfer function found characterizes the filter. In addition, other characteristics that define the filter, such as the filter order, its type of frequency response, etc, were characterized as well.

Although the input and output signals are in our case time signals, the transfer function can be mathematically expressed (in the time domain) as a fraction (H(z)). In this regard, if a signal X(z) passes through a system H(z), then the output will be: $Y(z) = H(z) \cdot X(z)$. Reorganizing the terms, the system can be characterized as the ratio between the output signal and the input signal: $H(z) = Y(z)/X(z)$. In addition, as we will see in our methodological approach, it is possible to express this equality in the frequency domain through suitable frequency transformations: H(f) = Y(f)/X(f). It is said that the values that make the numerator null are the zeros and those that make the denominator null are the poles. The number of poles expresses the order of the filter and its value determines the characteristics of the filter, such as its frequency response and stability.

9.1.4.2 Frequency response of the arterial wall: Bode diagrams

One of the classic ways to characterize the transfer function of a filter is to analyze it in terms of frequency (filter's frequency response). Frequency response is a representation of the relationship between the input of sine waves of different frequencies entering a filter (or any other system) and the output of such waves. The systems can modify both the phase and the modulus of each of the input sine waves and therefore the frequency response will be determined by the differences in magnitude and phase between the sinusoidal input and output.

As stated in chapters 4 and 5, due to their polyharmonic nature, the pressure and diameter periodic signals measured in the vascular system (real signals) can be decomposed into sine and cosine functions, that is, into their pure harmonics. As a result, the frequency response of the arterial wall can be analyzed by considering the pressure signal or, in other words, the different harmonics composing such a signal, as the input; and the different harmonics composing the diameter signal, as the output.

The frequency response of a system can be studied using two different approaches: Bode diagrams or Nyquist diagrams. Both methods provide the same information, but in a different way. In our work, we decided to use the 'magnitude' graphs or diagrams proposed by Hendrik Wade Bode ('Bode diagrams') for the graphic representation of the transfer function as a function of frequency.

A Bode diagram usually consists of two separate graphs, one corresponding to the magnitude of such a function and the other corresponding to the phase. The Bode magnitude diagram represents the transfer function modulus (gain) in decibels as a function of frequency using a logarithmic scale (figure 9.5). This magnitude diagram is typically used in signal processing to show the frequency response of a linear time-invariant system. In addition, it is a widely used tool in circuit analysis in electronics, being essential for the design and analysis of filters. Among other features, it can be used to analyze the frequency response of the arterial wall and quickly provide an intuitive idea of the system's behavior through simple observation.

Knowing these diagrams and how to analyze them is paramount for a proper interpretation of the filter's characteristics and thus to understand the scope of the results that will be presented later in this chapter. For this reason, the main characteristics to be considered when analyzing these diagrams will be described below, based on a typical Bode diagram (figure 9.5).

When interpreting a Bode diagram, it is important to notice that the scale corresponding to the frequency axis (abscissa) is logarithmic. Logarithmic scales are used to represent data whose values range across several orders of magnitude (in figure 9.5, for example, frequency varies between 1 rad s^{-1} and 10^3 rad s^{-1}). If a linear scale were used, only data corresponding to the higher frequencies would be

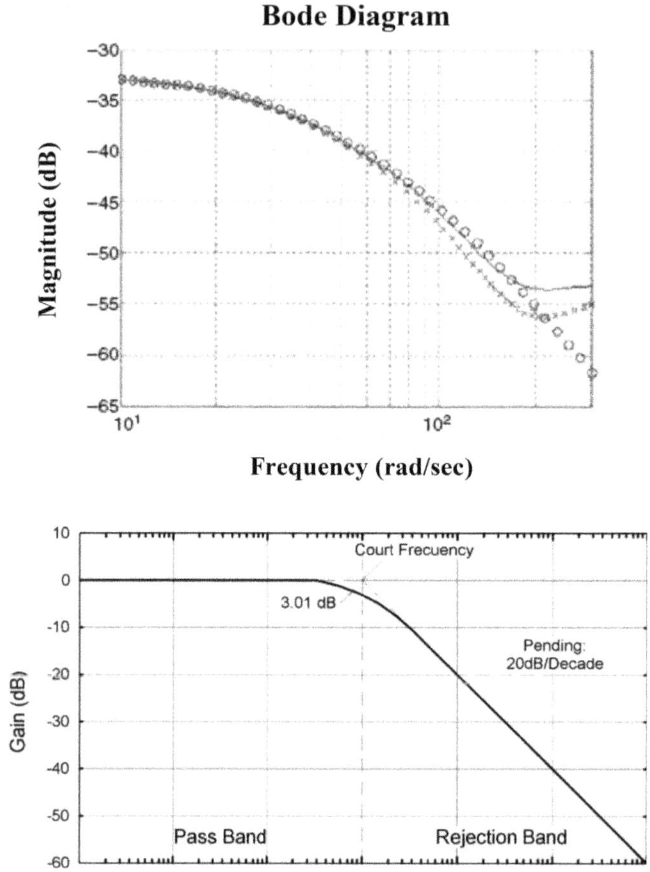

Figure 9.5. Top: Bode amplitude diagram showing the pressure–diameter transfer function of a sheep's aorta. Down: main characteristics to be considered when analyzing a Bode diagram.

properly appreciated while all points below $10^2\,\mathrm{rad\,s^{-1}}$ would be represented in a very small fraction of the abscissa axis. Logarithmic scales are thus used to avoid this problem since they allow data of different orders of magnitude to be represented in the same axis, separating them in decades. In order to do this, rather than marking the position of the datum we want to represent in the axis, the position of its decimal logarithm is marked instead. Now, representing data in logarithmic scale (e.g. as in the frequency axis of the Bode diagram) should not be confused with representing the data algorithm, or something proportional. When a logarithmic scale is used, the position of the points in relation to the linear scale is changed, but they are still labeled with their values. Another characteristic of the Bode diagram in relation to the modulus is that the ordinate axis is represented in dB. In other words, $20 \cdot \log|H(\omega)|$ is represented instead of $|H(\omega)|$. This is another way of visualizing transfer functions as well, which may vary by several orders of magnitude.

The arterial wall behaves as a 'frequency selective' filter. These filters are capable of blocking or permitting the passage of a certain range of frequencies, by modifying the relationship between the magnitudes of the input and output signals. Frequency selective filters are classified into four main types: lowpass, highpass, passband and stopband. Within this classification, the frequency response of the arterial wall behaves like a 'lowpass filter'. Lowpass filters permit the passage of lower frequencies and attenuate higher frequencies. More specifically, this type of filter allows low frequencies to pass, from frequency 0 (or continuous) to a certain frequency known as 'cutoff frequency', which is the frequency at which the filter starts to attenuate (reduce the amplitude of) the input signal. In general, the cutoff frequency corresponds to the frequency at which the output level has been attenuated (reduced) to the value of −3 dB = 70.1% in relation to a 0 dB = 100% reference level. Between frequency 0 and the cutoff frequency, we find the range of frequencies that the filter allows to 'pass' without attenuating the frequency components. This range is called 'dynamic range or passband', which is, in other words, the width (measured in Hz) of the frequency range which concentrates the largest part of the signal power. The frequencies within the dynamic range are known as 'effective frequencies'. In turn, the frequency range above the cutoff frequency is called 'attenuated range or stopband'.

A first order lowpass filter (e.g. 'RC' type), for example, has the following frequency response:

$$H(f) = \frac{1}{1 + j2\pi fRC}$$

in the case of the arterial wall, R would be its viscosity and $C = 1/E$, where E is the elasticity of the wall. Given that in these filters the cutoff frequency (f_c) has the following value

$$f_c = \frac{1}{2\pi RC}.$$

The cutoff frequency would be determined by the E/R relationship, that is, elasticity/viscosity.

In this case, the linear approximation of the Bode amplitude diagram has two lines: (a) for frequencies below the f_c, it is a horizontal line at 0 dB ('flat response', which means that the output is equivalent to the input); (b) for frequencies above the f_c, it is a line with a −20 dB/decade slope. These two lines meet at the cutoff frequency. The graph will show that at frequencies well below such a frequency, the circuit will have an attenuation of 0 dB. Above it, the signal will be attenuated, and the higher the frequency, the higher the attenuation.

A lowpass filter has 'zeros' at high frequencies (at infinity) and 'poles' at low frequencies. It should be remembered that considering the transfer function equation (input/output), the values that make the numerator zero are the zeros and those which make the denominator zero are the poles. The number of poles indicate the 'order of the filter' and its value determines the characteristics of the filter, such as its frequency and stability. It should be noted that the order of a filter describes the level of acceptance or rejection of frequencies above or below the respective cutoff frequency. A first order filter, with a cutoff frequency equal to (F) will have an attenuation of 6 dB in the first octave ($2F$), 12 dB in the second octave ($4F$), 18 dB in the third octave ($8F$) and so on. A second order filter would have a slope twice as steep (represented in a logarithmic scale). This is related to poles and zeros: poles make the slope go up with 20 dB and zeros make it go down. Therefore, poles and zeros may compensate their effect. The higher the order, the more complex the filter.

9.1.5 The arterial wall as an active and smart 'damper or filter'

One of the main hypotheses we have posed is that just like some industrial dampers or filters, the arterial wall may behave as a variable damper or filter (e.g. of a rheological type). A rheological variable damper is a damper of variable viscoelasticity capable of modifying its viscosity (e.g. modifying the viscosity of the liquid contained in it) so as to adjust the stiffness variation range or damping capacity, in a continuum, instead of being restricted to four or five fixed values. Therefore, the damping capacity, or the arterial wall 'damper stiffness' might adopt a continuous value between two limits (it does not have fixed positions).

Our hypothesis, verified after several works, established that the damping capacity of the arterial wall could be modulated mainly through the continuous adjustment of the levels of the wall's viscous and elastic responses, and these levels, in turn, would depend on the vascular smooth muscle tone and/or the number and type of extra- and intra-cellular components (Armentano *et al* 2006, 2007, Bia *et al* 2005a, 2005b, 2005c). Consequently, as we will see, modifications in the smooth muscle tone (e.g. during acute hypertensive states) and/or in the composition of the arterial wall (e.g. produced by a remodeling of the wall as a result of a chronic hypertensive state) might alter the damping capacity or function of the arterial wall.

In other words, far from being a 'passive' damping and suspension system, the arterial wall is capable of 'actively' regulating its damping capacities. Furthermore, the arterial wall, like some industrial dampers currently available, might be 'smart' and thus behave as a 'smart damper' (Armentano *et al* 2006, 2007). It should be pointed out that smart, active materials, also known as multi-functional, are those capable of responding in a reversible and controlled fashion to different external physical or chemical stimuli, modifying some of their properties. In our case, the 'smartness' of the materials composing the arterial wall (or some of them) would lie in the fact that they would allow the damping capacity of the arterial wall to adapt to the pulsatility conditions or oscillations it must face, by making adjustments in the characteristics of the spring (e.g. smooth muscle elasticity) and/or damper (e.g. smooth muscle viscosity) in the short (seconds), medium (minutes, hours) and long terms (days, months) in order to continuously reach a proper attenuation.

Consequently, the arterial wall, or some of its constituent elements, would be able to continuously 'self-diagnose' in relation to their damping capacity and thus 'auto-adapt' to the conditions they have identified as optimal or correct.

This type of smart damper is currently used in different elements created by man. In this sense, there are now automobile damping systems that can be electronically controlled when the car is moving, so as to adapt the damper's level of stiffness, manually or automatically, depending on the road and the driving dynamic conditions. Such adjustment can even be performed using the information from sensors installed in different parts of the vehicle, which can be used to provide feedback or make predictions in relation to the damper control system.

Why not think that nature, much more versatile and powerful than us, has created arterial walls with the ability to continuously adapt to the hemodynamic conditions they face, so as to always ensure an adequate level of wall damping?

9.1.6 Determinants of the wall damping or filtering function: wall elasticity and viscosity

From a mechanical point of view, the arterial wall behaves like a viscoelastic material (Nichols and O'Rourke 1998, O'Rourke 1995). By definition, a viscoelastic fluid or material has intermediate properties between a perfectly elastic solid and a perfectly viscous fluid (Nichols and O'Rourke 1998). As a result, the arterial wall exhibits both characteristics.

The viscous and elastic properties of the arterial wall have so far been generally characterized together, under the term 'viscoelasticity'. However, evidence showing that arterial viscosity and elasticity can change independently from one another under various physiological and pathological conditions (e.g. during wall remodeling processes (Armentano *et al* 1995)), during states with and without smooth muscle hyperactivity (Bia *et al* 2003, Armentano *et al* 2003, Barra *et al* 1997), and during the normal development of the individual (Wells 1998), requires the use of methods to quantify them separately.

In reference to this, several works have shown that each of these properties deal with different aspects of the arterial function (Pontrelli and Rossoni 2003).

9.2 Methodological approach

An alternative approach to that of the constitutive equation in the time domain presented in chapters 4 and 5 is the concept of the complex Young's modulus. Using stress–strain signals in the frequency domain, the quotient is defined as complex elastic modulus:

$$E^{*}(\omega) = \frac{\sigma(\omega)}{\varepsilon(\omega)}. \tag{9.1}$$

Assuming that the arterial system works around a mean pressure, with a linear response, the frequency response of arterial elasticity can be studied using the quotient harmonic to harmonic. If we separate the real from the imaginary part, the storage (E') and loss (E'') moduli can be defined. The first is associated with the ability to store elastic potential energy, while the second is related to the dissipation of energy as heat.

$$E^{*}(\omega) = E'(\omega) + iE''(\omega). \tag{9.2}$$

The first *in vitro* studies showing these frequency dependences (Bauer *et al* 1979) revealed that E' was relatively constant in the 1–20 Hz band. In turn, the loss modulus E'' increased up to 4 Hz and then reached a plateau at high frequencies. Several attempts were made to obtain integro-differential equations modeling this frequency behavior, maintaining a certain coherence with time stretching and relaxation studies.

The generalization of a model with parameters to be determined through least square methods was proposed by Westerhof and Noordergraaf (Westerhof and Noordergraaf 1970) in the following equation:

$$E^{*}(\omega) = \frac{\sum_{n=0}^{Q} c_n(i\omega)^n}{\sum_{m=0}^{P} a_m(i\omega)^m}. \tag{9.3}$$

Limiting the order of the model is essential since it is necessary to consider the number of parameters to be used, the computational cost and, particularly, the theoretical association of such parameters with measurable physiological variables. The minimum order established was of two coefficients in the numerator and two in the denominator. In this way, a reasonable time response, without oscillations and extra peaks, is ensured, as well as a frequency adjustment.

We have recently applied adaptive methods to find the model's coefficients, and at the same time, to try to relate them to the parameters of the constitutive equation (Gamero *et al* 2001). We primarily worked with digitized signals, the model in the normalized frequency domain and its conversion to the Laplace domain by means of a bilinear transformation. The coefficient adjustment was performed in the time domain (figure 9.6) through adaptive models of the black box with exogenous input (ARX) type. The order of the model was analyzed and established using the Akaike criterion (Akaike 1969). Unlike Fourier analysis, the results provide a continuous response in the frequency axis. Furthermore, this adaptive methodology could be implemented in real time, offering a beat-by-beat tracking of any changes in wall mechanical properties, which will be identified in the alteration of the coefficients.

The mechanical moduli of the wall were obtained using the adaptive filtering method, in which the input of an ARMA (auto regressive moving average) digital filter, more commonly known as IIR (infinite impulse response), is the instantaneous arterial pressure signal and the output is the instantaneous arterial diameter. From these magnitudes, we obtain the equivalent ones for stress–strain. The filter will try to adapt the polynomial coefficients of the numerator and denominator (which will determine the location of the poles and zeros in the arterial system). The equation to be adapted will be as follows:

$$P(t) = E \cdot D(t) + \eta \cdot \frac{dD(t)}{dt} + M \cdot \frac{d^2D(t)}{dt^2}. \tag{9.4}$$

The filter adapts its coefficients sample by sample, minimizing the error function until reaching a minimum variation. The transfer of the digital filter H(z) will be:

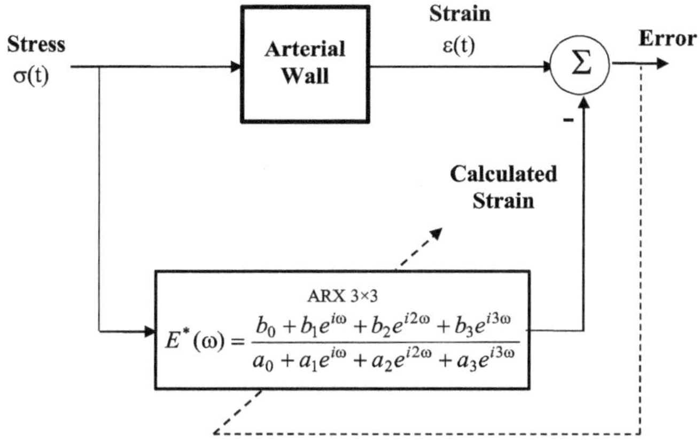

Figure 9.6. Schema of the adaptive modeling of the arterial wall. The parameters of the model are obtained from the stress–strain signals. The frequency response of Young's modulus uses a 3 × 3 model, thus minimizing the mean squared error.

$$H(z) = \frac{D(z)}{P(z)} = \frac{b_0 + b_1 \cdot z^{-1} + b_2 \cdot z^{-2} + b_3 \cdot z^{-3}}{a_0 + a_1 \cdot z^{-1} + a_2 \cdot z^{-2} + a_3 \cdot z^{-3}}. \tag{9.5}$$

Once the minimum is reached, the bilinear transform which related the Laplace transform with the Z transform is used, through the following expression:

$$s = \frac{2}{T_s}\frac{1 - z^1}{1 + z^{-1}}, \tag{9.6}$$

where T_s is the sampling time at which the pressure–diameter signals were acquired. As a result, the following system is obtained in the Laplace domain:

$$H(s) = \frac{D(s)}{P(s)} = \frac{s^3 + n_2 \cdot s^2 + n_1 \cdot s + n_0}{s^3 + m_2 \cdot s^2 + m_1 \cdot s + m_0}, \tag{9.7}$$

where the coefficients n_i and m_i of the transfer $H(s)$ are related to the coefficients a_i and b_i of the adaptive digital filter $H(z)$ in equation (9.5). Finally, we can find relationships between the coefficients n_i, m_i and the differential equation, from which the wall moduli are obtained: elasticity (E), viscosity (η) and inertia (M).

Modeling the vascular wall as a second order system, the filter's cutoff frequencies (f_{C1} and f_{C2}) are:

$$f_{C1,2} = \frac{1}{2\pi}\left[\frac{\eta}{2M} \pm \sqrt{\left(\frac{\eta}{2M}\right)^2 - \frac{E}{M}}\right]. \tag{9.8}$$

Assuming that f_{C2} (related to the inertial effects or the effects dependent on the mass modulus) is higher than f_{C1}, it is possible to accept that $2.\pi.f_{C1}$ is the dominant

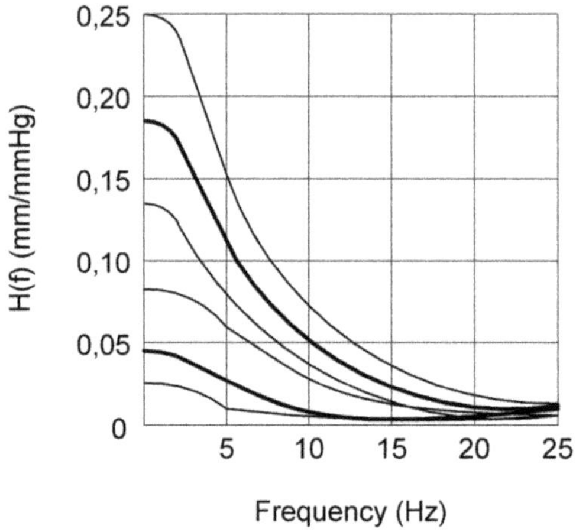

Figure 9.7. Amplitude frequency response of an ascending aortic artery (bottom lines) and main pulmonary artery. The mean values can be observed together with the standard errors, indicating a higher stiffness of the aorta, but with the same dynamic range as the pulmonary artery.

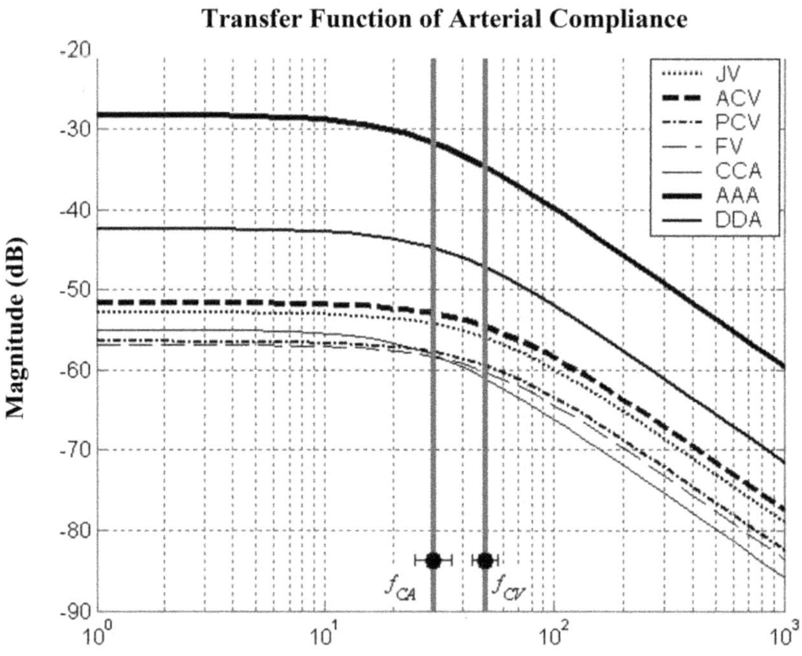

Figure 9.8. Frequency response (Bode graph) of all the veins (dotted and dashed lines) and arteries (solid lines). Observe the differences in the cutoff frequency between veins (FCV) and arterial segments (FCA). JV: jugular vein; ACV: anterior vena cava; PCV: posterior vena cava; FV: femoral vein; CCA: common carotid artery; AAA: ascending aortic artery; DDA: distal descending aortic artery.

pole of the transfer function $H(\omega)$. Considering this reduction, the cutoff frequency of the lowpass filter would be:

$$f_{C1} = \frac{1}{2\pi}\frac{E}{\eta} = \frac{1}{2\pi}\frac{1}{\eta C}. \tag{9.9}$$

With a flat response amplitude $C = 1/E$ in the passband of the frequency response.

In short, the foregoing constitutes only one of the major topics in arterial dynamics, but, in our opinion, has great theoretical, experimental and clinical relevance since this approach allows us to analyze not only the functional behavior of the wall but also morphological alterations of the vascular wall, which are very helpful for diagnosis.

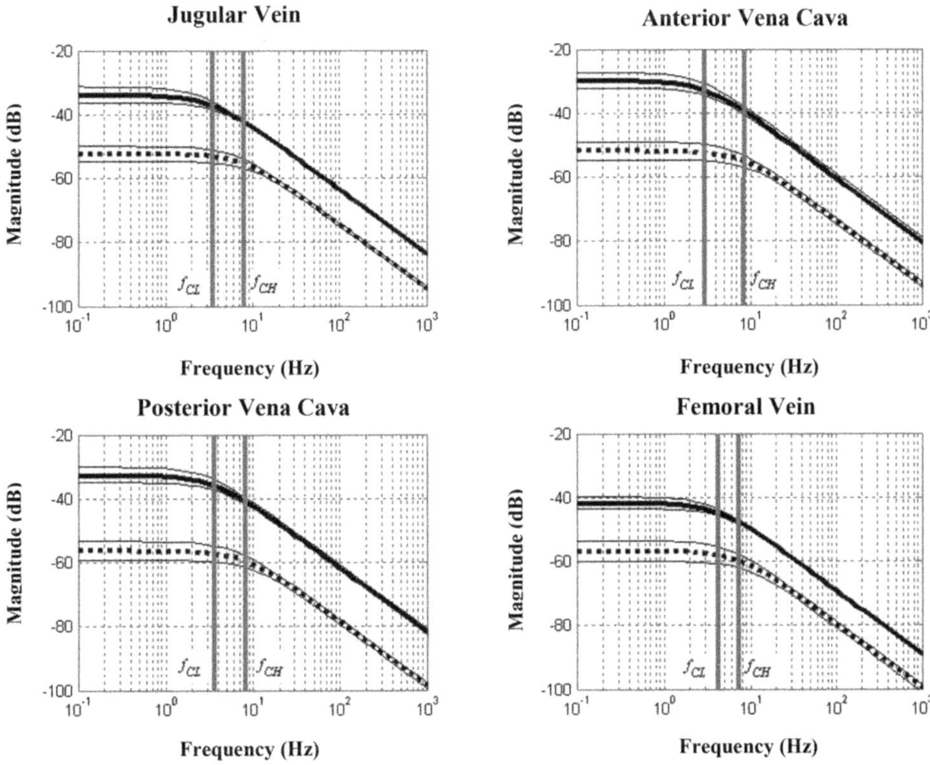

Figure 9.9. Bode diagrams of the first order frequency responses of veins under physiological hemodynamic conditions (solid lines) and under arterial hemodynamic conditions (dotted lines). The values were expressed as mean and standard deviation. The difference in amplitude at low frequencies (elasticity) for each vein under analysis should be noted. The difference in the filtering function (cutoff frequency of −3 dB, f_C) calculated for low pressures (physiological state, f_{Cp}) and high pressures (arterial substitutes, f_{Cg}) should also be observed. For each experimental condition (physiological situation or arterial substitute), different venous segments showed a similar filtering function and, in all cases, the amplitude at frequency 0 Hz was reduced and the cutoff frequency increased when passing from the physiological state to the arterial state or to the high pressure state.

9.3 Experimental applications

To finish this chapter, we present a series of results showing the frequency response of the arterial wall in an asymptotic Bode diagram. This diagram allows us to visualize the frequency response of the arterial wall, the half power cutoff frequency (−3 dB), the elastic response of the wall at low frequencies and its relationship with viscosity at high frequencies. Figure 9.7 represents the frequency response (amplitude in terms of the diameter-pressure transfer function) for the aorta and the pulmonary artery of the same animal (Pessana *et al* 2004).

Figure 9.8 presents the results of a mapping study of different arterial and venous segments (Zócalo 2006). This study showed that veins from different regions have different elasticity and viscosity but have a filtering function similar to that of arteries. Therefore, due to this difference in the viscous and elastic components, veins exhibit differences in their functional capacity when they are used as arterial substitutes. These differences are reduced in relation to the common carotid artery (the most peripheral and smallest artery analyzed in this study) and their elastic and viscous indexes show significant similarities.

Finally, in figure 9.9, the venous wall dynamics was compared with similar arterial hemodynamic conditions. These physiological conditions represent different changes depending on the venous segment under analysis. Femoral veins showed the fewest changes when subjected to arterial substitute conditions. The regional differences in venous dynamics in relation to arterial conditions and their relative changes might explain the different results found in the arterial substitutes when using venous segments.

References

Akaike H 1969 Fitting autoregressive models for prediction *Ann. Inst. Stat. Math.* **21** 243–7

Alarcón E, Álvarez R and Gómez S 1989 Sistemas de un grado de libertad *Cálculo Matricial de Estructuras* (Colección de matemática aplicada e informática) 1st edn ed F Michavila (Editorial Reverte S.A) pp 353–402

Armentano R L, Barra J G, Levenson J, Simon A and Pichel R H 1995 Arterial wall mechanics in conscious dogs: assessment of viscous, inertial and elastic moduli to characterize the aortic wall behavior *Circ. Res.* **76** 68–478

Armentano R L, Graf S, Barra J G, Velikovsky G, Baglivo H, Sanchez R, Simon A, Pichel R H and Levenson J 1998 Carotid wall viscosity increase is related to intima-media thickening in hypertensive patients *Hypertension* **31** 534–9

Armentano R L, Bia D, Craiem D, Gamero L, Levenson J, Grignola J C and Gines F F 2003 Respuesta en frecuencia de la pared arterial: inocente o culpable de las discrepancias entre filtrado sistémico y pulmonar? *Rev. Mex. Ing. Biomed.* **24** 45–54

Armentano R L, Barra J G, Bia Santana D, Pessana F M, Graf S, Craiem D, Brandani L M, Baglivo H P and Sanchez R A 2006 Smart damping modulation of carotid wall energetics in human hypertension: effects of angiotensin-converting enzyme inhibition *Hypertension* **47** 384–90

Armentano R L, Barra J G, Pessana F M, Craiem D O, Graf S, Santana D B and Sanchez R A 2007 Smart smooth muscle spring-dampers. Smooth muscle smart filtering helps to more efficiently protect the arterial wall *IEEE Eng. Med. Biol. Mag.* **26** 62–70

Barra J G, Levenson J, Armentano R L, Cabrera Fischer E I, Pichel R H and Simon A 1997 *In vivo* angiotensin II receptor blockade and converting enzyme inhibition on canine aortic viscoelasticity *Am. J. Physiol.* **272** H859–68

Bauer R D, Busse R, Schabert A, Summa Y and Wetterer E 1979 Separate determination of the pulsatile elastic and viscous forces developed in the arterial wall *in vivo Pflugers Arch.* **380** 221–26

Bia D, Armentano R L, Grignola J C, Craiem D, Zocalo Y A, Gines F F and Levenson J 2003 The vascular smooth muscle of great arteries: local control site of arterial buffering function? *Rev. Esp. Cardiol.* **56** 1202–9

Bia D, Aguirre I, Zocalo Y, Devera L, Cabrera Fischer E and Armentano R 2005a Regional differences in viscosity, elasticity and wall buffering function in systemic arteries: pulse wave analysis of the arterial pressure-diameter relationship *Rev. Esp. Cardiol.* **58** 167–74

Bia D, Barra J G, Grignola J C, Gines F F and Armentano R L 2005b Pulmonary artery smooth muscle activation attenuates arterial dysfunction during acute pulmonary hypertension *J. Appl. Physiol.* **98** 605–13

Bia D, Zócalo Y, Pessana F, Armentano R, Perez-Campos H, Saldias M and Alvarez I 2005c Femoral arteries energy dissipation and filtering function remain unchanged after cryopreservation procedure *Transpl. Int.* **18** 1346–55

Bia D *et al* 2006 Cryopreservation procedure does not modify human carotid homografts mechanical properties: an isobaric and dynamic analysis *Cell Tissue Bank* **7** 183–94

Bia D, Zócalo Y, Pessana F, Armentano R, Pérez H, Saldías M and Álvarez I 2007 Differential functional coupling between human saphenous cryoallografts and arteries: importance of the arterial type and the biomechanical parameter evaluated *Artif. Organs* **31** 809–18

Cornejo C J 2002 Elastodynamics with hysteretic damping *PhD Thesis* Delft University Technology

Gamero L H, Armentano R L, Barra J G, Simon A and Levenson J 2001 Identification of arterial wall dynamics in conscious dogs *Exp. Physiol.* **86** 519–28

Nichols W W and O'Rourke M F 1998 Properties of the arterial wall: practice ed W W Nichols and M F O'Rourke *McDonald's Blood Flow in Arteries: Theoretical, Experimental and Clinical Principles* (London: Arnold) pp 73–97

O'Rourke M F 1995 Mechanical principles in arterial disease *Hypertensión* **26** 2–9

Pessana F, Bia D, Perez Campos H, Craiem D, Graf S, Zocalo Y, Risk M and Armentano R 2004 Dynamics of cryopreserved human carotid arteries *Conf. Proc. IEEE Eng. Med. Biol. Soc.* **1** 730–3

Pontrelli G and Rossoni E 2003 Numerical modelling of the pressure wave propagation in the arterial flow *Int. J. Numer. Meth. Fluids* **43** 651–71

Rodríguez V M and Miramontes D 2001 Identificación del amortiguamiento histerético efectivo de algunos modelos cíclicos en variables generalizadas. 5as Jornadas de Investigación. Universidad Autónoma de Zacatecas TI/UI-12/09

Varanasi K K 2002 On the design of a precision machine for closed-loop performance *MS Thesis* (Massachusetts Institute of Technology)

Varanasi K K 2004 Vibration damping using low-wave-speed media with applications to precision machines *PhD Thesis* (Massachusetts Institute of Technology)

Wells S M, Langille B L and Adamson S L 1998 *In vivo* and *in vitro* mechanical properties of the sheep thoracic aorta in the perinatal period and adulthood *Am. J. Physiol.* **274** h1749–60

Westerhof N and Noordergraaf A 1970 Arterial viscoelasticity: a generalized model. Effect on input impedance and wave travel in the systematic tree *J. Biomech.* **3** 357–79

Zócalo Y, Pessana F, Santana D B and Armentano R L 2006 Regional differences in vein wall dynamics under arterial hemodynamic conditions: comparison with arteries *Artif. Organs* **30** 265–75

Zócalo Y, Bia D, Pessana F and Armentano R 2007 Changes in veins dynamics ranging from low to high pressure levels as determinant of the differences in veins adaptation to arterial haemodinamic conditions *Artif. Organs* (at press)

Chapter 10

Modeling of biological prostheses

Ricardo L Armentano and Leandro J Cymberknop

10.1 Introduction

Tissue engineering is a relatively new discipline that offers the potential to create replacement structures from cells and biodegradable scaffolds. Since these constructs contain living cells, they have the potential to grow, self-remodel and self-repair, which make them of interest as grafts for fine caliber blood vessels (Campbell and Campbell 2007). Bioartificial tissues are composed of a supporting cell-populated matrix that can be implanted into an organism to replace lost or damaged tissues. For the design of these grafts, it is necessary to grow cells in the above-mentioned matrix. Stem or progenitor cells, differentiated or even genetically manipulated cells can be used. The supporting matrix should allow the maintenance of the specialized function of the differentiated cells or should promote progenitor or stem cell differentiation (King 2007). The ideal matrix should be biodegradable in order to be finally replaced by a natural matrix generated after the graft is implanted into the host organism and the cell integration occurs (King 2007).

Collagen-based supporting matrices are the most common for bioartificial tissues and for the promotion of *in vivo* regeneration. Collagens are the most abundant proteins in human extracellular matrices. Other synthetic biodegradable polymers used in the design of matrices are: poly (lactic acid), poly (glycolic acid), polydioxanone, and polycaprolactone. In addition, other natural polymers are used such as: collagen, elastin, alginate, and gelatin, among others. Grafts to replace or repair tissues or organs can be classified into two categories: biological grafts and man-made grafts. Biological grafts are classified into three types according to their origin with respect to the receptor: autograft, allograft and xenograft.

The autograft consists of the extraction of healthy tissues from a given site of the patient's body to be transplanted to another part of the same patient. This type of graft generally yields the best clinical results and does not produce immune rejection. Nevertheless, it poses problems such as infections, pain in the area of extraction, etc. In addition, they may not be readily available. In the case of vascular bypass, the

doi:10.1088/2053-2563/aafb0dch10

autograft is considered the gold standard (Chlupac *et al* 2009). In general, all these types of grafts (biological or manufactured) pose a certain degree of infection and reduction of the clearance degree (Baguneid *et al* 2006). The allograft (or homograft) entails transplanting organs or tissues from individuals of one species to individuals of the same species. Two of the main problems for this type of graft are the rejection by the receptor's immunological system and the scarcity of donors (there are grafts that can only be obtained from recently deceased patients, such as the heart). In the case of vascular allografts, these can be fresh (cold preserved) or cryopreserved (Chlupac *et al* 2009). Xenografts entail the implant of tissues from one species to another. This type of implant requires a treatment to reduce the chance of rejection, thrombosis, etc. Particularly in the case of engineered vascular grafts, they can be categorized into three types: synthetic, biosynthetic/biohybrid and living grafts (living tissue-engineered vascular grafts—totally engineered blood vessels) (Chlupac *et al* 2009). Among vascular synthetic grafts are those manufactured from polyethylene terephthalate polymers (PET/Dacron), polytetrafluoroethylene (PTFE or Teflon and ePTFE or Gore-Tex) and polyurethanes (PU) (with fibril and spongy structure). The inner surface of these grafts can be treated so as to diminish the formation of thrombi (for example, Dacron with bound heparin). In some cases, these synthetic grafts are applied in combination with segments of veins (compound graft) (Chlupac *et al* 2009). This procedure improves compliance coupling and reduces the hyperplasia in the intima (Cabrera Fischer *et al* 2005). Biosynthetic/hybrid grafts emerge as an intent to obtain more biocompatible grafts than purely synthetic ones. In this type of graft, biological components are introduced in a substrate or engineered structure (scaffold). For example, these grafts are grown using endothelial cells in their lumen to obtain an antithromobotic surface. Tissue-engineered vascular graft construction requires a scaffold or structure that provides it with initial shape and resistance, an adhesive matrix and living cells. There are four types of them: permanent synthetic, decellurized tissues, biodegradable and without scaffold (Chlupac *et al* 2009, Campbell and Campbell 2007). The performance of the different biological or engineered grafts will depend on the vascular region where they must be grafted.

There is a worldwide need for vascular grafts, mainly for vascular bypass. Arteriovenous vascular grafts are also needed to allow access for dialysis in end-stage kidney disease patients. Some patients do not have any suitable tissues to be used as grafts due to diseases or because they have already been extracted in previous surgeries. In these cases, synthetic vascular conduits can be used, such as polytetrafluoroethylene (ePTFE) and polyethylene terephthalate (PET), which have been used since the 1950s and have been useful to substitute large-caliber arteries whose high flow and low resistance bring about low rates of thrombosis and high degrees of clearance in the long run (Rocco *et al* 2014). In the case of artificial vascular grafts of small caliber arteries (less than 6 mm), the results of their use in bypass show in some cases a clearance value of 40% after six months and 25% after three years (in reference to the initial state) (Sayers *et al* 1998). They are more vulnerable to failures due to the formation of thrombi or hiperplasia of the intima. Furthermore, these artificial substitutes are unable to grow or pose a chronic risk of infection. In particular, in the case of pediatric and young patients, these substitutes cannot accompany the patients' growth. Consequently, new surgeries must be performed, thus increasing the risks of morbidity and mortality (Rocco *et al* 2014). The ideal substitute should integrate to the patient's native tissue and should have the same physiological function as the vessel to be substituted in normal conditions. These functions range from the capacity to grow, remodel, respond to chemical and nervous stimuli and reconstruct if damaged. In addition, the substitute must be resistant to the formation of thrombi, it must not have blood leaks (but it should have the appropriate porosity to allow for angiogenesis), it must not be toxic, immunogenic, or carcinogenic, it must not destroy blood cells or enzymes, it must not alter plasma proteins or cause depletion of ions and it must be resistant to the formation of aneurisms and rupture when subjected to systemic pressures (Campbell and Campbell 2007). From the mechanical viewpoint, it must show suitable compliance (distensibility), resistance to the pressures to which it will be subjected and resistance to twisting and bending. It must endure sutures under circumferential and longitudinal stress. Finally, it should be easily manufactured according to the specifications required by each patient, at a reasonable cost and in a short period of time (Campbell and Campbell 2007).

The capacity to produce substitutes on demand, adapted to the needs of each patient in particular is one of the objectives pursued by the vascular substitute tissue engineering field. In nonbiodegradable synthetic substitutes, it was observed that the differences in elastic compliances (due to different properties and geometrical characteristics of the material) between the substitute and the native artery, either pre- or post-implantation have unfavorable consequences, such as promoting hyperplasia in the tunica intima. Among other aspects to consider, good coupling of compliances since the implantation should be one of the objectives of the design. It is possible to elaborate substitutes that, within certain limits, reproduce the mechanical response of the arteries.

A scaffold can be defined as a three-dimensional platform that is required to be able to perform actions ranging from cell–biomaterial interaction and cell adhesion, to having controlled rates of biodegradation equivalent to tissue regeneration rates (Thottappillil and Nair 2015). The porous polymeric matrix is eventually replaced by neotissue with similar characteristics to the tissue of native vessels. The substitutes that are not based solely on a porous polymeric matrix are produced from *in vitro* cellular cultures. Both solutions seek to achieve an implant capable of having the same physiological functions as the vessel to be replaced provided it does not present any pathology. Substitutes based on porous polymeric matrices must have a structure similar to that of the native extracellular matrix, reflecting the biomechanical properties of the vessel while serving as a platform for the fixation and the proliferation of cells. In general, the desired characteristics for the porous polymeric matrices are: capacity to maintain the clearance, compliance, porosity, sterility, resistance to localized twisting and curving, resistance to stretching and circumferential deformation, suturability and suitable biodegradation profile.

Considering the physiological aspect, the mechanical response of the arterial wall depends on the mechanical role of its passive (elastin and collagen fibers) and active components (smooth muscle cells). The mechanical properties of the vessel are determined by these components and it is possible to identify each component contribution to the final elastic response (Armentano *et al* 1991). Arterial wall mechanical properties produce nonlinear pressure–diameter relations (known as a J-shaped curve), particularly when vessel structure is examined over a wide range. Total elastic modulus can be decomposed, where contribution of elastin, collagen and smooth muscle can be quantified (Armentano *et al* 1995). The function of elastin and collagen fibers is to maintain a steady tension to hold the wall against the transmural pressure present in the vessel, while the activation of smooth muscle alters both viscosity as well as elasticity of the vessel wall (Barra *et al* 1993). An artery can largely expand and contract elastically mainly due to elastin fibers, when low pressure variations are applied, whereas collagenous fibers remain unstretched (Sonoda *et al* 2001). Furthermore, the amount of elastic components differs greatly between different types of normal vessels. A mathematical approach allows the individual characterization assuming a three-element Maxwell model (Barra *et al* 1993). The activation of smooth muscle indicates a greater expenditure of energy in the pulsatile expansion of the vessel with each heartbeat. Under physiological conditions, the artery can be considered essentially viscoelastic. This behavior can be perfectly appreciated in the hysteresis loop, evidenced by the pressure–diameter relationship (Armentano *et al* 1995). In this sense, elastic deformation is proportional to the potential energy stored during systole that will be yielded to the system during the diastole. On the other hand, viscosity quantifies the absorption of energy by the vessel wall (figure 10.1).

Presently, the design and construction of artificial grafts pose many open issues. Among these are: the mechanical decoupling between the native artery and the graft (in general for a diameter smaller than 6 mm), the gap between the absorption of the graft material and the growth of the arterial wall on the substituted area, the scarcity of models for predicting the performance of *in vivo* grafts. Among the existing techniques for the manufacture of porous polymeric matrices are gas foaming, salt

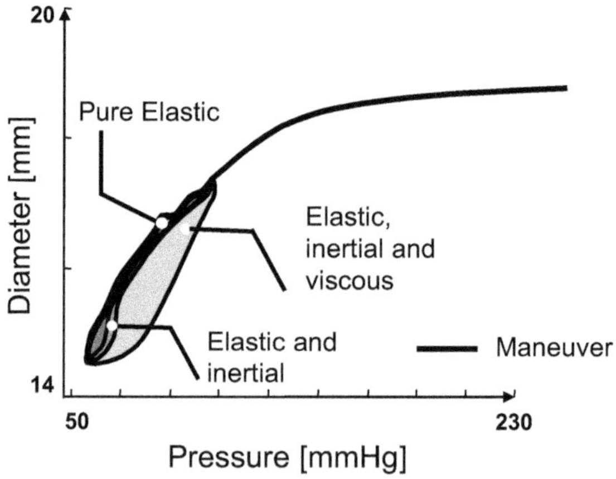

Figure 10.1. Schematic diameter versus pressure loop, where its elastic, inertial and viscous components are presented. A high pressure maneuver is also shown (solid line).

leaching, phase separation, freeze drying, electrospinning and 3D printing (Thottappillil and Nair 2015).

10.1.1 Electrospinning technique

Electrospinning is an electrohydrodynamic process. Electrospraying is also within this category. The electrospinning technique entails passing an electrically charged solution using an infusion pump through a capillary nozzle or nozzle to a grounded target. A difference potential develops between the nozzle and the target (generally between 10 and 30 kV). Figure 10.2 shows a scheme of an electrospinning system. At a certain critical tension, the electrostatic repulsion of the polymer solution drop exceeds the surface tension thereof, resulting in the formation of a micro jet of polymer solution. The jet accelerates in the electric field, suffering various instabilities and evaporating the solvent, depositing as a micro/nanometric fiber in the collector.

The electrospinning process is characterized by several parameters that can be modified as needed. These are: type of polymer and molecular weight, solvent, concentration and viscosity of the solution, flow, voltage, distance between nozzle and collector (target), collector design (Rocco *et al* 2014). In general, the production of uniform fibers is achieved from a certain critical concentration of the solution, with voltage being one of the parameters that controls their diameter. Below that concentration, fibers can be obtained with beads, spheres or collapsed particles (Zamani *et al* 2013). There are other factors that influence the process such as ambient temperature, humidity and air speed. This technique allows one to obtain nanofibers that can be as thin as 20–50 nm in diameter (figure 10.3.)

10.2 Biomechanical evaluation on electrospun vascular grafts

The design of small-diameter artificial artery grafts has several open problems. Most of these grafts apparently fail *in vivo* due to the differences between the mechanical properties of the graft and those of the native vessel. The arterial wall has a complex structure, capable of changing its properties and mechanical response in the short term due to the action of the smooth muscle and in the longer term due to remodeling and/or deterioration processes. The success of a vascular graft depends

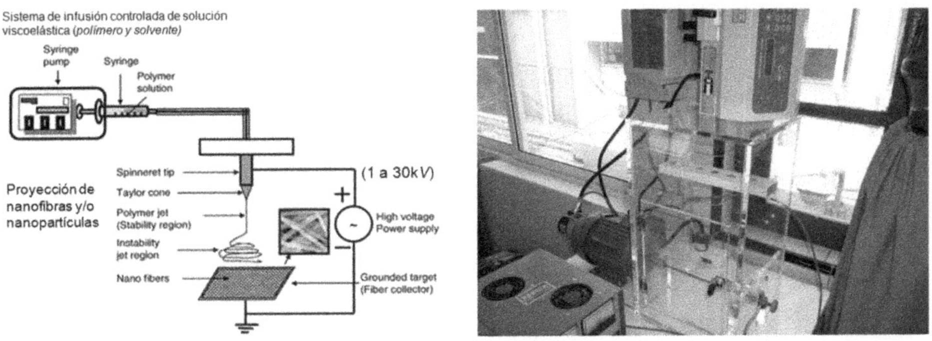

Figure 10.2. Left: electrospinning system scheme. Right: electrospinning system with rotary mandrel collector (INTEMA, Mar del Plata).

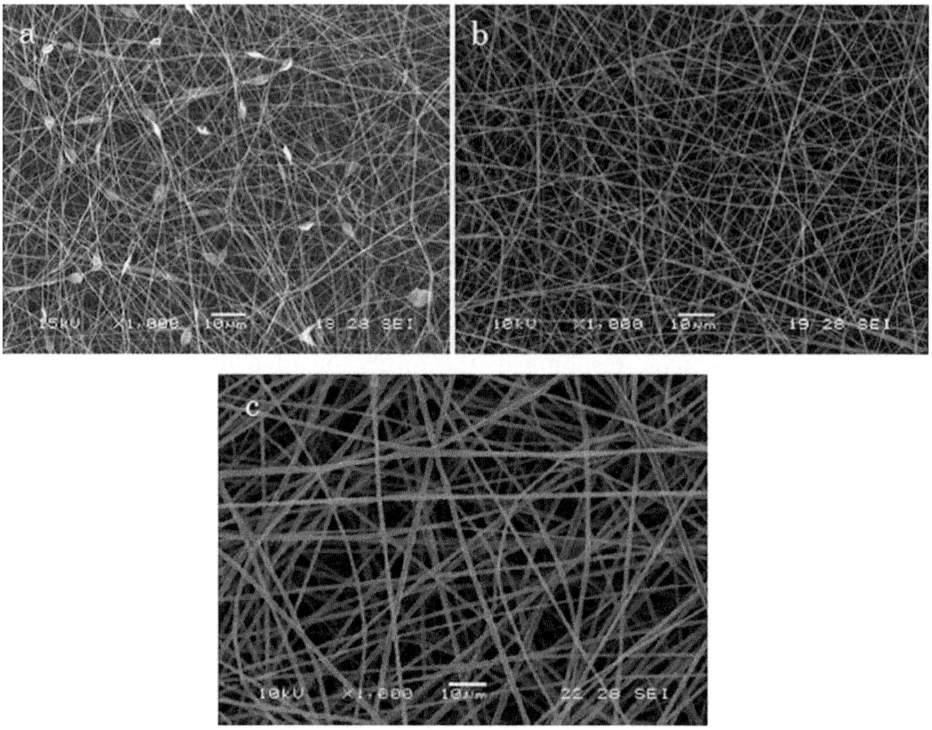

Figure 10.3. Photographs obtained through SEM of electrospun PLLA matrices from solutions at (a) 7%, (b) 10% and (c) 15% w/v. (Taken from Montini Ballarin *et al* 2015.)

in part on how well it can imitate the mechanical response of the adjacent area of the region it is replacing. The mechanical behavior of an arterial segment or a graft may be characterized by measuring its response when subjected to adequate controlled pressure and flow conditions.

Several experiments were conducted in order to study the behavior of bioresorbable nanofibrous polymeric structures which could be potentially used in vascular tissue engineering. The tubes were made using a 5 mm-diameter rotating cylindrical mandrel and three types of specimens were instrumented and measured: poly(L-lactic acid) (PLLA) and bioreabsorbable segmented poly(ester urethane) (SPEU, also named as PHD) and mixtures of both polymers PLLA/SPEU. PLLA was chosen as a representative bioresorbable polymer, commonly used in biomedical applications, such as drug delivery systems, tissue engineering, and biomedical devices. PLLA is an FDA approved biodegradable polyester that exhibits semicrystalline structure and good electro-spinability (Suarez Bagnasco *et al* 2014a). The degradation kinetics of PLLA was studied *in vitro*, showing a degradation period (into its monomers) of 6–12 months. This rate of *in vitro* and *in vivo* biodegradation can be adjusted by manipulating the crystallinity and copolymerization of isomers or other monomers (Sin *et al* 2013). SPEU was synthesized from aliphatic diisocyanate (HDI), aliphatic olyester (poly(ε-caprolactone) diol, PCL diol), and a novel aromatic chain extender as shown in Caracciolo *et al* (2009).

10.2.1 Distensibility test

A potential implantable vascular graft needs to be submitted to the so-called circumferential dynamic compliance (distensibility) test, in terms of the criteria established by the ANSI/AAMI/ISO7198:1998/2001/(R) 2010 Cardiovascular implants - Tubular vascular prostheses standard. In general terms, this standard specifies requirements relating to testing, packaging, labeling and terminology for sterile tubular vascular prostheses intended to replace, bypass or to form shunts between segments of the vascular system in humans.

One of the devices usually used to perform this type of evaluation consists of a *closed-loop hydraulic system* in which the sample is subjected to a variable pressure under different flow conditions. It consists basically of a specially designed programmable pump that pulses fluid into a hydraulic closed circuit, and a fluid pool where samples are placed in an adjustable sample fixing system and immersed in a physiological solution. The closed circuit is basically composed of silicone tubes, variable constrictions, the sample to be tested (a native vessel or a vascular graft) and a fluid reservoir (figure 10.4). Variable constrictions are used as a hydraulic resistance that allows one to generate pressure reflected waves. Pulse frequency can be adjusted in order to mimic the pulse rate of a normal adult human, which is generally between 60 and 80 beats per minute, considering basal conditions. Internal sample pressure can be measured using a high fidelity micro transducer (Konigsberg Inc., Pasadena, USA) placed near the center of each sample.

External graft diameter variations can be obtained using the sonomicrometry technique (Suarez Bagnasco *et al* 2014a). Since its first implementation in 1956 (Rushmer *et al* 1956) by Franklin and Rushmer, this procedure has been improved and refined, becoming a gold standard for *in vivo* physiological research. Sonomicrometry determines instantaneous external diameter by means of measuring the flight time of an ultrasound burst between a pair of small 5 MHz ultrasound transducers, fixed diametrally opposed on conduit external wall. The system (Triton Technology INC, SD, USA) needs to be calibrated using its internal time-diameter reference before each *in vitro* measurement. On the other hand, ultrasound

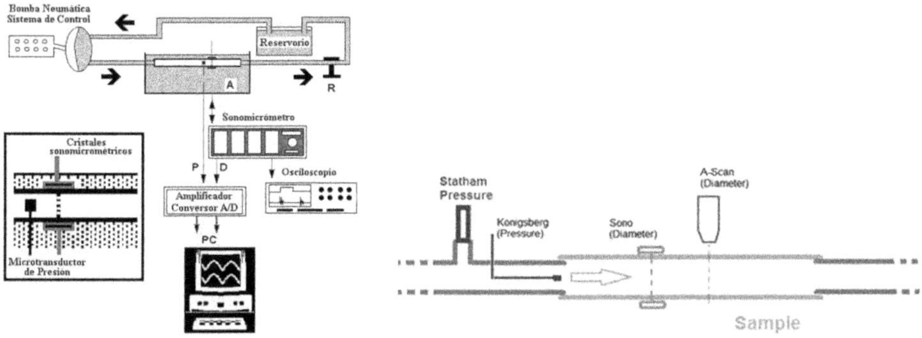

Figure 10.4. Left: closed-loop hydraulic system used for the evaluation of a native vessel or a vascular graft. Right: diagram showing the position of the sonomicrometry and pressure sensors. The ultrasound 'A-Scan' sensor can also be observed.

transducers have to be placed as close as possible to the pressure transducer in order to avoid any possible undesired viscous behavior.

Once the sample is attached to the circulating system (including attached sonomicrometry crystals), the wall thickness of each sample is calculated. The wall thickness of each sample can be also measured by means of high resolution ultrasound techniques, constituted by an ultrasound probe (Panametrics Inc., Massachusetts, USA), a graduated mechanical positioning system and a set of cross correlation processing algorithms (Balay *et al* 2010).

10.2.2 PLLA/SPEU evaluation protocol

In order to achieve a pressure variation similar to each of the intervals suggested by the standard, the reservoir's basal pressure and the hydraulic resistance of the circulating loop were adjusted. First, adjustments are made in order to subject the sample to be tested to a pressure cycling in the 50–90 mmHg interval. Once the adjustment was made, the recording was taken. Next, the same procedure is repeated for the 80–120 mmHg and 110–150 mmHg intervals. As can be observed, the pressure cycling intervals show an overlapping region of 10 mmHg. The 50–90 interval overlaps with the 80–120 interval and the latter, in turn, overlaps with the 110–150 interval. In figure 10.5, an example of pressure waves corresponding to the three intervals suggested by the standard and the variation of the external diameter can be visualized.

10.2.3 PLLA/SPEU mechanical properties assessment

The action of internal pressure determines different types of wall stress (Armentano *et al* 1995). In this sense, the corresponding circumferential mean value (σ_M) was approximated according to:

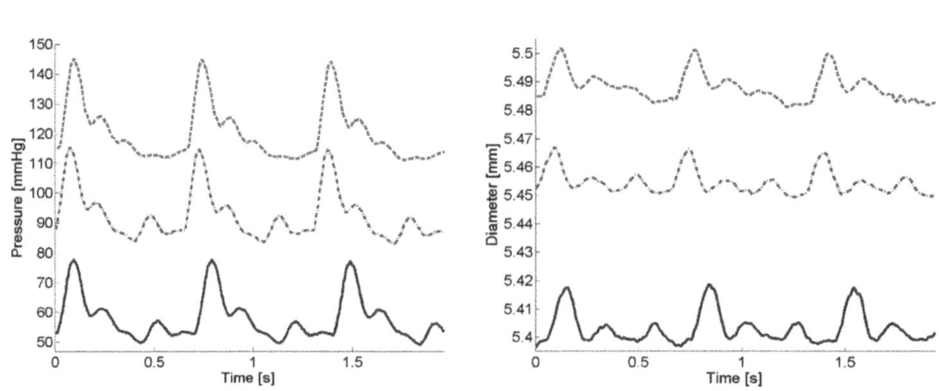

Figure 10.5. Left: example of pressure waveforms applied by approximating the 50–90 mmHg (solid line), 80–120 mmHg (dashed line), 110–150 mmHg (dotted line) intervals. Right: diameter waves measured for the intervals mentioned. The correspondence between the pressure and diameter waves is shown by the line pattern (solid, dashed, dotted).

$$\sigma_M = P_M \cdot (R_M/h),$$

where P_M is the internal applied pressure, R_M the corresponding mean radius and h the wall thickness. In addition, vessel (artery or graft) elastic response was evaluated by means of two parameters. Firstly, dynamic compliance was calculated as defined in the above-mentioned standard, as follows:

$$\%C = [(R_S - R_D) \cdot 10^4/R_D]/(P_S - P_D),$$

where P_S is the highest pressure value (systolic, mmHg) and P_D is the lowest pressure value (diastolic, mmHg). R_S and R_D are the corresponding internal radius (mm). The circumferential compliance (as calculated above) is expressed as a percentage of the diameter change per 100 mmHg. The wall was assumed to be elastic and incompressible, following the linear theory. If the thickness of the wall is lower than 5% of the internal radius, it is possible to approximate the internal radius r_i with the value of the external radius r_e (Nichols *et al* 2011). Moreover, and because estimated arterial diameter could be characterized as a continuous function of pressure by means of an interpolating method, the compliance pressure curve was calculated by deriving the diameter–pressure curve (dD/dP) to determine compliance for a given value of blood pressure. In all cases, the curve was obtained over pressures ranging from 50 to 150 mmHg, allowing comparison with other studies (Suarez Bagnasco *et al* 2014a). Secondly, incremental elastic modulus ($E_{P\varepsilon}$) was estimated at mean pressure, for each of the pressure ranges, according to (Armentano *et al* 1994):

$$E_{P\varepsilon} = dP/d\varepsilon \mid \text{mean pressure} \quad \varepsilon = D/D_0,$$

where P constitutes the transmural pressure and ε is the corresponding strain, obtained by referencing the diameter dynamic changes (D) to its unstressed value (D_0). Additionally, the diameter–pressure relationship for the entire set of vascular grafts was assessed.

The mechanical performance of synthetic PLLA grafts was compared to ovine femoral arteries in Suarez Bagnasco *et al* (2014a), using the methodology described before. It was concluded that the behavior of a PLLA graft could be associated to the collagen response in femoral arteries in the range of 100–130 mmHg (figure 10.6). Later, in Alfonso *et al* (2016), samples of electrospun nanofibrous PLLA and expanded polytetrafluoroethylene (ePTFE) vascular grafts were also subjected to pulsated pressure conditions using the experimental method. In this case, they were prepared with femoral and carotid arteries of normotensive male control subjects and ambulatory male patients, with mild to moderate hypertension. The obtained results verified the existence of important biomechanical differences between vascular grafts and human arteries. Under normal physiological conditions, the pressure–strain modulus $E_{P\varepsilon}$ of ePTFE and PLLA results were significantly higher than the carotid and femoral modulus values. During the hypertensive condition (higher pressure levels) ePTFE and PLLA increased their elasticity values with respect to an increase of carotid and femoral arteries. As was expected, ePTFE elasticity behaves markedly higher than that observed in native arteries (under normal physiological conditions). Concerning PLLA, the calculated modulus was

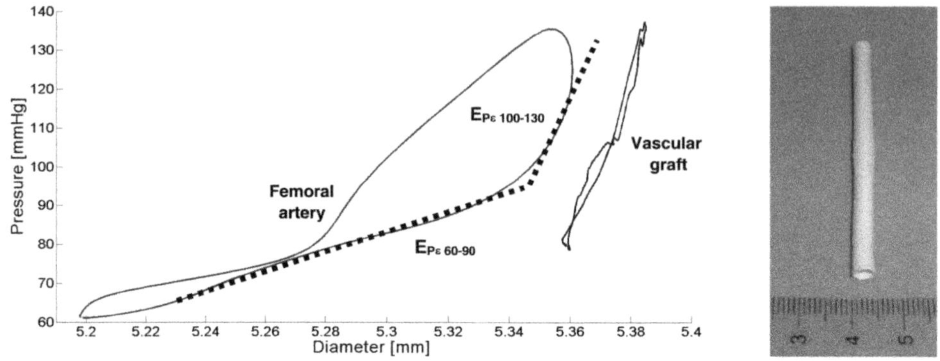

Figure 10.6. Left: diameter versus pressure loop of a femoral artery (solid, left) and a vascular graft (solid, right) for a typical case. Elastin ($E_{P\varepsilon\ 60\text{–}90}$) and collagen ranges ($E_{P\varepsilon\ 100\text{–}130}$) pressure–strain elastic modulus slopes are also presented (dashed). Right: obtained small-diameter PLLA electrospun vascular graft by means of the electrospinning technique.

also higher regarding the vascular conduits, but to a significantly lesser degree, manifesting a mechanical behavior that mimicked the response to pulsatile pressure regimes of *in vivo* femoral and carotid arteries, primarily under hypertensive conditions. The latter constitutes a highly desirable property in vascular tissue-engineered scaffolds.

In Montini Ballarin *et al* (2014, 2015), bilayered PLLA/PHU vascular grafts were instrumented and tested jointly with individual samples of PLLA and SPEU. Separation between layers of the PLLA/SPEU graft's structure was between 100 and 200 μm. The internal layer was constituted by a PLLA/SPEU (PHD) 50/50 ratio, with a higher percentage of SPEU than the external layer, which has a composition of PLLA/SPEU 90/10. The external layer is coupled to the internal one when a certain level of circumferential deformation is reached.

Individually, the PHD curve resembles the response of elastin, with an elastic behavior until rupture and a lack of yielding zone. PLLA showed a more rigid response (lower $\%C$ values), with a steeper slope similar to the one presented by collagen. Therefore, producing a small-diameter vascular graft with the proportions of both polymers in similar ratio as natural arteries could result in a biomimetic compliant structure. In figure 10.7, the $\Delta P = P - P_0$ versus D/D_0 loops were graphed for a pressure variation at the 80–120 mmHg interval both for a PLLA tube and a PHD one. In this case P is the instant pressure, P_0 is the minimum pressure, D is the instant diameter and D_0 is the minimum diameter. In this way, it is possible to compare the slope of both loops, which show little hysteresis.

Regarding bilayered PLLA/PHU vascular grafts, a J-shaped response when subjected to internal pressure (a PHD-like response for low pressure ranges and a PLLA-like response at high pressures) was observed as a cause of the nanofibrous layered structure, and the materials used, which was more pronounced than the one observed for monolayer grafts (Sonoda *et al* 2001, 2003, McClure *et al* 2010). Compared to native arteries, compliance values were in the order of natural

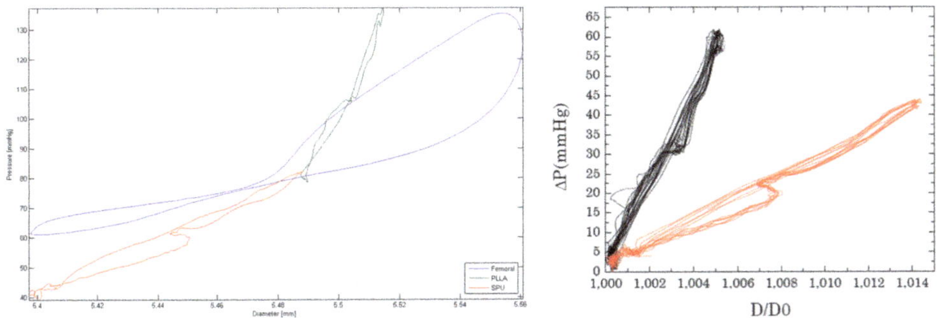

Figure 10.7. Left: comparison between a femoral native artery and SPEU (red, 50–90 mmHg interval) and PLLA (green, 80–120 mmHg interval) vascular grafts. Right: the pressure variation $\Delta P = P - P_0$ versus diameter variation D/D_0 loops with respect to their minimum values (P_0, D_0) for PLLA (black) and PHD (SPEU) (red) for a pressure variation close to the 80–120 mmHg interval.

coronary arteries and very close to the bypass gold-standard saphenous vein jointly with enough strength and stiffness to withstand elevated pressures.

Following this, scaffolds prepared with PLLA/SPEU blends were surface-modified with heparin following two different strategies that rely on the grafting of heparin to either PLLA or PHD functional groups (Caracciolo *et al* 2011). Both strategies afforded high heparin density, but higher for urethane methodology. Since the functionalized scaffolds did not cause hemolysis and inhibited platelet adhesion to a large extent, lysozyme/heparin-functionalized scaffolds obtained through urethane methodology achieved the highest platelet attachment inhibition. The increase in hydrophilicity and water absorption of the surface-functionalized nano-structures favored adhesion and proliferation of human adipose-derived stem cells. Additionally, heparinized surfaces conjugated with lysozyme presented microbial hydrolysis activity dependent on heparin content. Overall, scaffolds functionalized by this route may perform as advanced components of small-diameter vascular grafts, suitable for vascular tissue engineering, exhibiting biomimetic behavior, avoiding thrombi formation and providing antimicrobial features.

In conclusion, an arterial mechanics framework using sonomicrometry, extensively applied in the characterization of vascular conduits (Armentano *et al* 2013), has been used to characterize PLLA/SPEU vascular grafts *in vitro* and to compare them with native arteries, including other types of vascular prostheses. In particular, this technique allows the extension of its application directly to *in vivo* experiences, in conscious and chronically-instrumented animals, due to sonomicrometry having the unique ability to measure diameter variation under physiologically minimally invasive conditions. Furthermore, the mechanical response developed by multilayer grafts could be optimized, based on their *in vitro* and *in vivo* pressure–diameter evaluation.

References

Alfonso M, Cymberknop L, Armentano R, Pessana F, Wray S and Legnani W 2016 Arterial pulse pressure amplification described by means of a nonlinear wave model: characterization of human aging *J. Phys.: Conf. Ser.* **705** 012029

ANSI/AAMI/ISO, ANSI/AAMI/ISO7198:1998/2001/(R) 2010 Cardiovascular implants - Tubular vascular prostheses 2010 *Association for the Advancement of Medical Instrumentation: Arlington, VA*

Armentano R L, Barra J G, Levenson J, Simon A and Pichel R H 1995 Arterial wall mechanics in conscious dogs: assessment of viscous, inertial, and elastic moduli to characterize aortic wall behavior *Circ. Res.* **76** 468–78

Armentano R L, Cymberknop L, Montini Ballarin F, Balay G, Suarez D, Negreira C and Abraham G A 2013 A novel approach for assessment of the mechanical properties of synthetic arterial grafts *19th Congress of the European Society of Biomechanics (ESB2013)* (Patras, Grecia)

Armentano R L, Cabrera Fischer E I, Barra J G, Levenson J A, Simon A C and Pichel R H 1994 Single beat evaluation of circumferential aortic elastin elastic modulus in conscious dogs. Potential application in non-invasive measurements *Med. Prog. Technol.* **20** 91–9

Armentano R L *et al* 1991 Assessment of elastin and collagen contribution to aortic elasticity in conscious dogs *Am. J. Physiol.* **260** H1870–7

Baguneid M S, Seifalian A M, Salacinski I H J, Murray D, Hamilton G and Walker M G 2006 Tissue engineering of blood vessels *Br. J. Surg.* **93** 282–90

Balay G, Brum J, Bia D, Armentano R L and Negreira C 2010 Improvement of artery radii determination with single ultra sound channel hardware & *in vitro* artificial heart system *Conf. Proc. IEEE Eng. Med. Biol. Soc.* **2010** 2521–4

Barra J G, Armentano R L, Levenson J, Fischer E I, Pichel R H and Simon A 1993 Assessment of smooth muscle contribution to descending thoracic aortic elastic mechanics in conscious dogs *Circ. Res.* **73** 1040–50

Cabrera Fischer E I, Bia Santana D, Cassangelo G L, Zócalo Y, Crawford E V, Casas R F and Armentano R L 2005 Reduced elastic mismatch achieved by interposing vein cuff in expanded polytetrafluoroethylene femoral bypass decreases intimal hyperplasia *Artif. Organs* **29** 122–30

Campbell G R and Campbell J H 2007 Development of tissue engineered vascular grafts *Curr. Pharm. Biotechnol.* **8** 43–50

Caracciolo P C, Cortez Tornello P R, Buffa F, Montini Ballarin F, Cuadrado T R and Abraham G A 2011 Pequeñas fibras, grandes aplicaciones *Ciencia Hoy* **20** 121

Caracciolo P C, Buffa F and Abraham G A 2009 Effect of the hard segment chemistry and structure on the thermal and mechanical properties of novel biomedical segmented poly (esterurethanes) *J. Mater. Sci., Mater. Med.* **20** 145–55

Chlupac J, Filova E and Bacakova L 2009 Blood vessel replacement: 50 years of development and tissue engineering paradigms in vascular surgery *Physiol. Res.* **58** S119–39

King M 2007 Cellular development *Applied Cell and Molecular Biology for Engineers* ed G Waite and R Waite (New York: McGraw Hill)

McClure M J, Sell S A, Simpson D G, Walpoth B H and Bowlin G L 2010 A three-layered electrospun matrix to mimic native arterial architecture using polycaprolactone, elastin, and collagen: A preliminary study *Acta Biomater.* **6** 2422–33

Montini Ballarin F, Suarez Bagnasco D, Cymberknop L J, Caracciolo P C, Balay G, Negreira C, Armentano R L and Abraham G A 2014 Mechanical characterization of nanofibrous small-diameter vascular grafts *8vo Congreso Latinoamericano de Órganos Artificiales, Biomateriales e Ingeniería de Tejidos (COLAOB)* (Rosario, Argentina)

Montini Ballarin F, Calvo D, Caracciolo P C, Rojo F, Frontini P M, Abraham G A and Guinea-Totuero G 2015 Mechanical behaviour of bilayered small-diameter nanofibrous structures as biomimetic vascular grafts *J. Mech. Behav. Biomed. Mater.* **60** 220–33

Nichols W, O'Rourke M and Vlachopoulos Ch 2011 *McDonald's Blood Flow in Arteries: Theoretical, Experimental and Clinical Principles* (London: Hodder-Arnold)

Rocco K A, Maxfield M W, Best C A, Dean E W and Breuer C K 2014 *In vivo* applications of electrospun tissue-engineered vascular grafts: a review *Tissue Eng.* Part B **20** 628–40

Rushmer R F, Franklin D L and Ellis R M 1956 Left ventricular dimensions recorded by sonocardiometry *Circ. Res.* **4** 684–8

Sayers R D, Raptis S, Berce M and Miller J H 1998 Longterm results of femorotibial bypass with vein or polytetrafluoroethylene *Br. J. Surg.* **85** 934–8

Sin L T, Rahmat A R and Rahman W A W A 2013 Degradation and stability of poly(lactic acid) *Polylactic Acid* (Volume in Plastics Design Library) (William Andrew) pp 247–99

Sonoda H, Takamizawa K, Nakayama Y, Yasui H and Matsuda T 2001 Small-diameter compliant arterial graft prosthesis: Design concept of coaxial double tubular graft and its fabrication *J. Biomed. Mater. Res.* **55** 266–76

Sonoda H, Takamizawa K, Nakayama Y, Yasui H and Matsuda T 2003 Coaxial double-tubular compliant arterial graft prosthesis: time-dependent morphogenesis and compliance changes after implantation *J. Biomed. Mater. Res.* **65A** 170–81

Suarez Bagnasco D, Montini Ballarin F, Cymberknop L J, Balay G, Negreira C, Abraham G A and Armentano R L 2014 Elasticity assessment of electrospun nanofibrous vascular grafts: a comparison with femoral ovine arteries *Mater. Sci. Eng. Part C* **45** 446–54

Thottappillil N and Nair P D 2015 Scaffolds in vascular regeneration: current status *Vasc. Health Risk Manag.* **11** 79–91

Zamani M, Prabhakaran M P and Ramakrishna S 2013 Advances in drug delivery via electrospun and electrosprayed nanomaterials *Int. J. Nanomed.* **8** 2997–3017

IOP Publishing

Biomechanical Modeling of the Cardiovascular System

Ricardo L Armentano, Edmundo I Cabrera Fischer and Leandro J Cymberknop

Chapter 11

Arterial hypertension, chaos and fractals

Ricardo L Armentano and Leandro J Cymberknop

Fractal signals are those that show detail or structure at the moment of processing through all their time scales (Madisetti 2009). Formally, a fractal structure is an *irregular* geometric object that has self-similarity. It is composed of sub-units replicated iteratively so that under any scale of observation (considering ideal conditions), a structure similar to the whole set can be observed. Since this type of object is characterized by a fractional dimension, it is called *fractal dimension* (*FD*). Conceptually speaking, *FD* may also be considered a measure for irregularity. As *FD* increases, the dimension also increases its value, so it may be used as a measure for *roughness* or variation (Bassingthwaighte 1988). Natural structures are typically fractal. Their high irregularity can be observed in the contour of rock formations or in the structure of the leaves of a tree. The intense manifestation of deformations and holes places such objects in non-integer intermediate dimensions (figure 11.1). As a consequence, Euclidean geometry is unable to quantify the space occupied by a naturally-generated object (Barnsley 2000, Falconer 2003). Although it may be evident, clouds are not spheres, mountains are not cones and lightning bolts are not lines (Mandelbrot 1983). In physiological terms, fractal structures can be observed, for example, in arterial and venous branching, cardiopulmonary structures and bile ducts (Goldberger and West 1987). In this regard, one of the excluding aspects that differentiates geometric natural fractality is that in natural fractals, the invariance to the scale is appreciated only within certain limits (Goldberger *et al* 2002). In addition, the presence of self-similarity does not convert a geometric object into a fractal. Although this is a necessary condition, it needs additional contributions for the consolidation of the concept. To such effect, a fractal object is characterized in accordance with the following conditions (Falconer 2003):

- It shows self-similarity.
- It has a fine structure (detail is observed irrespective of scale).
- It is too irregular to be described by traditional geometry.

doi:10.1088/2053-2563/aafb0dch11

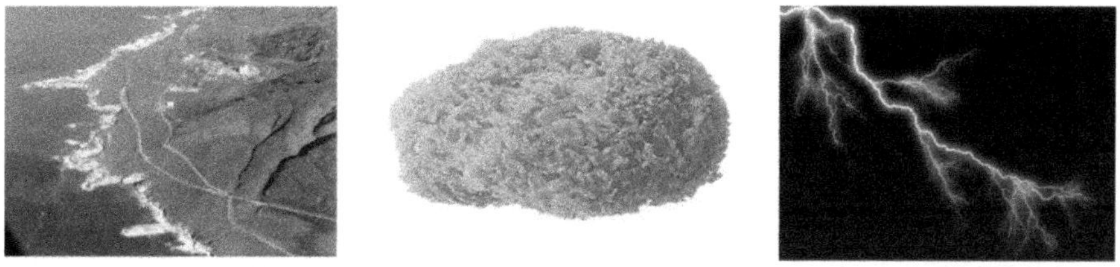

(a) *(b)* *(c)*

FD~1,20 ***FD~2,80*** ***FD~1,40***

Figure 11.1. Fractal dimension values (*FD*) corresponding to natural formations. (a) Irregular curve revealed by a coastline, which exceeds its topological dimension (*TD*) of units. (b) Irregular volume delimited by a sponge, whose holes place it dimensionally under $TD = 3$. (c) Manifestation of an electrical discharge embedded in $TD = 2$.

- Usually, its Haussdorf dimension exceeds its topological dimension.
- In some cases, it can be described through recursive procedures.

A classic example describing a non-fractal structure is the real line. Although it is self-similar (composed by reproductions of itself at different scales), the remaining imposed conditions cannot be attributed to it (Falconer 2003). As a consequence, the presence of characteristic qualities of fractal objects in time series does not necessarily mean that they can be considered fractal. However, the attribution of such quality makes them *candidates* for such behavior and they deserve deeper analysis. To accomplish this goal, tools that can provide quantitative measures are required, such as *FD*.

The fundamental goal of the systemic arterial network is to reach certain organs (or specific areas) in order to supply them with the correct amount of blood flow (Zamir 2001). This network consists of a series of vascular conduits which recursively bifurcate in a dichotomic fashion (a parent branch, two child branches) until they reach the arteriole level. At this last level, the process no longer continues in a dichotomic fashion; but the number of branches generated multiplies considerably (Bassingthwaighte *et al* 1994). Each bifurcation generated within the network implies the creation of a new scale or level. In particular, what makes the arterial tree different from other vascular structures (such as those observed in pulmonary cavities, the tracheobronchial tract, the His–Purkinje system or the kidneys) is the fact that the distribution of its branches and sub-branches is considerably uniform (Zamir 2001). The presence of repetitive patterns at different scales can be observed, for example, in the relationship that exists between the length of the generating artery and the diameter of the generated one. This relation remains constant if quantified using a double logarithmic scale, thus indicating the presence of a power law. This mechanism is consistent with a fractal recursive rule (Bassingthwaighte *et al* 1994). As a result, the *spatial* fractal properties of the arterial tree can be assessed in terms of the *FD*. Together with the structural aspects of the relationship among its ramifications, the dimension also includes the flow rate value (or its velocity) in relation to the level of diversification reached (Zamir 2001). There is previous evidence showing that the dimensional value acquired (between 1.2 and 1.4) results from the metabolic dependence of the tissue to be perfused and not from the tree structure itself (Karch *et al* 2003).

11.1 Complexity, health and disease

In general terms, the non-stationarity and nonlinearity in signals generated by living organisms challenge homeostasis-based approaches and conventional biostatistical methodologies (Goldberger *et al* 2002). In particular, the cardiovascular system shows an outstanding capacity to develop complex behaviors, which are generated from the interaction between the arterial conduits and the cardiac muscle. In this regard, physiological applications based on fractal geometry analysis comprise two clearly differentiated groups: the first one conducts a spatial assessment of the branching patterns, while the second one performs an assessment on the time variable parameters (Masters 2004). The latter approach was selected to be applied throughout this chapter. Similar to the self-similarity of anatomical nature (laws that govern vascular network branching), fractal processes produce fluctuations in the waveforms, which manifest in multiple scales. In addition to the characteristic morphological irregularity, non-stationary behaviors are frequently observed (Goldberger *et al* 2002). In essence, there is evidence showing that the fractal structure of an arterial network allows minimization of the transport task. Together with this phenomenon, the local regulation of vasomotor tone shows rhythmic variations which bifurcate between states of quasi-periodicity and chaos. Furthermore, vasodilating substances, which increase A_D and reduce A_P, keep the system under periodic dynamics (Sharma 2009). One of the greatest contributions of nonlinear dynamics to the understanding of the mechanisms that rule cardiovascular control consists of the processing of heart rate variability (HRV). This is defined as the instantaneous variation of the heart rate (H_R) and reflects the activity of the central nervous system. Traditionally, HRV spectral analysis (through the application of TF_D) shows the interaction between the parasympathetic system (whose action decreases H_R) and the sympathetic system (whose action increases H_R) (Nichols *et al* 2011). What is remarkable in relation to the above exposed, is that the HRV nonlinear analysis reveals the presence of self-affinity. It should be remembered that using this procedure, it is possible to reveal the structural composition of the signal and its behavior in multiple time scales. As a result of this finding, the information obtained from fractal measures on physiological time series is called *fractal complexity* and it essentially refers to the morphological structure of the signal under study.

In relation to acute cardiovascular events, such as arrhythmia or myocardial infarction, the *decrease* of fractal complexity in HRV is an efficient predictor of mortality, including traditional HRV indicators (Sharma 2009). An explanation to this phenomenon lies in the fact that *healthy* systems reveal a type of complex variability, related to multiscale nonlinear interactions of varied nature. The resulting time series show far-reaching correlations, revealing behaviors related to the presence of fractality. With the emergence of certain pathologies, complex series experience a transition oriented towards a differentiated dynamic, evidenced by a *rupture* of the above-mentioned correlation properties. This behavior, which entails a loss of complexity, may be related to both a pathological periodicity (the series are governed by specific frequency modes) and an uncorrelated randomization. Consequently, the approach proposed entails the analysis of the fractal complexity of the time series related to cardiovascular mechanics, both in healthy conditions and differentiated states that may be related to the presence of vascular pathologies, such as arterial hypertension *(AHT)*, diabetes mellitus *(DM)*, or atherosclerosis. In this regard, it should be considered that the result of estimating *FD* on a time series is inevitably a numerical value, *regardless of whether the signal is fractal or not*. Indeed, the *FD* value reflects the structural complexity of the series regardless of the presence of self-similarity (Raghavendra and Narayana 2010). Figure 11.2 shows two time series from sites of vital physiopathological relevance. The first one corresponds to the left ventricular pressure (LVP) waveform, initiator of the A_P pulse that will propagate throughout the arterial vascular bed. The second one represents the time variation of the arterial pressure in the ascending aorta (P_{AO}). With a simple examination, a substantial difference in its morphology can be observed, especially in terms of its associated roughness. Furthermore, the A_P wave will be subjected to subsequent variations as it progresses along its path. Consequently, the aim of future works will consist of determining whether *FD* is able to identify such variations, considering the *fractality, health and disease* conceptual framework as the trend for functional analysis.

The conception of the arterial system as a single close-ended conduit, with constant or variable properties along its length and a definite termination (Windkessel model) has generated acceptable results in relation to low frequency perturbations (Taylor 1966). However, in the case of high frequencies, the discrepancies are evident. The justification of this situation lies in the fact that although the arterial system is not a single conduit, it is made up of a set of tubular branches. In

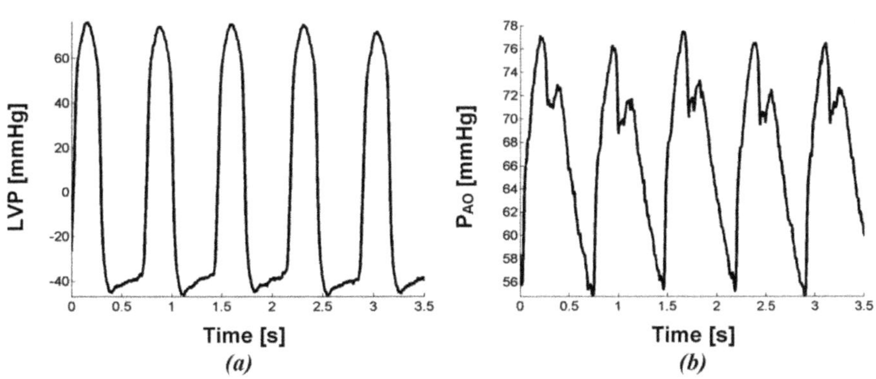

Figure 11.2. (a) Time series corresponding to left ventricular pressure (LVP). (b) Times series corresponding to aortic pressure P_{AO}.

addition, the attenuation effect, produced by arterial wall viscosity on the waves propagating through the network, must also be considered (Taylor 1966). One of the most relevant aspects is the inverse relationship that exists between frequency and wavelength since wavelengths corresponding to high frequencies will produce significant phase differences between the waves coming from different reflection sites. For this reason, the consideration of the stiffness gradient together with the distributed nature of the terminal branches significantly affects the overall behavior of the arterial system (Taylor 1966). In terms of nonlinear processing, such behavior may be expressed in multiple scales and thus evaluated through a fractal measure. The loss of high frequency components is a typical feature of the loss of complexity and can be associated with the presence of diseases. In fact, this idea is part of the *health/disease and FD* conceptual framework, adopted in this work. In this sense, the transmission network models based on fractality have been consistently applied in the study of circulation (Milnor 1989). In a paper by Brown (Brown 1996), arterial network simulations based on fractal rules were developed, where Taylor's proposed premises were extended. One of the most relevant findings is that regardless of the dichotomic distribution of the branches and of the application of a power law to the relationship between their dimensions, the characteristic asymmetry of the bifurcations plays a fundamental role. This phenomenon is responsible for a marked reduction in the reflection coefficient and therefore affects the spectral oscillations in the input impedance. Dispersion phenomena in physiological measurements are inevitable. The problem lies with the methodology used to quantify them, regardless of the size of the domain considered. Although a coincidence in the mean values is possible, this is not observed in the relative variance, since the latter depends on the measurement scale chosen to estimate the parameter. It is in these cases that the intervention of the concept of fractality cannot be disregarded (Bassingthwaighte 1988). This idea was first associated with physiological structures in Mandelbrot's book (Mandelbrot 1983). In that work, explicit reference to the creation of vascular networks from fractal rules was made. As a result, an acceptably consistent hypothesis was posed: If the geometry of vascular beds has a fractal structure, isn't it expected that perfusion pressure and flow will be governed by such geometry? (Bassingthwaighte 1988). The impact of this structure on A_P, its association with pathological states related to A_S, and the presence of peripheral reflections are the main premises of this chapter.

The dichotomous branching of the arterial tree reflects its first fractal characteristic though in a more basic form. Indeed, the result is an open structure consisting of vascular segments and bifurcations, which constitute the universal block of the arterial network (Zamir 2001). In view of the foregoing, the fractal genesis of the arterial network is unquestionable. For this reason, the temporal behavior of its associated hemodynamic variables was evaluated, using processing methodologies appropriate to such conception. However, although there are studies addressing the allocation of geometric parameters to each branch (Murray 1926, Pollanen 1992, Zamir 2001), no allocations related to intrinsic arterial wall features have been evaluated. As previously stated, the activity of the viscoelastic components of the arterial wall strongly determines arterial impedance. Therefore, the self-affine phenomenon observed in the A_P series can be modeled from the interaction of the reflected propagating components, whose distribution within the morphology is the result of local (or eventually systemic) biomechanical alterations of the arterial vascular structure.

11.1.1 Unwrinkling effect

The characterization of the morphological changes in the A_P waveform resulted in the coinage of the term *unwrinkling*. This effect was first observed in the invasive experimental protocols implemented in the coronary network. The increase in vascular stiffness, induced by the activation of *smooth muscle*, was concomitant to an increase and loss of roughness in the time series structure. This behavior was also observed in obstructive events of the descending aorta (absence of reflected peripheral waves) as well as in the pressure morphological variation analyses performed on the carotid and femoral arteries. The latter situation was associated with the effect produced by the *AF*, whose activity has been described according to similar terms. Therefore, the scaling phenomenon observed in mechanical waves in their path from the myocardium can be conceptualized as a *stretching* (unwrinkling), as shown in figure 11.3.

11.1.2 Influence of the reflected wave

It should be noted that in *in vitro* tests, the conduit's typical A_S variation was reflected in losses of structural complexity in A_P and A_D, in the absence of a distributed cardiovascular system *CVS*. In fact, the waves were structurally modified as a result of the presence of a liquid reservoir which acted as compliance and of a marked wave reflection site provided by hydraulic obstruction. For this reason, it has been suggested that the changes experienced by the vascular response caused by flow variations were essential in the formation of the fine structure of the generated

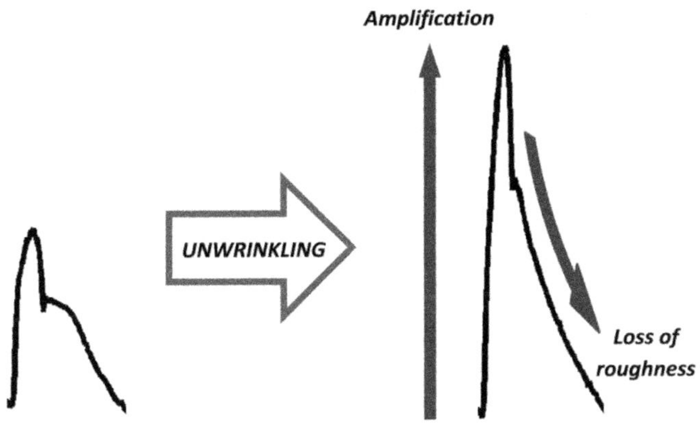

Figure 11.3. *Unwrinkling* (stretching) effect shown by the actions of amplification and loss of roughness in the waveform.

waves. Considering the systemic effects, the *CVS* uses the arterial damping effect (through the major arterial conduits) in order to attenuate the pulsatility of the fluid and ensure a quasi-stable regime at the capillary level.

In relation to this, a comparison of the structural complexity between a ventricular pressure wave and an aortic wave is presented above. Although the aortic wave is constrained in its frequency content (as a result of the damping effect), it shows a marked irregularity in terms of morphology. The presence of wave reflections, coming from the multiple vascular branching sites, modifies its contour significantly. It was already stated that under pathological states, such as *AHT*, an increase in A_S represents a decrease in the system's global compliance. As a result, the elimination of high frequency fluctuations is less efficient. In addition, the resulting increase in *PWV* generates an early return of the peripheral waves to the heart muscle, thus increasing the pressure in the abdominal aorta region (Westerhof *et al* 2010). In terms of fractality, the processing of P_{AO} waveforms shows that they have lower roughness values compared to normal states. Consequently, it may be inferred that the *dispersion* of reflections in relation to the structure plays a fundamental role. The early return of the reflected wave not only increases A_P maximum value during its systolic excursion, but also has an impact on the *distribution of singularities* that are part of heartbeat morphology. Such alterations are clearly differentiated by *FD* variation, which in fact presents the *unwrinkling* phenomenon.

11.2 Fractal dimension: a holistic index

In previous paragraphs, *FD* was proposed as a *holistic* indicator directly related to A_S and wave reflection. As can be observed, the *in vitro* experiments revealed a relationship between *FD* and A_S at the local vascular level. This consideration is valid due to the absence of branches distributed in the circuit design of the blood circulation simulator used. The results obtained from the processing subsequently conducted on the morphology of ventricular thickness in ischemic events were consistent with the observations of the parietal response. Then, structural trials on the coronary bed (a *reduced* arterial network) revealed the presence of morphological changes in the aortic A_P in activation states of the vascular smooth muscle. For this reason, the processing of *in vivo* experiments with total reflection maneuvers allowed a structural evaluation of the whole arterial network and its impact on A_P morphology. Unlike the experiments performed on the coronary arterial bed, where the activation process caused A_S to increase, a similar effect was replicated by means of an obstructive maneuver. As a result of it, the reflected components coming from the peripheral bed were eliminated, while during the activation state such reflections were present. In both situations, the *FD* decrease was concomitant to both the vascular response and the influence of the reflected waves. For this reason, the detection of a stretching in A_P with a loss of complexity (*unwrinkling*) can be attributed to both an increase in A_S (*conductive factor*) and to structural alterations typical of the arterial tree (*obstructive factor*). In addition, as already stated, the *FD* evaluations performed on *PP* only show significant differences in the presence of

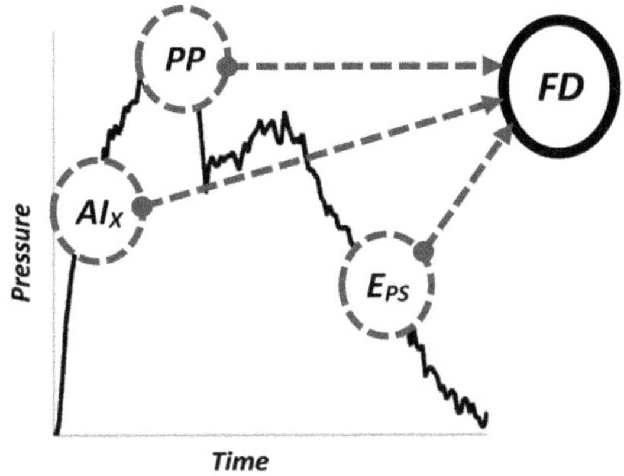

Figure 11.4. Definition of the fractal dimension (*FD*) as a holistic indicator, since it accounts for variations in parameters related to wave pulsatility (pulsatile pressure, *PP*), vascular elasticity (pressure versus strain index, E_{PS}) and wave reflection (augmentation index, AI_X).

nonlinear processes. The loss of morphological roughness means that the *AF* has different impacts on pulsatility frequency components, making the waveform less complex and taking it to its pure oscillatory levels. This phenomenon may, in some aspects, be associated with the concept of oscillatory disease (figure 11.4) (Cymberknop *et al* 2013a, 2013b, Politi *et al* 2016).

In view of the foregoing, proposing *FD* as a holistic indicator is appropriate from more than one point of view. The holism concept entails the presence of non-linearity, where the whole is not the sum of its parts, thus not complying with the superposition principle. In addition, the *FD* has intrinsic behaviors based on multiscale information, which are not specifically related to any particular magnitude or biological system. Moreover, the calibration of the signal acquired in its determination is not required and therefore the measurement is independent of specific units. It should be stressed that the non-invasive determination of A_P systo-diastolic variations (by means of the applanation tonometry technique) requires additional sphygmomanometric measurements, where the invariance of the mean and diastolic pressures throughout the vascular network are assumed. In this sense, the *FD* estimation is not affected at all by the values of such pressures.

11.3 Conclusion

The various analyses performed indicated the presence of morphological variations in hemodynamic variables of the vascular mechanics, induced by the presence of pathological states. Such variations were quantified through nonlinear processing based on fractal geometry. The main finding shows a decreased *FD*, concomitant to both the changes in A_S and the absence of wave reflections. As a result, it may be inferred that the information provided by the measurement is systemic since it is influenced by both factors simultaneously. The *FD* observational analysis, associated with a potential marker, is significantly consistent in terms of health and disease. Through the adoption of this conceptual framework it was possible to use the quantification of fractal complexity to detect underlying pathological states, associated with descriptive parameters of cardiovascular mechanics.

References

Barnsley M F 2000 *Fractals Everywhere* 2nd edn (Morgan Kaufmann)

Bassingthwaighte J B 1988 Physiological heterogeneity: fractals link determinism and randomness in structures and functions *News Physiol. Sci.* **3** 5–10

Bassingthwaighte J B, Liebovitch L S and West B J 1994 *Fractal Physiology* (New York: Oxford University Press)

Brown D J 1996 Input impedance and reflection coefficient in fractal-like models of asymmetrically branching compliant tubes *IEEE Trans. Biomed. Eng.* **43** 715–22

Cymberknop L J, Legnani W, Barra J G, Pessana F M and Armentano R L 2013a Fractal dimension as an index of left ventricular ischemia: a pilot study *Physiol. Meas.* **34** 83–97

Cymberknop L J, Armentano R L, Legnani W, Pessana F M, Craiem D, Graf S and Barra J G 2013b Contribution of arterial tree structure to the arterial pressure fractal behavior *J. Phys.: Conf. Ser.* **477** 012030

Falconer K 2003 *Fractal Geometry: Mathematical Foundations and Applications* 2nd edn (New York: Wiley)

Goldberger A L and West B J 1987 Fractals in physiology and medicine *Yale J. Biol. Med.* **60** 421–35

Goldberger A L, Peng C K and Lipsitz L A 2002 What is physiologic complexity and how does it change with aging and disease? *Neurobiol. Aging* **23** 23–6

Karch R, Neumann F, Podesser B K, Neumann M, Szawlowski P and Schreiner W 2003 Fractal properties of perfusion heterogeneity in optimized arterial trees *J. Gen. Physiol.* **122** 307–22

Madisetti V 2009 *The Digital Signal Processing Handbook* 2nd edn (Boca Raton, FL: CRC Press)

Mandelbrot B 1983 *The Fractal Geometry of Nature* (New York: Freeman)

Masters B R 2004 Fractal analysis of the vascular tree in the human retina *Annu. Rev. Biomed. Eng.* **6** 427–52

Milnor W R 1989 *Hemodynamics* 2th edn (Baltimore, MD: Williams & Wilkins)

Murray C D 1926 The physiological principle of minimum work applied to the angle of branching of arteries *J. Gen. Physiol.* **9** 835–41

Nichols W W, O'Rourke M F and Vlachopoulus C 2011 *McDonald's Blood Flow in Arteries: Theoretical, Experimental and Clinical Principles* 6th ed (London: Hodder Arnold)

Politi M T, Wray S, Fernández J, Gaudric J, Ghigo A, Lagrée P-Y, Capurro C, Fullana J M and Armentano R 2016 Impact of arterial cross-clamping during vascular surgery on arterial stiffness measured by the augmentation index and fractal dimension of arterial pressure *Health Technol.* **6**

Pollanen M S 1992 Dimensional optimization at different levels of the arterial hierarchy *J. Theor. Biol.* **159** 267–70

Raghavendra B S and Narayana D 2010 Computing fractal dimension of signals using multiresolution box-counting method 2010 *Int. J. Inform. Math. Sci.* **6** 50–65

Sharma V 2009 Deterministic chaos and fractal complexity in the dynamics of cardiovascular behavior: perspectives on a new frontier *Open Cardiovasc. Med. J.* **3** 110–23

Taylor M G 1966 The input impedance of an assembly of randomly branching elastic tubes *Biophys. J.* **6** 29–51

Westerhof N, Stergiopulos N and Noble M I M 2010 *Snapshots of Hemodynamics: An Aid for Clinical Research and Graduate Education* 2nd edn (Berlin: Springer)

Zamir M 2001 Arterial branching within the confines of fractal L-system formalism *J. Gen. Physiol.* **118** 267–76

Chapter 12

Mathematical blood flow models: numerical computing and applications

Ricardo L Armentano and Leandro J Cymberknop

The general phenomenon of flow in the arterial systems will be studied in order to model arterial flow and to try to identify the mechanisms underlying experimental or clinical observations, whether in normal or pathological blood circulation conditions. Modeling allows different kinds of relations to be established, resulting in a set of equations which are currently solved using numerical methods.

Blood circulation in the arterial or venous vessels includes two biomechanical phenomena, blood flow (governed by fluid mechanics) and the deformation of the arterial wall (governed by solid mechanics). Both are coupled in such a way that there is an inherent interdependence that can only be disregarded in a few circumstances in order to consider them independently. The aim of this chapter is to review some of the most significant existing numerical models, which provides a sufficiently precise and practical interpretation of vascular biomechanics.

The development of cardiovascular pathologies is a complex multiscale process involving a combination of geometrical, mechanical, hemodynamical and biological factors. 3D blood flow models are the numerical counterpart to *in vitro* models, in the sense that they enable a complete description of all relevant scales. As such, they have been solved using a variety of fluid–structure interaction (FSI) numerical methods coupling the motion of blood and the deformation of the arterial wall (Hughes *et al* 1981, Farhat *et al* 2001, Tezduyar 2003, Figueroa *et al* 2006, Tezduyar *et al* 2007, Mayr *et al* 2015).

Fortunately, there is now a widespread recognition that mathematical models and numerical simulations can help to better understand physiological and pathological processes. More than complementing data obtained by non-invasive measurements and medical imaging, they provide a means to analyze and predict hemodynamics at a wide variety of vascular scales. However, the relevance and accuracy of the numerical predictions of a mathematical blood flow model are inherently conditioned by its modeling limits; and unfortunately all cardiovascular blood flow

doi:10.1088/2053-2563/aafb0dch12

models have their limits. With the advent of medical imaging and computer sciences, clinicians are renewing the idea of cardiovascular models to represent hemodynamics at different vascular scales. While mathematical blood flow models were initially developed to complement clinicians' understanding of the cardiovascular system, they have now outgrown this purpose and are being used as predictive tools for patient-specific clinical studies (Formaggia *et al* 2009).

Understanding of the pulsatile flow in vascular vessels can benefit at least the following aspects:

1. To help investigate the pathology of diseases. Surely, cardiovascular diseases are related to many factors. But a lot of studies show that arterial wall remodels in response to the mechanical stimuli imposed by the blood. Quantities of the flow field, e.g. wall shear stress (WSS), turbulence, etc, are directly related to the initiation and progression of atherosclerosis, stenosis and aneurysms (Nichols *et al* 2011). Previous computational fluid dynamics (CFD) studies have assumed a steady flow or/and rigid walls (Formaggia *et al* 2009). However, in many scenarios, the unsteadiness and wall movement may have significant influence on the predictions of CFD simulation. It is necessary to model the pulsatile flow within distensible vessels to predict more reliably or to justify the aforementioned simplified assumptions on walls and inflow and outflow boundary conditions.
2. To develop non-invasive diagnosis tools. The most well-known quantities of blood flow used for diagnosis purposes are heart rate and the systolic/diastolic pressure. These biomarkers can be measured easily and are reliable regarding some diseases. Recently, additional tools based on the analysis of pulse waves have been proposed for early detection of vascular disorders, such as pulse wave velocity (PWV), augmentation index, brachial ankle vascular index and pulse wave separation method (Saito 2011), among others. The development of techniques to estimate parameters from flow rate and pressure make applications in this direction promising (Leguy *et al* 2010, Lombardi 2014).
3. To optimize the design of intravascular prostheses and surgery planning. Simulations of bypass graft surgery in both coronary and peripheral vascular systems have been addressed (Sankaran *et al* 2012, Huberts *et al* 2012a, 2012b, Marchandise *et al* 2009, Willemet *et al* 2013). The insertion of a stent changes the local compliance of the vessel. The pressure reflection and WSS alterations incurred by the stent can be predicted by computing an unsteady blood flow field with moving boundaries (Smith *et al* 2002).

In terms of the above-mentioned, models with various complexities have been developed for the pulsatile flow, which can be briefly summarized as follows:

Three-dimensional (3D) models: In these models, the mass conservation equations, time-dependent Navier–Stokes equations and equations of elasticity of the vessel wall are solved with proper boundary conditions (Gerbeau *et al* 2005). Based on medical imaging, a patient-specific simulation of the largest arteries of a whole body have recently proven to be a useful complementary tool (Xiao *et al* 2013).

Nevertheless, due to this simulation providing specific details regarding the flow field, it is very 'expensive' to compute. Moreover, there are a lot of parameters to set in this model, which makes it difficult for clinical applications. At the current stage, such simulations are only suitable for the purpose of research when a system with a considerable amount of computational power is available. The most feasible approach is to model only one or several segments of interest with the 3D model, while the rest of the network is described by proper boundary conditions.

Two-dimensional (2D) models: When the flow through a pipe is modeled and the turbulence phenomenon is not considered, the velocity at the circumferential direction can be neglected, and only velocities in the axial and radial directions are computed. Additionally, the nonlinear convective term is also neglected, and solutions are obtained in the frequency domain.

One-dimensional (1D) models: In addition to the assumption of axial symmetry, the long-wave assumption is always satisfied for the blood flow waves. With those two main assumptions, the pressure at the local cross-sections is considered constant and thus radial velocity is neglected. In this model, the velocity (V) is described by $V(t; r; x)$, where t is time, r is radius and x is axial distance. This model is sometimes called the 1.5 dimensional model (Čanić *et al* 2006, Lagree 2000, Ling and Atabek 1972). If a proper axial velocity profile $\phi(r)$ is defined such that $V(t; r; x) = V(t; x).\phi(r)$, the governing equations can be integrated over r. Thus, the conservation of mass and balance of momentum can be expressed as partial differential equations in time and axial distance. This system is closed by a constitutive law of the mechanical properties of the wall. Since they do not provide detailed information on the distribution of blood flow, recirculation, tangential stresses in the wall, etc. However, in these models, boundary conditions corresponding to mean flow, mean pressure, resistance, impedance, etc, can be easily imposed. By coupling these 1D models with 3D models, through suitable algorithms that maintain flow and pressure continuity, the effect of the downstream arterial network on the three-dimensional model can be efficiently represented. Both *in vitro* (Alastruey *et al* 2011, Saito *et al* 2011, Wang *et al* 2012) and *in vivo* (DeVault *et al* 2008, Olufsen *et al* 2000, Reymond *et al* 2009, 2011, Steele *et al* 2003, Willemet *et al* 2013) observations have shown that they can capture all of the features of propagated waveforms along the arterial system. The 1D models are well balanced between complexity and computational cost, thus they become very suitable for many applications. According to this, it will be possible in the near future to achieve fast, accurate, patient-specific and clinically applicable solutions supported by the simulation of complete circulating systems.

Zero-dimensional (0D) models: Zero-dimensional models are described by ordinary differential equations that depend only on time. Due to a spatial variable not being involved (thus the name 0D or 'lumped' models), the wave propagation in space cannot be evaluated. In this sense, these models impose a low computational cost and can describe the main characteristics of a vascular network (also known as 'Windkessel' models), relating the blood pressure and blood flow in terms of concentrated parameters such as the arterial compliance (elasticity and extensibility of arteries) and the peripheral resistance (flow resistance encountered by the blood as it flows). They are usually integrated with 3D or 1D models to provide the inflow and outflow boundary conditions with a limited computational cost (Bertoglio *et al* 2012, Vignon and Taylor 2004, Vignon-Clementel *et al* 2010).

12.1 Towards a patient-specific modeling for clinical applications

It is well known that hemodynamics of large arteries is too complex to be apprehended using only non-invasive measurements and medical imaging techniques. For this reason, patient-specific numerical simulations of blood flow have therefore been developed to provide clinicians with valuable insights on pathogenesis and the outcome of surgeries. As 3D models can only be used in small portions of the cardiovascular system due to their high modeling and computational costs, reduced-order models have gained attention to reproduce complex wave propagation behaviors in large networks of arteries.

One-dimensional blood flow models can be obtained by integrating the 3D equations governing blood flow over the cross-sectional area of an artery, assuming that the characteristic axial length scale is much longer than the radial one and that the flow is axisymmetric. In this integration process, only the radial dependence is lost, and 1D blood flow models still retain the ability to propagate elastic waves. Indeed, their hyperbolic nature is well adapted to reproduce the wave propagation phenomena in the systemic arterial tree. These 1D models give accurate predictions of pressure and flow waveforms in all the main arteries at a low computational cost, which offers a distinct advantage for clinical applications using patient-specific data. In fact, Leonhard Euler was the first to write, in 1755, the 1D equations for the conservation mass and the continuity of momentum describing blood flow (Euler 1844). Unfortunately, he was unable to properly solve them.

Actually, the main focus for 1D models is to develop novel approaches based on considering the non-Newtonian behavior of blood and the viscoelastic response of the arterial wall. Regarding blood flow, a suitable numerical treatment must be incorporated to avoid the instability originated by the convective terms in the Navier–Stokes equations, and especially in this case, to consider the interaction between blood flow and the nonlinear deformation of the vascular wall. In relation to vascular wall tissue, they must deal with a strongly nonlinear behavior due to diverse sources: on the one hand, the intrinsic response of the tissue itself due to the progressive recruitment of the collagen fibers in the mechanical response; on the other hand, the typical large material deformations and rotations of soft tissues. In addition, a key factor is the anisotropy and a suitable physiological characterization of the tissue, which, in turn, exhibits properties that evolve through time in response to different stimuli and biological processes, as living material.

The pressure and flow waves caused by the pumping of a heart travel along the main arteries damping and reflecting themselves due to the change of diameter in blood vessels, the branching and the neighboring tissues. Consequently, it is essential to impose realistic boundary conditions to obtain realistic results. The usual boundary conditions correspond to certain velocity profiles defined through a pressure time series of constant profile in cross-sections. From the experimental point of view, it is feasible to quantify the velocities of blood flow through techniques ranging from simple ultrasound-based measurements to complex measurements with cardiac magnetic resonance. Although arterial pressure is easy to measure, the precise measurement of blood pressure requires highly invasive techniques. The main problem of these boundary conditions is that the velocities and pressures calculated through computational simulation are determined only by the blood flow resistance of the domain that has been modelized. Diverse solutions have been proposed to overcome this problem, among which are the distributed models that represent the rest of the downstream circulatory system through its resistance or impedance values (Vignon-Clementel *et al* 2006, Steele *et al* 2003), and the coupling of the realistic three-dimensional geometry models with unidimensional models that solve the Navier–Stokes equations considering flow–arterial wall interaction (Formaggia *et al* 2003). The resistance-based boundary conditions establish a constant relation between the mean pressure and the flow rate: $P = QxR$ (Milnor 1982). This condition, though it implies an advancement on the boundary conditions corresponding to imposed pressures, results in extremely high-pressure pulses and establishes that, at the output, pressure and flow are in phase. The impedance-based boundary conditions (Milnor 1982) define the relation between the mean pressure and flow in relation to frequency. In this case, the flow rate at an instant t depends on the history of pressures in a complete period. The impedances to be imposed in the 3D model can be obtained from experimental measurements (Kelly and Fitchett 1992) or through numerical algorithms based on the definition of binary fractal trees used to calculate the impedances applying Womersley's linear wave theory (Taylor 1966, Olufsen 1999, Steele *et al* 2003). These boundary conditions provide realistic peak and mean pressure values. Another numerical problem is associated with the incompressibility of blood flow. This phenomenon imposes the constraint that the velocity field must have a null divergence. The pressure field, which remains free in the formulation because it is not associated with any constitutive equation, is interpreted as an additional unknown field that is necessary to meet the incompressibility condition. In the weak formulation, pressure plays the role of a Lagrange multiplier associated with the incompressibility constraint, and thus the velocity and pressure fields remain coupled. Diverse formulations have been proposed to deal with the incompressible flow problem, based on the so-called *mixed elements* that incorporate velocities and pressures as primary variables (Hughes 2000).

During the last few years, the progress of mathematics (solution of hyperbolic systems) and computer sciences has enabled one to solve the 1D equations for blood in single arteries as well as in large networks (Sherwin *et al* 2003, Sherwin 2007, Formaggia *et al* 2003) using a wide variety of numerical methods (Delestre and Lagrée 2013, Boileau *et al* 2015, Wang *et al* 2015, Puelz *et al* 2017). To obtain physiological waveforms in 1D systemic network models, much effort was put into obtaining realistic boundary conditions accurately modeling the behavior of the heart (Mynard and Nithiarasu 2008), the flow in junctions (Fullana and Zaleski 2009, Mynard and Valen-Sendstad 2015, Contarino *et al* 2016, Müller *et al* 2016b, Chnafa *et al* 2017) and the vascular network distal to the terminal vessels (Olufsen *et al* 2000, Alastruey *et al* 2007, Cousins and Gremaud 2012, Perdikaris *et al* 2015,

Guan *et al* 2016). These 1D models have then been extensively used to study the flow in the main systemic arteries, from the ascending aorta to the upper and lower limbs (Matthys *et al* 2007, Müller and Blanco 2015, Müller *et al* 2016a). Other studies have considered the cerebral circulation in detail (Zagzoule and Marc-Vergnes 1986, Alastruey *et al* 2007). More recently, simulation of the complete systemic circulation (Liang *et al* 2011, Reymond *et al* 2009, 2011, Watanabe *et al* 2013, Blanco *et al* 2014, 2015) and the complete cardiovascular system (Müller and Toro 2014) have been performed. Some studies have gone beyond reproducing healthy networks and have considered pathological networks with stenoses and aneurysms (Müller *et al* 2013, Delestre and Lagrée 2013, Murillo and García-Navarro 2015, Ghigo *et al* 2017b, Sazonov *et al* 2017) and have modeled their treatment using endovascular or extracorporeal surgeries (Willemet *et al* 2013, Drzisga *et al* 2016, Ghigo *et al* 2017a, Strocchi *et al* 2017). In time, these 1D models will be integrated in daily clinical practice to provide clinicians with rapid information on hemodynamics in patient-specific networks and on the possible outcome of surgical treatments.

12.2 Interaction between blood flow and the arterial wall: fluid–structure coupling

The computational modeling of blood flow coupling with the arterial wall has caught the attention of several researchers in the last few years, as a tool for the diagnosis and prognosis of diverse pathologies in the cardiovascular system, which in some way offers a more complete insight than the models that simulate blood flow phenomena only (Formaggia *et al* 2009). From the conceptual point of view, in the flow–arterial wall interaction models, the domain in which the fluid is defined (generally the arterial lumen) is not fixed, and therefore its boundaries must adapt to the arterial wall motion. The classical formulations of solid computational mechanics, based on Lagrangian finite element meshes that get deformed as they move in the same way as the solid, are suitable. However, for flow analysis, the classical Eulerian formulations that use fixed meshes are not valid due to the motion of the fluid domain. The so-called ALE (arbitrary Lagrangian–Eulerian) formulation is a suitable method to model the motion of a fluid with mobile boundaries. In this case, the mesh is neither fixed nor does it accompany the fluid motion, but rather has an arbitrary motion. In the case of blood flow, a restriction is imposed on this arbitrary motion of the mesh so that its boundary must accompany the motion of the solid.

The fluid–structure interaction problems include three models that must be solved in a coupled fashion: the flow model, the solid model and the model that determines the fluid–structure interface. The manner in which the solutions are coupled results in two main groups of coupling techniques. *Monolithic methods* provide a strong coupling in which the problem is globally stated, using Newton or quasi-Newton methods to iteratively solve the whole problem (Fernández and Moubachir 2005). *Partitioned methods* solve the fluid mechanics model and solid mechanics model separately, using different software and applying different techniques so that the solutions provided by the two models are compatible in terms of the global equilibrium of the full model (Calvo 2006). In turn, partitioned methods can be classified into *weak coupling* (or explicit or sequential methods) or *strong coupling* ('implicit' or 'iterative' methods). In the explicit methods, time integration progresses in time without internal iterations of the equilibrium between the solid and the fluid: both systems simply exchange information at the end of each time step, and that information is used in the next step. In hemodynamics, these schemes do not work well due to the so-called added mass effect, which implies that when the fluid and solid densities have the same order of magnitude, the solution is unstable (Causin *et al* 2005). Consequently, the equilibrium between the solid and fluid mechanics models is achieved through iterations based on the fixed-point theorem, by means of Block–Jacobi and Block–Gauss–Seidel schemes. The solutions obtained with these methods are similar to those obtained using monolithic methods in terms of coupling, but they require a considerably higher number of iterations. This loss of computational efficiency may be compensated by the higher level of generality of the problems that can be addressed. By modeling the solid and the fluid separately, the calculation code capabilities can be leveraged in relation to boundary conditions, constitutive models, etc.

As a result of that mentioned above, there are many factors that may influence the validity of the 1D models and should be taken into account for the simulation:

a) **Incompressible flow**: The computational simulation of incompressible flow through the Navier–Stokes equations exhibits several numerical problems that must be corrected for reliable results. In the first place, the convective term is a nonlinear concept and thus the equation system must be solved iteratively through some Newton–Raphson-like scheme. In addition, the convection matrix associated with such a term is not symmetric, making the computational solution of the equation system highly costly, especially in three-dimensional models with a high number of nodes and elements. Finally, the convective term causes the standard finite element formulation based on Bubnov–Galerkin methods to yield unstable numerical solutions for high values of the Reynolds number. This requires the use of efficient stabilization methods (Codina 1998, Harari and Hughes 1994), among which are the SUPG techniques (streamline upwind Petrov–Galerkin), GLS (Galerkin least squares), SGS (sub-grid scale) and the multiscale variational methods.
b) **Lateral leakage and tapering**: The aorta is tapered from the proximal to the distal end. The tapering wall will increase the pulse pressure by continuous reflection. It is also observed that there are tiny side branches at the aorta. Some studies show that the effect of the tapering wall is compensated by the blood loss to the side branches. In net effect, it is more like a flow in a straight tube with no lateral leakage (Nichols *et al* 2011). However, both the branches and tapering can be modeled by the 1D models.
c) **Wave length is much longer than vessel radius**: In the aorta, the wave speed is about $5\,\mathrm{m\,s^{-1}}$ and the radius is about 10 mm (Nichols *et al* 2011). If we assume the period of one pulse is 1 s, the ratio between the wave length and the radius is 500. In smaller arteries, the wave speed increases and the radius

decreases, the ratio becomes even bigger. Thus, the long-wave assumption is fully justified.

d) **Blood rheology:** Rheology consists of the study of the flow properties of fluids that are subjected to shearing forces. The viscous nature of the fluid is related to microscopic phenomena occurring in the fluid volume. When shear stress is applied on the fluid, it sets the fluid in motion. However, the presence of boundary conditions or the molecular characteristics of the fluid in the same external conditions limits such motion, resulting in specific responses. The idealized presentation of the motion of a fluid in laminar and isothermal flow stationary conditions, with homogeneous and isotropic fluid, can be expressed through an equation that relates the shear stress applied with the shear rate (γ) or velocity gradient resulting from such stress. From the so-called rheograms expressed by $\tau = f(\gamma)$, it can be observed that a slope of the characteristic curves of each fluid can be obtained. This slope is named 'viscosity' (η), and represents the resistance of the fluid to deformation:

$$\eta = \frac{\partial \tau}{\partial \gamma}.$$

Fluids that show a constant value of η are known as 'Newtonian'. Although some fluids show increased viscosity with γ, others have a completely opposite behavior. The rheological response determines the properties of the fluid, including its elastic, viscous or time-dependent behavior according to each case. Blood, in particular, is a fluid that consists of plasma with high water content (78%), proteins (7%), other solutes (8%) and macromolecular components (7%) such as red cells or erythrocytes (99.9%), and white cells or leukocytes and platelets (0.1%). However, although plasma is considered a Newtonian fluid, the presence of particles turns the fluid into a nonlinear one. Thus, the higher the number of hematocrits, the greater the viscosity. Sometimes, the relation proposed by Einstein is used for spherical particle suspensions considering, in this case, a suspension of hematocrits:

$$\eta = \eta_{plasma}(1 + 2.5H_t),$$

where H_t corresponds to the concentration of hematocrits. Over a γ of 100 (1/sec), it is worth considering blood as a Newtonian fluid. From that value, it can reach a viscosity five times that of water.

To summarize, blood is considered to be a homogenous, Newtonian and incompressible fluid. About 45% of blood in volume is taken by blood cells, of which the majority are red blood cells (hemocyte). The disc-like red blood cells have a diameter $Dr \simeq 0.007$ mm. There are some white blood cells with a slightly larger size. But the number of white blood cells is very small compared to the red blood cells. In Smith *et al* (2002), vessels with diameters $Dv \geqslant 0.1$ mm were simulated by the 1D model. If we assume that the minimum vessel for the 1D model is 0.1 mm in diameter, then the ratio between the two diameters $Dv = Dr$ is larger than 14.3. In fact, the blood is a well-known non-Newtonian fluid with a shear-thinning property. But only in vessels with an internal diameter of less than 1 mm, is the apparent viscosity significantly dependent on the shear rate (Nichols *et al* 2011). However, in vessels smaller than this value, we can tune the friction coefficient to account for the changed viscosity. Within each particular vessel segment, we consider that the viscosity is constant, i.e. the blood is a Newtonian fluid. The bulk Young's modulus of water is about 2.2×10^9 Pa and that of a vessel volume to internal pressure is about 2.2×10^4. The ratio between the two moduli is 10^5, thus the incompressibility of blood is obvious.

e) **Profile of axial velocity**: One crucial step in deriving a 1D model is to prescribe a proper axial velocity profile. The fluid friction coefficient and the correction factor of the convection term in the momentum balance equation are dependent on this profile. The ratio between the transient inertia force and the viscous force can be estimated by the 'Womersley number' (α), the inertia forces being bigger than the viscous forces in larger vessels. In this case, the profile is essentially in the central part and there is a thin viscous boundary layer to match the no-slip boundary condition near the wall. When α is very small (small vessels), the profile is closer to a parabolic or Poiseuille flow. In small arteries, the Reynolds number drops a lot because both the velocity and the diameter of the vessels become smaller. Given that α is also much smaller in small arteries, laminar flow is very likely to appear in small arteries. That gives justification to Poiseuille's theory in estimating the peripheral resistance. In medium-sized arteries, there may be complex transition conditions between turbulent and laminar flow. The 1D models, in particular, neglect the velocity components in the circumferential direction and thus a laminar flow is an implicit assumption. However, the dissipating effect of turbulence on energy can be lumped into the skin friction term.

The Womersley model (Nichols *et al* 2011) is a particular case of the Navier–Stokes equation. However, when an approximation to the real case is carried out, the applied pressure gradient is pulsatile, that is, it has a spatial variation in relation to the transverse axis of a rigid conduit of radio R and infinite length. The reason for this infinite length is to avoid reflections, which should be taken into account when working with pressure wave transmission. However, when considering a rigid tube, pulse wave velocity is considered infinite. The fluid inside the conduit has a certain viscosity η and density ρ. The Womersley model must be applied when a profile $v = v(r, t)$ (where v is the axial velocity inside the conduit, r the axial coordinate, and t the time) is considered, and the artery is subjected to a periodic and pulse pressure gradient in relation to the longitudinal motion. If a harmonic motion of angular frequency ω ($Ae^{j\omega t}$) of the pressure gradient in relation to the longitudinal motion (z) of the conduit (dP/dz) is assumed, the solution to the differential equation will be a Bessel function of order zero and complex argument given by the following expression:

$$v(y,\ t) = \frac{AR^2}{j\eta\alpha^2} \cdot \left[1 - \frac{J_0\left(\alpha\ y\ j^{\frac{3}{2}}\right)}{J_0\left(\alpha j^{\frac{3}{2}}\right)}\right] \cdot e^{jwt} \quad \alpha = R\left(\frac{\omega}{v}\right)^{\frac{1}{2}},\ v = \frac{\eta}{\rho}\ y = \frac{r}{R},$$

where ν is known as the kinematic viscosity, α the Womersley number and y the normalized radius.

The solution for the generic case in which the pressure gradient is not represented by a simple harmonic motion, but rather consists in overlapping harmonics of angular frequency $\omega_n = n \cdot \omega_0$, gives the axial velocity profile, which will be a superposition of the stationary solution (Poiseuille model for stable flow) plus the harmonics, that is:

$$v = v(r,\ t) = v_e(r) + \sum_n v_n(v,\ t).$$

Replacing the above-mentioned results of the Fourier series expansion of $v(r,t)$, the following velocity profile is obtained:

$$v(\ y,\ t) = V_0(0)(1 - r^2) + 2\,\mathrm{Re}\left\{\sum_{n=1}^{\infty} V_n(0). \left[\frac{J_0\left(\alpha_n\, j^{\frac{3}{2}}\right) - J_0\left(\alpha_n\ y\ j^{\frac{3}{2}}\right)}{J_0\left(\alpha_n\, j^{\frac{3}{2}}\right) - 1}\right] \cdot e^{jn\omega_0 t}\right\},$$

where $V_n(0)$ are the coefficients of the Fourier series expansion of the 'center line' velocity of the artery, that is, of $v = v(0,\ t)$, ω_0 is the angular frequency of the cardiac cycle; and $J_0()$ are the coefficients of the Bessel polynomial of order zero and complex variable (Nichols *et al* 2011, Milnor 1982).

f) **Constitutive equation of vessel wall:** There is great interest in understanding the constitute equation of blood vessels in the human body. Many basic functions of the cardiovascular system depend on them such as blood distribution and the equilibrium in the pressure values. In particular, arterial mechanics determines not only the mean pressure values but also the pulsatile values, which determine blood flow and are partly responsible for the fatigue effect affecting the vessels. The challenge to describe the biomechanics of the arterial wall may be complex. Not because there are no composite materials like those forming the wall of a vessel, but because it is a biological tissue and it is necessary to consider the structural configuration and the active behavior of its constituent elements as well. Despite this additional complexity, the methods used to describe a biological material are similar to those employed to describe any other material. In general, the techniques include static and dynamic tests. In the latter, long time responses (low frequency) and short time responses (high frequency) are analyzed. The underlying purpose is to describe the mechanical response of the arterial wall through a mathematical model with few parameters that are representative of its structure and physiology.

The constitutive equation of the wall is derived from thin shell theory. The ratio between the thickness of the wall and the radius of the vessel is 0.1. The wall shows nonlinear elasticity properties in high pressure and the inertia of the wall may affect the pulse wave as well. But in most cases, a linear one is enough for a first approximation. Some recent studies show that viscoelastic property has a considerable effect on the pulse waves. Firstly, constitutive laws for biological tissue can be derived using integer-order differential equations that model stress–strain relations using additive combinations of purely elastic and viscous elements. The simplest integer-order models of linear viscoelasticity are the Voigt and standard linear solid (SLS or Kelvin–Zener) models (Armentano *et al* 1995, 2018a). The Voigt model can be constructed by the parallel combination of a spring and a dashpot and it is the simplest model that accounts for creep and hysteresis phenomena. Similarly, the SLS model is constructed using the parallel combination of a spring with a spring and a dashpot in series, and it accounts for creep, hysteresis and stress relaxation phenomena. Due to their simplicity, these models have been used in several 1D blood flow studies to describe arterial wall viscoelasticity. The success of the Kelvin–Voigt viscoelastic model is greatly due to its mathematical and modeling simplicity (it has only two parameters). Unfortunately, when confronted with experimental data, the Kelvin–Voigt model fails to capture the nonlinearities in the response of the arterial wall. Therefore, in this chapter we propose a modified Kelvin–Voigt model in which a nonlinear viscoelastic component is added. A similar nonlinear viscoelastic term is used in Erbay *et al* (1992) to study wave propagation in nonlinear viscoelastic tubes, and the theoretical basis of the approach is described in Bird *et al* (1977).

On the other hand, quasi-linear models relate the strain and stress in the arterial wall through a convolution between a normalized relaxation (or creep) function and a nonlinear elastic function (Holenstein *et al* 1980, Fung 1993). In this sense, linear and nonlinear viscoelastic models were used to predict biomechanical properties of the thoracic descending aorta and the carotid artery under *ex vivo* and *in vivo* conditions in ovine and human arteries (Valdez-Jasso *et al* 2009, 2011). The models analyzed included a four-parameter (linear) Kelvin viscoelastic model and two five-parameter nonlinear viscoelastic models (an arctangent and a sigmoid model) that relate changes in arterial blood pressure to the vessel cross-sectional area (via estimation of vessel strain). These models were developed using the framework of 'quasi-linear viscoelasticity' theory and were validated using measurements from the thoracic descending aorta and the carotid artery obtained from human and ovine arteries. Results showed that the Kelvin and sigmoid models were able to predict the zero-pressure vessel radius; that under *ex vivo* conditions vessels are more rigid, and comparatively, that the carotid artery is stiffer than the thoracic descending aorta.

Finally, fractional-order models describe the viscoelastic properties of the arterial wall using fractional-order differential equations (Craiem and

Armentano 2007, Craiem *et al* 2008) A 'fractal order', which may be understood as an infinite distribution of elements in a tree or a staircase shape, leads to the design of this type of models. The interesting thing is that fractional models correctly adjust the mechanical time and frequency responses and use a reduced number of parameters. The natural response to the fractional element is represented by a power-law curve that is consistent with the time relaxation curves and with the frequency response of the arterial wall. A fractional model is based on a mechanical element called a *spring–pot*, a combination of a viscous spring and a dashpot. The essence of this element is that it represents a derivative between stress and strain that is not necessarily of whole order. In other words, there is a theory of fractional calculus that admits intermediate-order derivatives rather than whole order derivatives. The possibility of having the fractional order of this derivative as a new parameter will pave the way for new interpretations on the structural organization of the arterial wall and on its active mechanical response, providing information on the current state of the vessel but also helping to predict its behavior in different pathological situations. Identifying a tissue through its parameters may be also useful for its classification within an organ bank. The main drawback until now has been that the models of arterial walls presented include a large number of parameters or require nonlinear complex relations that make them difficult to adjust numerically.

As mentioned previously, one of the more direct ways of modeling a material is by using springs and dashpots. The spring is a purely elastic element. Its only parameter E relates stress $\sigma(t)$ to strain $\varepsilon(t)$ proportionally:

$$\sigma(t) = E.\ D^0\varepsilon(t),$$

where D^0 represents the zero-order derivative. In a viscous dashpot, viscosity is proportional to the changes in stress through its first order derivative:

$$\sigma(t) = \eta.\ D^1\varepsilon(t).$$

By combining these elements in series and in parallel, the elastic curves can be adjusted, in time and frequency, thus obtaining the desired model. However, as mentioned, this combination is not trivial and, more often than not, the number of parameters grows without a direct relationship with the structural element composing the material. So, the adjustments may be appropriate but they become a large set of values without a particular sense. As is known, the larger the number of parameters, the better the adjustments but the more complicated the interpretations.

The fractional calculus theory proposes to fuse the spring and the dashpot into a new element called a *spring–pot* where stress and strain are related through a fractional-order derivative:

$$\sigma(t) = K.\ D^v\varepsilon(t), \ \ 1 > v > 0.$$

This new element gives a new versatility to the systems through the fractional-order parameter. For an extreme case in which $\upsilon = 0$, it behaves as a purely elastic spring without memory. But when $\upsilon = 1$, it becomes a viscous dashpot that dissipates energy proportionally to strain changes.

In further investigations of the behavior of fractional viscoelastic models it was demonstrated that wall viscoelasticity has only minor effects on flow rate wave propagation, while pressure waves and resulting wall displacements present variability in their phase and magnitude depending on the amount of viscoelastic dissipation introduced by the fractional order (Pérez Zerpa *et al* 2014). In Pérez Zerpa *et al* (2015), the accuracy of fractional models was improved through the use of a modified version of the spring–pot element, called a high-order spring–pot (HOSP). A numerical characterization method was applied, which consisted of minimizing the misfit among experimental measures of strains or stresses and the respective values predicted by the model, even in presence of noise in the data.

12.3 Implementing 1D models in arterial simulations

In the development of 1D models, difficulties arise when performing patient-specific simulations as the number of model parameters increases with the number of simulated arterial segments. This is especially true for quasi-linear models, as their parameters can exhibit dynamic variations during a cardiac cycle. Additionally, the parameters describing the viscoelasticity of the arterial wall are difficult to measure and are often hard to distinguish from those characterizing the viscoelastic properties of blood. For these reasons, most existing 1D blood flow simulations adopt an elastic wall model. Nonetheless, quasi-linear models have been successfully used in combination with a 1D blood flow model.

In Reymond *et al* (2009, 2011, 2012), comparison between numerical results and *in vivo* measurements revealed a considerable impact of the viscoelasticity on the pulse waves. In Battista *et al* (2016), a 1D fluid dynamics arterial network model with 14 vessels was developed to assimilate *ex vivo* 0D temporal data for pressure–area dynamics in individual vessel segments from 11 male Merino sheep, in combination with a four-parameter Kelvin viscoelastic model. In Perdikaris and Karniadakis (2014), a fractional-order model is used to compute blood flow in a patient-specific cranial network and the sensitivity of the model to the fractional order is quantified. A simpler integer-order model has also been used in 1D blood flow simulations. In Alastruey *et al* (2011), Montecinos *et al* (2014), Müller *et al* (2016b), Ghigo *et al* (2017a), a Kelvin–Voigt model was adopted and used to simulate the pulsatile flow in an *in vitro* experimental setup.

There are several factors that contribute to the global damping function of pressure and flow waves in large arteries and this effect can be modeled using a Kelvin–Voight model. However, in most of the 1D models found in the literature, the viscosity of the arterial wall was usually neglected (Azer *et al* 2007), essentially due to the complexity of its evaluation in humans. This term is responsible for the nonlinearity of the stress–strain relationship in large arteries and for the hysteresis phenomenon observed in the pressure–diameter loop, which also represents energy dissipation (London and Pannier 2010). In a recent work of Gabaldon Castillo *et al* (2016), and Cymberknop *et al* (2016), central blood pressure waveforms were introduced as an input of a simplified 1D viscoelastic model (i.e. tapered, but with no bifurcations), in order to reproduce the behavior of peripheral blood pressure variations. The influence of wall viscosity on the morphology of the simulated waveforms was then evaluated, using non-invasive radial artery measurements, constricted and expanded tubes. The implemented model perfectly reproduced the amplification factor as a consequence of the stiffness increase due to the tapering nature of the structure. The obtained results showed an improvement in the fit between the real and simulated data, due to the presence of wall viscosity mechanical property (in comparison to a pure elastic conduit) into the model calculations. Following this line of research, elastic mismatch between expended polytetrafluoroethylene (ePTFE) and poly-L-lactic acid (PLLA) vascular grafts in relation to femoral and carotid arteries in humans was evaluated in Alfonso *et al* (2016). The elastic mismatch generated by the interposition of both grafts between native arteries (carotid or femoral) was quantified by means of computational 1D simulations. PLLA tubular structures manifested a mechanical behavior that mimics the response to pulsatile hypertensive pressure regimes (pressure levels higher than those of the physiological range), which constitutes a highly desirable property for vascular tissue-engineered scaffold production.

Viscoelastic properties of the arterial wall play a significant role in normal and pathological vessels (Azer *et al* 2007). Pressure wave propagation in arteries depends on both elastic and viscous parameters, which counterbalance possible structural instabilities (Bouchut 2004). Arterial wall viscosity and elasticity are strongly influenced by changes in the local smooth muscle, independently of the prevailing pressure (Azer *et al* 2007). Using a viscoelastic model, i.e. the Kelvin model, is important in order to understand pressure–diameter dynamics. Consequently, in order to obtain a complete characterization of arterial behavior, viscous properties need to be used in simulations. For these reasons, the effect of viscoelasticity has a great significance in the implementation of 1D computational models, since a better fit between simulated and experimental data is achieved (Ghigo *et al* 2017c, Wang *et al* 2013).

In a recent work, an alternative approach was used where long-wave and perturbation theories allow them to derive a nonlinear dispersive and/or diffusive equation, like the Korteweg–de Vries (KdV) equation, starting from the Navier–Stokes equations (Cascaval 2012, Laleg *et al* 2007, Misra and Patra 2007, Yomosa 1987). Behind this model is the idea that blood pressure (BP) waves can be considered as combinations of solitons. The nonlinear representation of BP waves through the overlapping of two or three solitons is described in detail by Laleg *et al* (2007). This model captures many of the phenomena observed in BP propagation, such as peaking (increase in amplitude), steepening (decrease in width) and changes in wave propagation velocity. Furthermore, McDonald found that an amplitude increase of arterial pulse is concomitant with a decrease in pulse-width during the propagation of flow and pressure waveforms from the aorta to the saphenous artery in dogs (Nichols *et al* 2011), indicating a nonlinear rather than a linear behavior. Consequently, a 1D arterial network was constructed in order to simulate the behavior of synthesized pulse pressure waveforms as a combination of solitons throughout the arterial tree (Alfonso *et al* 2014, 2016, 2018). To this end, the pressure in each segment was computed using the KdV equation (KdVe), where vascular dimensions and elastic constants were obtained from the existing literature (Avolio 1980, Formaggia *et al* 2009, Reymond *et al* 2009). The main objective was to evaluate the propagation of acquired pulse pressure waves through a human-like arterial tree and quantify the ability of our model to capture changes in pulse pressure amplification (PPA) due to variations in arterial elasticity. Previously acquired central blood pressure (CBP) and peripheral blood pressure (PBP) waveforms were used, acquired from individuals separated into four well differentiated groups: young age group, adult age group and hypertensive type I and II groups.

To finalize, a two-dimensional (2D) nonlinear 'multi-ring' model for blood flow in axisymmetric elastic arteries has been proposed. It was designed to overcome the numerical difficulties of three-dimensional fluid–structure interaction simulations of blood flow without using the over-simplifications necessary to obtain one-dimensional models of blood flow. This multi-ring model is derived by integrating over concentric rings of fluid simplified long-wave Navier–Stokes equations coupled to an elastic model of the arterial wall. The resulting system of balance laws provides a unified framework in which both the motion of the fluid and the displacement of the wall are dealt with simultaneously. The mathematical structure of the multi-ring model allows us to use a finite volume method that guarantees the conservation of mass and the positivity of the numerical solution and can deal with nonlinear flows and large deformations of the arterial wall. We show that the finite volume numerical solution of the multi-ring model provides at a reasonable computational cost an asymptotically valid description of blood flow velocity profiles and other averaged quantities (wall shear stress, flow rate, ...) in large elastic and quasi-rigid arteries. This multi-ring model was validated against well-known solutions such as the Womersley or the Poiseuille solutions as well as against steady boundary layer solutions in quasi-rigid constricted and expanded tubes.

References

Alastruey J, Khir A W, Matthys K S, Segers P, Sherwin S J, Verdonck P R, Parker K H and Peiró J 2011 Pulse wave propagation in a model human arterial network: Assessment of 1-D viscoelastic simulations against *in vitro* measurements *J. Biomech.* **44** 2250–8

Alastruey J, Parker K H, Peiro J, Byrd S M and Sherwin S J 2007 Modelling the circle of Willis to assess the effects of anatomical variations and occlusions on cerebral flows *J. Biomech.* **40** 1794–805

Alfonso M R, Cymberknop L J, Legnani W, Pessana F and Armentano R L 2014 Conceptual model of arterial tree based on solitons by compartments, *Conf. Proc. IEEE Eng. Med. Biol. Soc.* pp 3224–7

Alfonso M, Cymberknop L, Armentano R, Pessana F, Wray S and Legnani W 2016 Arterial pulse pressure amplification described by means of a nonlinear wave model: characterization of human aging *J. Phys.: Conf. Ser.* **705** 012029

Alfonso M, Cymberknop L J, Suárez D, Castillo F G and Armentano R L 2016 Elastic mismatch between ePTFE and PLLA vascular grafts in relation to femoral and carotid arteries in humans: *in vivo*, *in vitro* and in silico assessment *Health Technol.* **6** 181–7

Alfonso M R, Armentano R L, Cymberknop L J, Ghigo A R, Pessana F M and Legnani W E 2018 A novel interpretation for arterial pulse pressure amplification in health and disease *J. Healthc. Eng.* **2018** art. no. 1364185

Armentano R L, Barra J G, Levenson J, Simon A and Pichel R H 1995 Arterial wall mechanics in conscious dog's assessment of viscous, inertial, and elastic moduli to characterize aortic wall behavior *Circ. Res.* **76** 468–78

Armentano R L and Cymberknop L J 2018a Quantitative vascular evaluation: From laboratory experiments to point-of-care patient (experimental approach) *Curr. Hypertens. Rev.* **14** 76–85

Avolio A P 1980 Multi-branched model of the human arterial system *Med. Biol. Eng. Comput.* **18** 709–18

Azer K and Peskin C S 2007 A one-dimensional model of blood flow in arteries with friction and convection based on the womersley velocity profile *Cardiovasc. Eng.* **7** 51–73

Battista C, Bia D, Germán Y Z, Armentano R L, Haider M A and Olufsen M S 2016 Wave propagation in a 1D fluid dynamics model using pressure-area measurements from ovine arteries *J. Mech. Med. Biol.* **16** 1650007

Bertoglio C, Moireau P and Gerbeau J-F 2012 Sequential parameter estimation for fluid-structure problems: Application to hemodynamics *Int. J. Numer. Method Biomed. Eng.* **28** 434–55

Bird R B, Armstrong R C, Hassager O and Curtiss C F 1977 *Dynamics of Polymeric Liquids* vol 1 (New York: Wiley) p 32

Blanco P J, Watanabe S M, Dari E A, Passos M A R F and Feijóo R A 2014 Blood flow distribution in an anatomically detailed arterial network model: criteria and algorithms *Biomech. Model. Mechanobiol.* **13** 1303–30

Blanco P J, Watanabe S M, Passos M A R F, Lemos P A and Feijóo R A 2015 An anatomically detailed arterial network model for one-dimensional computational hemodynamics *IEEE Trans. Biomed. Eng.* **62** 736–53

Boileau E, Nithiarasu P, Blanco P J, Müller L O, Fossan F E, Hellevik L R, Donders W P, Huberts W, Willemet M and Alastruey J 2015 A benchmark study of numerical schemes for one-dimensional arterial blood flow modelling *Int. J. Numer. Method Biomed. Eng.* **31**

Bouchut F 2004 *Nonlinear Stability of Finite Volume Methods for Hyperbolic Conservation Laws: And Well-Balanced Schemes for Sources* (Basel: Springer)

Calvo F 2006 Simulación del flujo sanguíneo y su interacción con la pared arterial mediante modelos de elementos finitos *Tesis doctoral* Universidad Politécnica de Madrid

Čanić S, Hartley C J and Rosenstrauch D *et al* 2006 Blood flow in compliant arteries: an effective viscoelastic reduced model, numerics, and experimental validation *Ann. Biomed. Eng.* **34** 575–92

Cascaval R C 2012 A Boussinesq model for pressure and flow velocity waves in arterial segments *Math. Comput. Simul.* **82** 1047–55

Causin P, Gerbeau J F and Nobile F 2005 Added-mass effect in the design of partitioned algorithms for fluid–structure problems *Comput. Methods Appl. Mech. Eng.* **194** 4506–27

Chnafa C, Valen-Sendstad K, Brina O, Pereira V M and Steinman D A 2017 Improved reduced-order modelling of cerebrovascular flow distribution by accounting for arterial bifurcation pressure drops *J. Biomech.* **51** 83–8

Codina R 1998 Comparison of some finite element methods for solving the diffusion-convection-reaction equation *Comput. Methods Appl. Mech. Eng.* **156** 185–210

Contarino C, Toro E F, Montecinos G I, Borsche R and Kall J 2016 Junction-generalized Riemann problem for stiff hyperbolic balance laws in networks: An implicit solver and ADER schemes *J. Comput. Phys.* **315** 409–33

Cousins W and Gremaud P-A 2012 Boundary conditions for hemodynamics: The structured tree revisited *J. Comput. Phys.* **231** 6086–96

Craiem D and Armentano R L 2007 A fractional derivative model to describe arterial viscoelasticity *Biorheology* **44** 251–63

Craiem D, Rojo F J, Atienza J M, Armentano R L and Guinea G V 2008 Fractional-order viscoelasticity applied to describe uniaxial stress relaxation of human arteries *Phys. Med. Biol.* **53** 4543

Cymberknop L J, Castillo F G, Alfonso M R, Sartore M M and Armentano R L 2016 1D blood pressure wave propagation modeling in young individuals *IEEE Biennial Congress of Argentina, ARGENCON 2016* pp 12100–1

Delestre O and Lagree P Y 2013 A 'well-balanced' finite volume scheme for blood flow simulation *Int. J. Numer. Methods Fluids* **72** 177–205

DeVault K, Gremaud P A, Novak V, Olufsen M S, Vernieres G and Zhao P 2008 Blood flow in the circle of Willis: Modeling and calibration *Multiscale Model Simul.* **7** 888–909

Drzisga D, Köppl T, Pohl U, Helmig R and Wohlmuth B 2016 Numerical modeling of compensation mechanisms for peripheral arterial stenoses *Comput. Biol. Med.* **70** 190–201

Erbay H A, Erbay S and Dost S 1992 Wave propagation in fluid filled nonlinear viscoelastic tubes *Acta Mech.* **95** 87–102

Euler L 1844 Principia pro motu sanguinis per arterias determinando, *Opera posthuma mathematica et physica anno* pp 814–23

Farhat C, Geuzaine P and Grandmont C 2001 The discrete geometric conservation law and the nonlinear stability of ALE schemes for the solution of flow problems on moving grids *J. Comput. Phys.* **17** 669–94

Fernández M A and Moubachir M 2005 A Newton method using exact Jacobians for solving fluid-structure coupling *Comput. Struct.* **142** 83–127

Figueroa C A, Vignon-Clementel I E, Jansen K E, Hughes T J R and Taylor C A 2006 A coupled momentum method for modeling blood flow in three-dimensional deformable arteries *Comput. Methods Appl. Mech. Eng.* **195** 5685–706

Formaggia L, Lamponi D and Quarteroni A 2003 One-dimensional models for blood flow in arteries *J. Eng. Math.* **47** 251–76

Formaggia L, Quarteroni A and Veneziani A (ed) 2009 *Cardiovascular Mathematics: Modeling and Simulation of the Circulatory System* vol 1 (Milan: Springer)

Fullana J-M and Zaleski S 2009 A branched one-dimensional model of vessel networks *J. Fluid Mech.* **621** 183–204

Fung Y C 1993 *Biomechanics: Mechanical Properties of Living Tissues* (New York: Springer)

Gabaldon Castillo F, Cymberknop L J, Alfonso M R, Martinez Sartore M and Armentano R L 2016 Evaluation of the impact of arterial wall viscosity in pressure morphology by means of a simplified 1D model *Conf. Proc. IEEE Eng. Med. Biol. Soc.* **2016** 2656–8

Gerbeau J-F, Vidrascu M and Frey P 2005 Fluid structure interaction in blood flows on geometries based on medical imaging *Comput. Struct.* **83** 155–65

Ghigo A R, Abou Taam S, Wang X, Lagrée P-Y and Fullana J-M 2017a A one-dimensional arterial network model for bypass graft assessment *Med. Eng. Phys.* **43** 39–47

Ghigo A R, Delestre O, Fullana J-M and Lagrée P-Y 2017b Low-Shapiro hydrostatic reconstruction technique for blood flow simulation in large arteries with varying geometrical and mechanical properties *J. Comput. Phys.* **331** 108–36

Ghigo A R, Wang X-F, Armentano R, Fullana J-M and Lagrée P-Y 2017c Linear and nonlinear viscoelastic arterial wall models: application on animals *J. Biomech. Eng.* **139**

Guan D, Liang F and Gremaud P-A 2016 Comparison of the Windkessel model and structured tree model applied to prescribe outflow boundary conditions for a one-dimensional arterial tree model *J. Biomech.* **49** 1583–92

Harari I and Hughes T J R 1994 Stabilized finite element methods for steady advection-diffusion with production *Comput. Methods Appl. Mech. Eng.* **115** 165–91

Holenstein R, Niederer P and Anliker M 1980 A viscoelastic model for use in predicting arterial pulse waves *J. Biomech. Eng.* **102** 318–25

Huberts W, Bode A S, Kroon W, Planken R N, Tordoir J H M, Van de Vosse F N and Bosboom E M H 2012a A pulse wave propagation model to support decision making in vascular access planning in the clinic *Med. Eng. Phys.* **34** 233–48

Huberts W, Van Canneyt K, Segers P, Eloot S, Tordoir J H M, Verdonck P, van de Vosse F N and Bosboom E M H 2012b Experimental validation of a pulse wave propagation model for predicting hemodynamics after vascular access surgery *J. Biomech.* **45** 1684–92

Hughes T J R, Liu W K and Zimmermann T K 1981 Lagrangian-Eulerian finite element formulation for incompressible viscous flows *Comput. Methods Appl. Mech. Eng.* **29** 329–49

Hughes T J R 2000 *The Finite Element Method: Linear Static and Dynamic Finite Element Analysis* (New York: Dover)

Kelly R and Fitchett D 1992 Noninvasive determination of aortic input impedance and external left ventricular power output: a validation and repeatability study of a new technique *J. Am. Coll. Cardiol.* **20** 952–63

Lagree P-Y 2000 An inverse technique to deduce the elasticity of a large artery *EPJ Appl. Phys.* **9** 153–64

Laleg T-M, Crepeau E, Papelier Y and Sorine M 2007 Arterial blood pressure analysis based on scattering transform I, *Conf. Proc. IEEE Eng. Med. Biol. Soc.* pp 5326–9

Leguy C A D, Bosboom E M H, Gelderblom H, Hoeks A P G and van de Vosse F N 2010 Estimation of distributed arterial mechanical properties using a wave propagation model in a reverse way *Med. Eng. Phys.* **32** 957–67

Liang F, Fukasaku K, Liu H and Takagi S 2011 A computational model study of the influence of the anatomy of the circle of Willis on cerebral hyperperfusion following carotid artery surgery *Biomed. Eng. Online* **10** 84

Ling S C and Atabek H B 1972 A nonlinear analysis of pulsatile flow in arteries *J. Fluid Mech.* **55** 493–511

Lombardi D 2014 Inverse problems in 1d hemodynamics on systemic networks: A sequential approach *Int. J. Numer. Method Biomed. Eng.* **30** 160–79

London G M and Pannier B 2010 Arterial functions: how to interpret the complexity physiology *Nephorl. Dial. Transplant.* **25** 3815–23

Matthys K S, Alastruey J, Peiró J, Khir A W, Segers P, Verdonck P R, Parker K H and Spencer J 2007 Pulse wave propagation in a model human arterial network: assessment of 1-D numerical simulations against *in vitro* measurements *J. Biomech.* **40** 3476–86

Marchandise E, Willemet M and Lacroix V 2009 A numerical hemodynamic tool for predictive vascular surgery *Med. Eng. Phys.* **31** 131–44

Mayr M, Klöppel T, Wall W A and Gee M W 2015 A temporal consistent monolithic approach to fluid-structure interaction enabling single field predictors *SIAM J. Sci. Comput.* **37** B30–59

Milnor W R 1982 *Hemodynamics* (Baltimore, MD: Williams & Wilkins)

Misra J C and Patra M K 2007 A study of solitary waves in a tapered aorta by using the theory of solitons *Comput. Math. Appl.* **54** 242–54

Montecinos G I, Müller L O and Toro E F 2014 Hyperbolic reformulation of a 1D viscoelastic blood flow model and ADER finite volume schemes *J. Comput. Phys.* **266** 101–23

Müller L O and Blanco P J 2015 A high order approximation of hyperbolic conservation laws in networks: application to one-dimensional blood flow *J. Comput. Phys.* **300** 423–37

Müller L O and Toro E F 2014 A global multiscale mathematical model for the human circulation with emphasis on the venous system *Int. J. Numer. Method Biomed. Eng.* **30** 681–725

Müller L O, Blanco P J, Watanabe S M and Feijóo R A 2016a A high-order local time stepping finite volume solver for one-dimensional blood flow simulations: application to the ADAN model *Int. J. Numer. Methods Biomed. Eng.* **32**

Müller L O, Leugering G and Blanco P J 2016b Consistent treatment of viscoelastic effects at junctions in one-dimensional blood flow models *J. Comput. Phys.* **314** 167–93

Müller L O, Parés C and Toro E F 2013 Well-balanced high-order numerical schemes for one-dimensional blood flow in vessels with varying mechanical properties *J. Comput. Phys.* **242** 53–85

Murillo J and García-Navarro P 2015 A Roe type energy balanced solver for 1D arterial blood flow and transport *Comput. Fluids* **117** 149–67

Mynard J P and Nithiarasu P 2008 A 1D arterial blood flow model incorporating ventricular pressure, aortic valve and regional coronary flow using the locally conservative Galerkin (LCG) method *Commun. Numer. Methods Eng.* **24** 367–417

Mynard J P and Valen-Sendstad K 2015 A unified method for estimating pressure losses at vascular junctions *Int. J. Numer. Method Biomed. Eng.* **31** e02717

Nichols W, O'Rourke M and Vlachopoulos C 2011 *Mcdonald's Blood Flow in Arteries: Theoretical, Experimental and Clinical Principles* (Boca Raton, FL: CRC Press)

Olufsen M S 1999 Structured tree outflow condition for blood flow in larger systemic arteries *Am. J. Physiol. Heart. Circ. Physiol.* **276** H257–68

Olufsen M S, Peskin C S, Kim W Y, Pedersen E M, Nadim A and Larsen J 2000 Numerical simulation and experimental validation of blood flow in arteries with structured-tree out flow conditions *Ann. Biomed. Eng.* **28** 1281–99

Perdikaris P and Karniadakis G E 2014 Fractional-order viscoelasticity in one-dimensional blood flow models *Ann. Biomed. Eng.* **42** 1012–23

Perdikaris P, Grinberg L and Karniadakis G E 2015 An effective fractal-tree closure model for simulating blood flow in large arterial networks *Ann. Biomed. Eng.* **43** 1432–42

Pérez Zerpa J M, Canelas A, Sensale B, Bia Santana D and Armentano R L 2015 Modeling the arterial wall mechanics using a novel high-order viscoelastic fractional element *Appl. Math. Model.* **39** 4767–80

Puelz C, Canic S, Rivière B and Rusin C G 2017 Comparison of reduced models for blood flow using Runge–Kutta discontinuous Galerkin methods *Appl. Numer. Math.* **115** 114–41

Raghu R, Vignon-Clementel I E, Figueroa C A and Taylor C A 2011 Comparative study of viscoelastic arterial wall models in nonlinear one-dimensional finite element simulations of blood flow *J. Biomech. Eng.* **133** 081003

Reymond P, Bohraus Y, Perren F, Lazeyras F and Stergiopulos N 2011 Validation of a patient-specific one-dimensional model of the systemic arterial tree *Am. J. Physiol. Heart. Circ. Physiol.* **301** H1173–82

Reymond P, Merenda F, Perren F, Rufenacht D and Stergiopulos N 2009 Validation of a one-dimensional model of the systemic arterial tree *Am. J. Physiol. Heart Circ. Physiol.* **297** H208–22

Reymond P, Perren F, Lazeyras F and Stergiopulos N 2012 Patient-specific mean pressure drop in the systemic arterial tree, a comparison between 1-D and 3-D models *J. Biomech.* **45** 2499–505

Saito M 2011 Non-invasive assessment of arterial stiffness by pulse wave analysis: *in vivo* measurements and one-dimensional theoretical model *PhD Thesis* Doshisha University

Saito M, Ikenaga Y, Matsukawa M, Watanabe Y, Asada T and Lagree P-Y 2011 One-dimensional model for propagation of a pressure wave in a model of the human arterial network: Comparison of theoretical and experimental results *J. Biomech. Eng.* **133** 121005

Sankaran S, Moghadam M E, Kahn A M, Tseng E E, Guccione J M and Marsden A L 2012 Patient-specific multiscale modeling of blood flow for coronary artery bypass graft surgery *Ann. Biomed. Eng.* **40** 2228–42

Sazonov I, Khir A W, Hacham W S, Boileau E, Carson J M, van Loon R, Ferguson C and Nithiarasu P 2017 A novel method for non-invasively detecting the severity and location of aortic aneurysms *Biomech. Model. Mechanobiol.* **16** 1225–42

Sherwin S J 2007 Pulse wave propagation in a model human arterial network: assessment of 1-D numerical simulations against *in vitro* measurements *J. Biomech.* **40** 3476–86

Sherwin S J, Formaggia L, Peiro J and Franke V 2003 Computational modelling of 1D blood flow with variable mechanical properties and its application to the simulation of wave propagation in the human arterial system *Int. J. Numer. Methods Fluids* **43** 673–700

Smith N P, Pullan A J and Hunter P J 2002 An anatomically based model of transient coronary blood flow in the heart *SIAM J. Appl. Math.* **62** 990–1018

Steele B N, Wan J, Ku J P, Hughes T J R and Taylor C A 2003 *In vivo* validation of a one-dimensional finite-element method for predicting blood flow in cardiovascular bypass grafts *IEEE Trans. Biomed. Eng.* **50** 649–56

Strocchi M, Contarino C, Zhang Q, Bonmassari R and Toro E F 2017 A global mathematical model for the simulation of stenoses and bypass placement in the human arterial system *Appl. Math. Comput.* **300** 21–39

Taylor M G 1966 Wave transmission through an assembly of randomly branching elastic tubes *Biophys. J.* **6** 697–716

Tezduyar T E 2003 Computation of moving boundaries and interfaces and stabilization parameters *Int. J. Numer. Methods Fluids* **43** 555–75

Tezduyar T E, Sathe S, Cragin T, Nanna B, Conklin B S, Pausewang J and Schwaab M 2007 Modelling of fluid–structure interactions with the space–time finite elements: Arterial fluid mechanics *Int. J. Numer. Methods Fluids* **54** 901–22

Valdez-Jasso D, Bia D, Zócalo Y, Armentano R, Haider M and Olufsen M 2011 Linear and nonlinear viscoelastic modeling of aorta and carotid pressure-area dynamics under *in vivo* and *ex vivo* conditions *Ann. Biomed. Eng.* **39** 1438–56

Valdez-Jasso D, Haider M A, Banks H T, Santana D B, German Y Z, Armentano R L and Olufsen M S 2009 Analysis of viscoelastic wall properties in ovine arteries *IEEE Trans. Biomed. Eng.* **56** 210–9

Vignon I E and Taylor C A 2004 Out flow boundary conditions for one-dimensional finite element modeling of blood flow and pressure waves in arteries *Wave Motion* **39** 361–74

Vignon-Clementel I E, Figueroa C A, Jansen K E and Taylor C A 2010 Out flow boundary conditions for 3d simulations of non-periodic blood flow and pressure fields in deformable arteries *Comput. Methods Appl. Mech. Eng.* **13** 625–40

Vignon-Clementel I E, Figueroa C A, Jansen K E and Taylor C A 2006 Outflow boundary conditions for three-dimensional finite element modeling of blood flow and pressure in arteries *Comput. Methods Appl. Mech. Eng.* **195** 3776–96

Wang X-F, Fullana J-M and Lagrée P-Y 2015 Verification and comparison of four numerical schemes for a 1D viscoelastic blood flow model *Comput. Methods Biomech. Biomed. Eng.* **18** 1704–25

Wang X-F, Fullana J-M, Lagrée P-Y and Armentano R L 2013 Effect of viscoelasticity of arterial wall on pulse wave: A comparative study on ovine *Comput. Methods Biomech. Biomed. Eng.* **16** 25–6

Watanabe S M, Blanco P J and Feijóo R A 2013 Mathematical model of blood flow in an anatomically detailed arterial network of the arm *ESAIM: Math. Model. Numer. Anal.* **47** 961–85

Willemet M, Lacroix V and Marchandise E 2013 Validation of a 1D patient-specific model of the arterial hemodynamics in bypassed lower-limbs: simulations against *in vivo* measurements *Med. Eng. Phys.* **35** 1573–83

Wang X, Delestre O, Fullana J-M, Saito M, Ikenaga Y, Matsukawa M and Lagree P-Y 2012 Comparing different numerical methods for solving arterial 1d flows in networks *Comput. Methods Biomech. Biomed. Eng.* **15** 61–2

Xiao N, Humphrey J D and Figueroa C A 2013 Multi-scale computational model of three-dimensional hemodynamics within a deformable full-body arterial network *J. Comput. Phys.* **244** 22–40

Yomosa S 1987 Solitary waves in large blood vessels *J. Phys. Soc. Jpn.* **56** 506–20

Zagzoule M and Marc-Vergnes J-P 1986 A global mathematical model of the cerebral circulation in man *J. Biomech.* **19** 1015–22

Zerpa J M P, Canelas A, Sensale B, Santana D B and Armentano R L 2014 A high-order viscoelastic fractional element applied to modeling ovine arterial wall behavior, *11th World Congress on Computational Mechanics, WCCM 2014, 5th European Conf. on Computational Mechanics, ECCM 2014 and 6th European Conf. on Computational Fluid Dynamics, ECFD 2014* pp 935–46

Lightning Source UK Ltd.
Milton Keynes UK
UKHW051328190220
358970UK00003B/124

9 780750 312820